INQUIRY AND LEADERSHIP

A RESOURCE FOR THE DNP Project

KATHY REAVY, PhD, RN

Professor
Boise State University
Boise, ID

F.A. Davis Company • Philadelphia

F. A. Davis Company
1915 Arch Street
Philadelphia, PA 19103
www. fadavis. com

Printed in the United States of America

Last digit indicates print number: 10 9 8 7 6 5 4 3 2 1

Acquisitions Editor, Nursing: Susan Rhyner
Developmental Editor: Jennifer Schmidt
Content Project Manager: Christina L. Snyder
Design and Illustration Manager: Carolyn O'Brien

As new scientific information becomes available through basic and clinical research, recommended treatments and drug therapies undergo changes. The author(s) and publisher have done everything possible to make this book accurate, up to date, and in accord with accepted standards at the time of publication. The author(s), editors, and publisher are not responsible for errors or omissions or for consequences from application of the book, and make no warranty, expressed or implied, in regard to the contents of the book. Any practice described in this book should be applied by the reader in accordance with professional standards of care used in regard to the unique circumstances that may apply in each situation. The reader is advised always to check product information (package inserts) for changes and new information regarding dose and contraindications before administering any drug. Caution is especially urged when using new or infrequently ordered drugs.

Library of Congress Cataloging-in-Publication Data

Names: Reavy, Kathleen, author.
Title: Inquiry and leadership : a resource for the DNP project / Kathy Reavy.
Description: Philadelphia, PA : F. A. Davis Company, [2016] | Includes bibliographical references and index.
Identifiers: LCCN 2015051403 | ISBN 9780803642041
Subjects: | MESH: Education, Nursing, Graduate | Nurse Clinicians–education | Nurse Practitioners–education | Leadership
Classification: LCC RT75 | NLM WY 18. 5 | DDC 610. 73071/1–dc23 LC record available at http://lccn. loc. gov/2015051403

Preface

Enthusiasm about the Doctor of Nursing Practice (DNP) degree is evidenced by the phenomenal growth in programs and student enrollments. Rapid growth, however, created a need for evaluation. In August 2015, an AACN Task Force released a report clarifying issues and making recommendations that address characteristics of the DNP degree and DNP project. The AACN clarifications are pertinent for our current healthcare system that is changing and adjusting to meet today's needs. Recommendations related to the DNP project are reflected in this new book. *Inquiry and Leadership* is an evidenced-based book that focuses on quality and rigor for successful completion of a DNP project. This book was written in the spirit of Miles and Huberman's 1994 classic resource for qualitative research. The intent of this new book is to enhance rigor in the construction and implementation of the DNP project by providing detailed information and rationale about process and actions. The book also contains scholarly tools and forms to assist organization and structure of the DNP project.

Inquiry and Leadership is well organized with four distinct sections. Section I is titled *Foundations* and provides foundational knowledge in preparation for planning and implementing a quality DNP project. Chapter 1 provides an overview of the DNP project and frames the DNP project within the model of translational science. Knowing the direction in which one will travel as he or she builds a DNP project contributes to strategy, effectiveness, and efficiency of the plan. Chapter 2 introduces the underpinnings for thinking about the DNP project. The underpinnings are correlated with AACN (2006) essentials. The intent of Section I is to provide a solid foundation on which to build the DNP project.

Inquiry, the title of Section II, is about investigation and creativity. The aim of the section is to provide detailed information regarding structure and process in planning and organizing the DNP project from idea to searchable question to evidence-based practice (EBP) recommendations for practice. Chapter 3 presents conceptual frameworks and models for EBP in order to enhance meaningfulness of the EBP linear process. Chapter 4 is about harnessing an idea and turning it into a searchable question or statement. Beginnings are difficult, so a good beginning is essential for a quality DNP project. The chapter begins by analyzing the components of an idea before writing a searchable question using the PICO(T) format. Chapter 5 introduces the student to the nature of evidence and what constitutes best evidence for a DNP project. Search strategies and organizational plans for finding best evidence are presented in Chapter 6. Organization is essential for orderliness of thought and is best demonstrated with an evidence table. The importance of critiquing evidence leading to establishment of trust in the evidence is the focus of Chapter 7. Chapter 8 directs the reader in writing a synthesis of the evidence findings. A well-written synthesis addresses the EBP searchable question and provides the basis for making EBP recommendation(s) for practice.

Section III focuses on *Leadership* for planning and implementing the EBP recommendation(s) for practice. Planning and evaluating are complex processes and actions that require quality leadership and management skills (Rycroft-Malone, 2012). Chapter 9 provides conceptual models and frameworks for consideration in thinking about the complexity of implementation. Chapter 10 begins the explanation about planning for implementation by focusing on building a detailed logic model showing relationships of actions, resources, and outcomes. Chapter 11 continues the focus on planning, specifically planning for evaluation. A review of quantitative and qualitative evaluation methods for clinical practice is provided in Appendixes A and B at the end of the book. Chapter 12 continues the focus on planning by examining the details of cost management considerations (e.g., budgets), economic analyses, and risk management. Chapter 13 targets creation of the written proposal for the DNP project team. The written proposal is based on planning as described in Chapters 9 through 12 and builds on the EBP synthesis and recommendations for practice. Chapter 14, the last chapter in Section III, focuses on review of project management and leadership skills for actualization of the implementation plan. Planning for all segments of the DNP project is complex, iterative, and time consuming. Yet the value of time spent planning contributes to quality, rigor, and success of the DNP project.

Looking Forward, the title of Section IV, focuses on professional responsibility for post-graduate scholarly activities in practice. Section IV is a reminder that completion of the DNP degree is only the beginning. The topics of Chapter 15 are dissemination and collaboration. Dissemination is grounded in communication and leads to collaboration within a structure of translational science. Dissemination of the final report from the DNP project is a beginning of new collaborations within the healthcare organization. Chapter 16 focuses on the structure of translational science. Translational science effectively models a cyclic nature of creating, finding, and using evidence in practice. The statement attributed to Green and Ottoson (2004), "If we want more evidence-based practice, we need more practice-based evidence" (Leeman & Sandelowski, 2012) emphasizes the need for translational science.

REFERENCES

AACN. (August 2015). *The Doctor of Nursing Practice: Current issues and clarifying recommendations.* Washington, DC: AACN. Retrieved from http://www.aacn.nche.edu/news/articles/2015/dnp-white-paper

AACN. (October 2006). *The essentials of doctoral education for advanced nursing practice.* Retrieved from http://www.aacn.nche.edu/publications/position/DNPEssentials.pdf

Green, L.W., & Ottoson, J.M. (2004). From efficacy to effectiveness to community and back: Evidence-based practice vs. practice-based evidence. Paper presented at *From Clinical Trials to Community: The Science of Translating Diabetes and Obesity Research,* January 12–13, 2004, Bethesda, MD.

Leeman, J., & Sandelowski, M. (2012). Practice-based evidence and quality inquiry. *Journal of Nursing Scholarship, 44*(2), 171–179. DOI: 10.1111/j.1547-5069.2012.01449.x

Rycroft-Malone, J., Harvey, G., Seers, K., Kitson, A., McCormack, B., & Titchen, A. (2004). An exploration of the factors that influence the implementation of evidence into practice. *Journal of Clinical Nursing, 13,* 913–924.

Acknowledgments

Writing a textbook is a journey wherein awareness and understanding increase along the way. Continuous reading, actively analyzing and synthesizing evidence, and the enrichment of conversations with old and new friends made the journey a valuable experience. Indeed, this textbook could not have been written without the contributions, assistance, and support from faculty and clinical peers, working DNPs, and student scholars. Thank you.

A very special thank you goes to Dr. Suzie Kardong-Edgren, the Jody DeMeyer Endowed Chair at Boise State University from 2011 through 2014. I am forever grateful for her positive influence and motivation from the initial outline to the final product. Thank you also to Dr. Edgren for selecting student scholars and training them as undergraduate research assistants. Thank you to the Jody DeMeyer Endowed Chair fund for supporting Melissa Vera, student scholar, as my research assistant and manuscript reviewer. Melissa shares my enthusiasm for this book and has become a good friend.

My faculty friends and peers at Boise State University were supportive during the time spent writing the text. Thank you to Kelley Connor, PhD; Pam Gehrke, EdD; Pam Strohfus, DNP; Jane Grassley, PhD; Ann Butt, EdD; Mary Hereford, PhD; Marty Downey, PhD; Shoni Davis, PhD; Molly Prengaman, PhD; and Cindy Clark. PhD. A special thank you to Cecile Evans, PhD, for your valued input. Finally, Dr. Denise Seigart, Chair of the Undergraduate and Master's Programs, is acknowledged and thanked for sharing her knowledge while encouraging our individual scholarly projects. A special thank you to Kelly Pesnell, DNP and faculty member at Idaho State University. Kelly's written contributions are incorporated into chapters in the textbook. And thank you to Cherese Severson, DNP and expert clinician, for her ideas and enthusiasm in getting this textbook started.

Acknowledgments and recognitions would be remiss without focusing on student scholars. In addition to Melissa Vera and Amanda Erickson, this book benefited from student questions and my time working with students. Additional acknowledgments go to my colleagues in the Education Department at Saint Alphonsus Regional Medical Center. We made a great team with evidence-based practice. Thank you to Catie Prinzing, Jill Anderson, and Renae Dougal.

The journey of writing this book would not have been possible without the support, patience, and encouragement from my expert editors at F.A. Davis Company: Joanne DaCunha, Susan Rhyner, Sean West, and Jennifer Schmidt.

Looking back, writing a textbook has been a positive adventure because of the encouragement and support of my family. Thank you to my wonderful husband, Jim, and our boys, Pat, Sean, and Brad – and their families. Without you, life would be boring and lack meaning. You make me happy.

To Jim, my husband,

for his continuous support

and encouragement

Contributors

This book would not be possible without help from faculty peers, working DNPs, and student scholars. Following is an alphabetized list of contributors who deserve recognition and heartfelt thanks for their time and efforts in writing and/or reviewing portions of the textbook. These contributors brought richness, diversity, and understanding to this textbook because of our differing academic histories. For that reason, academic degrees and universities where the degree was earned are provided.

Kelley Connor, PhD, RN

Degree from University of Kansas

Amanda Erickson, MSN, RN

Degree from Boise State University

Cecile Evans, PhD, RN

Degree from University of Tennessee

Cara Gallegos, PhD, RN

Degree from University of New Mexico

Jane Grassley, PhD, RN

Degree from Texas Woman's University

Kelly Pesnell, DNP, RN

Degree from University of Alabama

Cherese Severson, DNP, RN

Degree from University of Alabama

Pam Strohfus, DNP, RN

Degree from Rush University

Melissa Vera, BA, BSN, RN

BA from University of Washington
BSN from Boise State University

Contents

I

Foundations

PURPOSE

The aim of this section is to increase understanding of the essential foundations of the DNP project and to conceptually frame the structure and process for planning and implementation.

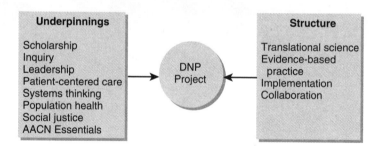

Foundational knowledge is preparatory for planning and implementing a rigorous DNP project. Section I focuses on the meaningfulness of the foundation.

Chapter 1 provides an overview of the purpose for the DNP project. Beginning this book with a vision of outcome assists the reader in thinking about the plan and structure of his or her DNP project. Knowing the direction in which one travels contributes to strategy, effectiveness, and efficiency. Chapter 2 introduces the underpinnings for thinking about the project. The underpinnings are correlated with American Association of Colleges of Nursing (2006) essentials. Having a solid foundation from the beginning strengthens the building of the DNP project.

REFERENCE

American Association of Colleges of Nursing (AACN). (October 2006). *The essentials of doctoral education for advanced nursing practice.* Retrieved from http://www.aacn .nche.edu/publications/position/DNPEssentials.pdf

1

What Is a DNP Project?

Scholarly activity includes perpetual curiosity, a focused commitment, and a willingness to risk challenge.

PARSE, 1994, p 143

OUTCOME OBJECTIVES

- Differentiate roles and scholarly outcomes for a practice doctorate and a research doctorate.
- Reflect on the academic goals for completing a DNP project.
- Assess the importance of program and intervention evaluations.
- Describe the purposes for quality improvement projects.
- Discuss policy revision and utilization as a potential DNP project.
- Discuss ideas that might lead to a nursing informatics project.

TERMS

Continuous quality improvement (CQI)	DNP project Evidence-based practice (EBP)	Nursing informatics Policy revision

Continued

TERMS—cont'd

Program or intervention evaluation	Practice-focused degree (DNP)	Total quality management (TQM)
Quality improvement (QI)	Research-focused degree (PhD)	Translational science (T1 through T4)

Understanding the purpose and constructs of a DNP project is essential before beginning your personal journey. This chapter provides an overview of the intent for the DNP project. Specifically, this chapter differentiates the histories and purposes between a practice project and a research dissertation, thereby assisting the DNP student to envision a scholarly plan that meets practice needs. A good beginning contributes to strategy, effectiveness, and efficiency.

DIFFERENTIATING PRACTICE AND RESEARCH DEGREES

Doctoral degrees recognized by nursing fall into two categories: research focus (PhD, EdD, DNSc, DSN) and practice focus (DNP). The two types of doctoral programs differ historically and in expected outcomes of graduates. The importance of understanding the differences helps you focus on your role as a DNP in the creation of a practice project that has meaningful use.

Modern history of the **research doctorate** credits its origin to educational reforms in Germany during the early 19th century. By the middle of the 19th century, scholars around the world went to Germany to study for a Doctor of Philosophy (PhD) degree in the sciences or humanities. By the 1890s, Johns Hopkins University, Harvard University, Columbia University, the University of Michigan, and the University of Wisconsin offered a PhD degree in their newly created graduate programs. The long history of the research doctorate began in an era when education was mainly available to wealthy students. The term *philosophy*, meaning *love of learning*, seems appropriate for students with extended time to focus only on learning (Diehl, 1978; Geitz, Heideking, & Herbst, 1995). Today, the research doctorate is the expected terminal degree for tenure track professors. Currently, the average time to complete a PhD is 6 to 8 years: 3 to 4 years to complete course work followed by 3 to 4 years to complete the dissertation (Townsend, 2006). The purpose of a dissertation is to add new evidence to the general body of knowledge. To achieve this goal, research is described as *examining carefully*. "Research is the diligent, systematic inquiry or investigation to validate and refine existing knowledge and generate new knowledge" (Grove, Burns, Gray, 2013, p 1).

Florence Nightingale is credited with the beginning of nursing research. Nightingale's leadership of 38 volunteer nurses and their services during the Crimean War (1853 to 1856) contributed to substantial change in unsanitary hospital conditions. Diseases, including typhoid, cholera, and rampant infections, killed soldiers at a rate 10 times that of war casualties. Nightingale introduced change to these poor hospital conditions and kept scrupulous written notes about her actions. Following the war and her return to England, Nightingale prepared an 800-page report based on evaluation of her notes. Nightingale's transformational leadership to improve sanitary conditions, her detailed epidemiological notes, and dissemination of her findings made a huge impact. Her 1859 publication, *Notes on Nursing*, contributed to improvements in public health, including safe water and sanitation. The result was better physical and mental health for all British people (Burns & Grove, 2011; Fee & Garofalo, 2010; Palmer, 1977; Polit & Beck, 2012).

Nightingale's influence, however, was limited. It was not until the 1960s that nursing leaders confronted the scarcity of research related to nursing. Growth in nursing journals to publish scholarly findings and recognition of the need for research funding specifically for nurses subsequently occurred (Grove, Burns, & Gray, 2013; Polit & Beck, 2012). As of 2013, there were 131 research-focused nursing programs, an increase of 28 new programs over the previous 7 years (AACN, 2014a).

Nursing leaders also realized the importance of practice as a main context for a terminal nursing degree. Theorist Margaret Newman (1975) wrote a position paper encouraging creation of a practice doctorate. The first **practice doctorate** for nursing is credited to Boston University and was labeled Doctor of Nursing Science (DNSc). The University of Alabama followed with a Doctor of Science in Nursing (DSN) degree. Both degrees focused on clinical research, but the curricula were similar to that of the PhD. The degrees failed to attract adequate numbers of students and were subsequently designated by the AACN (2004) as research degrees. However, the idea of a practice degree remained active. In 1979, Case Western Reserve University addressed the challenge and introduced the Nursing Doctorate (ND) degree. The focus was on the clinical leader, not the researcher. The University of Colorado, Rush University, and South Carolina University introduced their own ND programs shortly afterward. Approximately 700 nurses completed the ND degree. Unfortunately, coursework for the ND degree was inconsistent and lacked uniformity. In 2002, the AACN phased out the ND degree, but the Doctor of Nursing Practice

(DNP) degree started. The first graduating class of 6 students in 2005 was credited to the University of Kentucky. As of 2015, there were 264 DNP programs enrolling students with an additional 60 programs in the planning stages (AACN, 2004; AACN 2015; Chism, 2011; Case Western Reserve University, 2013; Udlis & Mancuso, 2012).

Why has the practice doctorate been successful this time? AACN (2014b) identifies rapid growth in practice knowledge, increased complexity of patient care, and the increasing emphasis on quality care and patient safety. The National Academy of Sciences, in a 2005 report *Advancing the Nation's Health Needs*, recommended a nonresearch clinical doctorate in nursing (NAP, 2005). Today, nursing's leadership and decision-making skills are increasingly recognized in the transformation of healthcare delivery, administration, and education (AACN, 2004). The Institute of Medicine (2011) advocated for nurses to work to the full extent of their education. The DNP provides the pathway for practice.

The differences in roles and scholarly activities between a practice-focused and a research-focused prepared nurse are important (Table 1.1). The importance of difference does not imply division and competition among terminal degrees. Rather, difference implies depth and rigor of each degree contributing to intraprofessional complementary and collaborative approaches to care (AACN, 2006; AACN, 2010a; Edwardson, 2010). The differing yet collaborative roles are best described within the model of translational science.

WHAT IS TRANSLATIONAL SCIENCE?

This textbook is framed within the model of translational science (Table 1.2). Translational science is a 21st century movement begun by the medical profession to decrease the lag between doing research and applying research. The lag had been noted to be as long as 15 or more years. The initial idea of translational science was viewed as a two-phased process that promoted the implementation of new bench research (e.g., drugs, devices, patient treatment options). The two-phased process was referred to as *bench-to-bedside* clinical research. However, the two-phased option for translational science lacked clarity, especially in the application and evaluation stages. The medical interpretation focused on laboratory research and developing applications for human trials. At the same time, public health leaders interpreted translational science to mean integration of new knowledge into practice settings at the population level (ITHS, 2015). Dr. Steven Woolf (2008) wrote that "translational science means different things to different people, but it seems important to almost everyone."

TABLE 1.1 Differences Between Practice-Focused and Research-Focused Programs of Study

	DNP	PhD/EdD/DNSc
Program of Study	*Objectives:* Prepare nurse leaders at the highest level of nursing practice to improve patient outcomes and translate research into practice *Competencies:* See AACN's (2006) *Essentials of Doctoral Education for Advanced Nursing Practice*	*Objectives:* Prepare nurses at the highest level of nursing science to conduct research to advance the science of nursing *Content:* See AACN's (2010b) *The Research-Focused Doctoral Program in Nursing: Pathways to Excellence*
Students	Commitment to practice career Oriented toward improving outcomes of patient care and population health	Commitment to research career Oriented toward developing new nursing knowledge and scientific inquiry
Program Faculty	Practice or research doctorate in nursing and expertise in area teaching Leadership experience in area of role and population practice High level of expertise in practice congruent with focus of academic program	Research doctorate in nursing or related field Leadership experience in area of sustained research funding High level of expertise in research congruent with focus of academic program
Resources	Mentors and/or preceptors in leadership positions across practice settings Access to diverse practice settings with appropriate resources for areas of practice Access to financial aid Access to information and patient-care technology resources congruent with areas of study	Mentors and/or preceptors in research settings Access to research settings with appropriate resources Access to dissertation support dollars and financial aid Access to information and research technology resources congruent with program of research
Program Assessment and Evaluation	*Program outcome:* Healthcare improvements and contributions through practice, policy change, and practice scholarship Receives accreditation by nursing accreditor	*Program outcome:* Contributes to healthcare improvements through the development of new knowledge and scholarly products that provide the foundation for the advancement of nursing science Oversight by the institution's authorized bodies (i.e., graduate school) and regional accreditors

Adapted from AACN. (2014b). Doctor of Nursing Practice (DNP) Talking Points. *Retrieved from www.aacn.nche.edu/ContrastGrid.pdf*

TABLE 1.2 Overview of Translational Science for the DNP

Discovery BASIC RESEARCH Translational Phase 1 (T₁) (Basic Research)	Inquiry EVIDENCE-BASED FINDINGS TO PRACTICE RECOMMENDATIONS Translational Phase 2 (T₂) (Practice)	Leadership PILOT IMPLEMENTATION OF RECOMMENDATIONS INTO SINGLE PRACTICE CONTEXT Translational Phase 2 (T₂): (Practice)	Collaboration DISSEMINATION RESEARCH Translational phase 3 (T₃) (Collaborative Research)	Collaboration POPULATION HEALTH RESEARCH Translational Phase 4 (T₄) (Collaborative Research)
Definition: "A systematic inquiry that uses disciplined methods to answer questions or solve problems. The ultimate goal of research is to develop, refine, and expand a base of knowledge" (Polit and Beck, 2006, p 4).	*Definition:* "Evidence-based practice is the conscientious and judicious use of current best evidence in conjunction with clinical expertise and patient values to guide health care decisions" (Titler, 2010, p 36).	*Definition:* T₂ is about implementing, adjusting or refining, and establishing the value of EBP guidelines, quality improvement, or developmental projects that were identified through an EBP process (Sampselle, 2010; Titler, 2008; Woods & Magyary, 2010; Woolf, 2008).	*Definition:* Focus is on large-scale RCTs related to dissemination and effectiveness; the study of how to promote or disseminate adoption of intervention and methods in multiple sites (Khoury et al., 2007; Woods & Magyary, 2010).	*Definition:* Focus is on large-scale RCTs related to population health research: comparative-effectiveness; quality of life cost analysis (Sampselle, 2010).

Bench-to-bedside research; Intradisciplinary or Interdisciplinary	Creation of EBP recommendations for practice; Creating and leading an EBP team	Leading a pilot implementation and evaluation project of EBP recommendations for practice	RCTs of T_2 intervention methods	RCTs of intervention effects; comparative-effectiveness research, cost effectiveness
Process: Linear; Iterative	*Process: Linear; Iterative*	*Process: Complex; Contextual*	*Roles: T_3 Research*	*Roles: T_4 research process; Intradisciplinary and Interdisciplinary research*
• Identification of an idea	• Identification of an idea based on observation, experience, knowledge	• Building a logic model for implementing EBP guidelines or recommendations	*Process: Intradisciplinary and Interdisciplinary RCTs*	*Process: Linear; CER; RCTs*
• Introduction: Identification of:	• Identification of stakeholders	• Designing and leading an implementation plan	*Process: Linear; Iterative* • RCT research methods	• RCT research methods
1. Problem area	• Formation of an EBP team	• Designing and leading an evaluation plan		
2. Background and importance of problem	• Creating a searchable question:			
3. Purpose statement	1. Background questions			
Literature review:	2. Writing a searchable question or statement			
(1) 1. Identifies what is known and not known	• Searching for best evidence			
(2) 2. Identifies framework (biological, technical, pharmacological, socioeconomic, theoretical, etc.)	• Organizing and screening evidence			
• Methodology	• Critiquing best evidence			
(1) 1. Research questions, statements, or hypotheses	• Synthesizing evidence			
(2) Description of research design and methods	• Creating EBP practice recommendations			

Continued

TABLE 1.2 Overview of Translational Science for the DNP—cont'd

Discovery BASIC RESEARCH Translational Phase 1 (T_1) (Basic Research)	Inquiry EVIDENCE-BASED FINDINGS TO PRACTICE RECOMMENDATIONS Translational Phase 2 (T_2) (Practice)	Leadership PILOT IMPLEMENTATION OF RECOMMENDATIONS INTO SINGLE PRACTICE CONTEXT Translational Phase 2 (T_2): (Practice)	Collaboration DISSEMINATION RESEARCH Translational phase 3 (T_3) (Collaborative Research)	Collaboration POPULATION HEALTH RESEARCH Translational Phase 4 (T_4) (Collaborative Research)
• Data analysis 1. Statistical analysis • Discussion of results 1. Limitations of the study 2. Recommendations for use of research findings 3. Recommendations for new research				
Objective for DNP: Understanding the research process to critique and use the findings; establish trust in research methods	**Outcome objectives for DNP:** Creation of EBP recommendations for practice	**Outcome for DNP:** Contextual implementation and evaluation of recommendations for practice	**Outcome for DNP:** Collaboration with scientists for RCTs of implementation and dissemination science carried out in multiple sites	**Outcome for DNP:** Collaboration with scientists for comparative effectiveness research and population impact research

EBP, evidence-based practice; RCT, randomized controlled trial.

Translational science was in need of a scale. A 2007 publication by Khoury et al. (2007) proposed a framework of four translational phases, emphasizing collaborative research among academic disciplines and professions. The four phases are viewed as bidirectional, iterative, and overlapping. The glue that holds the model together consists of communication and collaboration.

Translational phase 1 (T_1) consists of basic research and development. Translational phase 2 (T_2) is identified as the phase for the DNP project. T_2 received the nickname *Translating Research Into Practice* or *TRIP* (AHRQ, 2001; Titler & Everett, 2001). The *T* in the acronym *TRIP* implies using evidence-based practice (EBP) and implementing practice improvements within the framework of *Translational Science.* Other interpretations for *T* observed in the literature include *transforming, transitioning,* or *turning.*

Translational science phases 3 and 4 (T_3 and T_4) build on T_2 evaluations from one setting and a small sample size. T_3 and T_4 are large-scale dissemination and population studies conducted with randomized controlled trials (RCT). Chapter 16 presents additional details of T_3 and T_4 within the concept of intraprofessional and interprofessional collaboration.

WHAT IS A DNP PROJECT?

A DNP project is a scholarly effort that addresses identified issues or ideas and is supported by best evidence. Contextually, a DNP project is acceptable to stakeholders and is implemented systematically and ethically. The project is analytically planned, implemented, evaluated, and disseminated. The hope is that the DNP project is a rewarding and scholarly experience for both students and faculty (Kirkpatrick & Weaver, 2013).

The DNP project may focus on a program, an intervention, a policy, a quality improvement (QI) project, a nursing informatics project, or another creative entity that promotes improvement or change related to the health of individuals or populations (AACN, 2004). Settings to implement your scholarly plan may be within an academic or a healthcare system, a clinical setting within an organization, or the community. Given the breadth of DNP practice roles and the variety of issues addressed in a specified context, your DNP project has multiple options. Whatever structure and process the final DNP project takes, it should serve as a foundation for future scholarly practice. Above all, it is important that the DNP project is adequately rigorous to meet the requirements for a practice doctorate degree and that it is recognized as a practice project, not a research dissertation (AACN, 2006; Burton, 2011; Moran, Burton, & Conrad, 2014; National Organization of Nurse Practitioner Faculties, 2013).

Purposes of the DNP Project

The purposes of the DNP project are many. First and foremost are the goals to provide the DNP student with an opportunity to "launch into scholarly practice" and demonstrate advanced knowledge in his or her area of expertise (Moran et al., 2014, p 7). The project provides the necessary knowledge, structure, and experience to position the DNP to lead practice change and improve the practice infrastructure. This challenge was proposed by the Institute of Medicine in the 2001 publication *Crossing the Quality Chasm: A New Health System for the 21st Century* (Institute of Medicine, 2001). The DNP project also positions students to demonstrate efficiency and effectiveness of costs and resources (Brown & Crabtree, 2013, p 333). The DNP project rigorously applies scholarship in using evidence at its highest level (Kirkpatrick & Weaver, 2013).

Structure of the DNP Project

The structure of a DNP project begins with an EBP process that develops a practice issue into a question or statement. The EBP question or statement provides the search terms for the literature search. Evidence findings are then screened for relevance and critiqued to ascertain strength and trust of the evidence, followed by a written synthesis of evidence and concluding with recommendations for practice. Decisions about implementation and evaluation of recommendations occur next with creation of a logic model. In all aspects of the DNP project, rigor and quality are expected. There are growing expectations that DNP projects should result in written manuscripts and public presentations, either before or after graduation (Kirkpatrick & Weaver, 2013). The following are short explanations and examples of categories of DNP projects.

Program or Intervention Project

A *program* is described as a "set of resources and activities toward one or more common goals" (Wholey, Hatry, & Newcomer, 2010, e-book). A program is generally under the direction of one manager within an organization. An *intervention* may be a trial of a product, curricular development, or evaluation of actions and processes within an identified program. Whether your project involves a program, an intervention within a program, or a stand-alone intervention, implementation and evaluation follow similar steps (Melnyk, 2013). Credible evaluations of a program or an intervention use systematic methods grounded in social science to answer specific questions about operations, processes, actions, or outcomes. Findings are used to increase understanding and improve an organization's provision of capacity and services. Evaluation is a useful learning strategy that contributes to understanding the logic of programs and interventions, as well as influencing policy and management decisions (Wholey et al., 2010).

An **example of a program intervention and evaluation** involved a new clinic model for pregnant refugee women. The idea grew from clinic observations following a large influx of refugees from camps in Africa and the Middle East. Refugees speaking multiple languages and dialects were relocated to a western state in the United States that has the designation of a resettlement area. Arriving to the new setting with increased food security and safety provided pregnant refugee women with a better context for sustaining a pregnancy. Cultural and language differences, however, initially caused confusion. Whereas health care in refugee camps required long hours waiting in lines, health care in the United States required expectations of timely appointments to see a provider. The women sometimes brought friends to their individual prenatal appointments with the expectation that all of them would receive care.

To address these issues, a prenatal care program was funded for a 2-hour group clinic of 15 to 20 women per clinic. The clinic provided group education about prenatal care, parenting, mental health, nutrition, and timeliness. Individual examinations were provided by a nurse midwife while the education classes were being held. Several interventions within the new program contributed to an overall, smooth-running, cost-effective clinic. One intervention within the program was an evidence-based project for group appointment scheduling, insurance reimbursement, and patient timeliness. The project included a format and database for patient appointment reminders, patient teaching about appointment times, meeting patient transportation needs (i.e., taxi services for small groups partially reimbursed by Medicaid), and patient completion of Medicaid insurance documents. Evaluation of the project demonstrated increased patient compliance, cost effectiveness, and patient satisfaction. Findings were shared with stakeholders (Reavy, Hobbs, Hereford, & Crosby, 2012).

Quality Improvement Projects

Quality improvement (QI) is a term increasingly connected with DNP projects. QI is aligned for value because it is "the combined and unceasing efforts of everyone—healthcare professionals, patients and their families, researchers, payers, planners, and educators—to make the changes that will lead to better patient outcomes [health], better systems performance [care] and better professional development [learning]" (Batalden & Davidoff, 2007, p 2). QI is about quality in delivery systems, processes, and outcomes for best patient care. QI is not an end-product but consists of ongoing cycles of improvement (Batalden & Davidoff, 2007). The Donabedian (1988) model identified three dimensions for the process of QI: (1) structure, or attributes of the care delivery setting; (2) process, or healthcare practices that are followed; and (3) outcome, or impact of care on health status. Successful QI is based on the following four principles: (1) QI works as systems and processes; (2) the focus is on patients; (3) health care is a team approach; (4) collected QI data are used for improvement (Batalden & Davidoff, 2007).

Continuous QI (CQI) is a category within QI. CQI is cyclical and data driven with the intent to be proactive, not reactive. CQI is an ongoing or periodic evaluation process (HRSA, 2011).

Total quality management (TQM) is another category within QI. The foci of TQM are management processes. Underlying philosophies relate to the processes, not the people, and the system should look for a cure to the problem, not a treatment for a symptom. Quality is a long-term financial investment and must be measurable (Harris, 2011).

Policy Revision Projects

Policy revision may be grouped under the broad heading of QI initiatives or program evaluation because policies are present in all systems within an organization, including clinical patient units, information technology, and management. Indeed, analyses of hospital-collected data and evidence-based patient care drive revisions and changes in policy (Desouza & Lin, 2011; Harris, 2014).

Policies are powerful because they contribute to lasting changes in terms of the healthcare environment and individual behavior. As such, policies have a greater reach and impact than individual interactions for implementing improvement or change. Policies also require less effort for sustainability (Chappelle & Wooster, 2011).

Organizational policies are revised on an ongoing basis because of the complexity and changes or improvements in the practice settings. In such dynamic environments, changes in values (which determine the outcome goals) are adapted according to best evidence and need. "Any new policy will only achieve part of the expected consequences and always produce some unanticipated outcomes" (Desoza & Lin, 2011, p 5). Policies, therefore, are consistently revised and updated, as needed. Equally important is communication between policy makers and stakeholders regarding implementation and evaluation. "Assessing a new policy before implementation is particularly important for complex adaptive systems due to the complexity of problems, high cost of policy implementation and the lag of feedback" (Desouza & Lin, 2011, p 6).

Nursing Informatics Projects

Nursing informatics is described as "the specialty that integrates nursing science with multiple information, management, and analytical sciences to define, manage, and communicate data, information, knowledge, and wisdom in nursing practice" (ANA, 2015). Informatics is about meaningful use of technology for healthcare information and healthcare management. **Nursing informatics** works with technology systems to improve efficiency, reduce costs, and improve overall patient care. Technology can also assist in policy evaluation, modeling, and prediction (Nursing Informatics, 2013). Examples of opportunities and settings for scholarly projects in the area of nursing informatics might include the following: a clinical decision-making program for nursing staff, patient education for improved home use of telehealth, QI analysis of patient access to personal healthcare records, analysis of hospital electronic health records (EHRs) for management and decision making, creation of a database for online patient education, creation of games or applications as patient teaching tools or student review tools.

CHAPTER SUMMARY AND AFTERTHOUGHTS

Completion of a DNP project is an essential component of demonstrating competence for the practice doctorate in nursing. The DNP project encompasses advanced knowledge acquisition in making decisions and highlights leadership skills. The DNP project also launches scholarly position papers and leads change through EBP. Completion of a DNP project addresses the Institute of Medicine's (2001) challenges to improve healthcare infrastructure and lead change. The DNP project is an "ongoing, systematic investigation of questions about practice and therapeutics with the intent to evaluate and translate, as appropriate, all forms of best evidence into practice and to evaluate the influence on healthcare outcomes" (Magyary, Whitney, & Brown, 2006, p 143).

DISCUSSION QUESTIONS

- Consider your desired DNP role and the context of your desired practice. Reflect on practice issues or ideas. Then discuss potential project ideas with peers.

- Discuss basic project designs (e.g., QI, program evaluation, policy revision) for your idea or ideas.

- What additional information do you need?

WRITING REMINDERS...

The Importance of Writing

* Writing is the basis on which your work, your learning, and your intellect will be judged.

  * Writing helps you express who you are.

  * Writing helps your thinking be visible.

  * Writing helps explain a complex position to your readers and to yourself.

  * Writing helps others give you feedback; feedback helps you refine your ideas.

  * Writing helps you think about your readers' needs. This is a demonstration of intellectual flexibility.

  * Writing your ideas saves them so you can reflect on them later.

  * Writing helps you assess the effectiveness of your argument.

  * Writing is an essential job skill. (Rebecca Nowacek, 2011)

REFERENCES

Agency for Healthcare Research and Quality (AHRQ). (2001). Translating research into practice (TRIP): II. AHRQ pub. no. 01-P017. Retrieved from http://archive.ahrq.gov/research/findings/factsheets/translating/tripfac/trip2fac.pdf

American Association of Colleges of Nursing (AACN). (2004). *AACN position statement on the practice doctorate in nursing.* Retrieved from http://www.aacn.nche.edu/publications/position/DNPpositionstatement.pdf

American Association of Colleges of Nursing (AACN). (2006). *The essentials of doctoral education for advanced nursing practice.* Retrieved from http://www.aacn.nche.edu/publications/position/DNPEssentials.pdf

American Association of Colleges of Nursing (AACN). (2010a). *The future of higher education in nursing: 2010 annual report.* Retrieved from http://www.aacn.nche.edu/publications/annual-reports/AR2010.pdf

American Association of Colleges of Nursing (AACN). (2010b). *The research focused doctoral program in nursing: Pathways to excellence.* Retrieved from http://www.aacn.nche.edu/education-resources/PhDPosition.pdf

American Association of Colleges of Nursing (AACN). (2014a). *Annual report 2014: Building a framework for the future.* Washington, DC: AACN. Retrieved from http://www.aacn.nche.edu/aacn-publications/annual-reports/AnnualReport14.pdf

American Association of Colleges of Nursing (AACN). (2014b). *Doctor of Nursing Practice (DNP) talking points.* Retrieved from http://www.aacn.nche.edu/leading-initiatives/dnp/dnp-tool-kit/DNP-Talking-Points.pdf

American Association of Colleges of Nursing (AACN). (2015). *DNP fact sheet.* Retrieved from http://www.aacn.nche.edu/media-relations/fact-sheets/dnp

American Nurses Association (ANA). (2015). *Nursing informatics: Scope and standards of practice* (2nd ed.). Silver Springs, MD: American Nurses Association, Inc.

Batalden, P.B., & Davidoff, F. (2007). What is "quality improvement" and how can it transform healthcare? *Quality Safety and Healthcare, 16*(1), 2–3. Retrieved from http://www.ncbi.nlm.nih.gov/pmc/articles/PMC2464920/#!po=10.0000

Brown, M.A., & Crabtree, K. (2013). The development of practice scholarship in DNP programs: A paradigm shift. *Journal of Professional Nursing, 29*(4), 330–337.

Burns, N., & Grove, S.K. (2011). *Understanding nursing research: Building an evidence-based practice* (5th ed.). Maryland Heights, MO: Elsevier.

Burton, R. (2011). DNP scholarly project survey. In C. Conrad, R. Burton, & K. Moran (Eds.). *The doctor of nursing practice scholarly project: A framework for success* (pp. 75–78). Burlington, MA: Jones & Bartlett Learning.

Case Western Reserve University. (2013). *History of the DNP at FPB.* Retrieved from http://fpb.case.edu/DNP/history.shtm

Chappelle, E., & Wooster, J. (2011). CDC coffee break: Evaluating policy. *National Center for Chronic Disease and Prevention and Health Promotion.* Retrieved from http://www.cdc.gov/dhdsp/pubs/docs/cb_june_14_2011.pdf

Chism, L. (2011). The roots of the DNP: This movement began a long time ago. *Advance Healthcare Network for NPs and PAs.* Retrieved from http://nurse-practitioners-and-physician-assistants.advanceweb.com/Column/DNP-Perspectives/The-Roots-of-the-DP.aspx

Desouza, K.C., & Lin, Y. (2011). Towards evidence-driven policy design: Complex adaptive systems and computational modeling. *The Innovation Journal: The Public Sector Innovation Journal, 16*(1), Article 7. Retrieved from http://www.innovation.cc/scholarly-style/desouza_lin_policy_informatics_v16i1a7.pdf

Diehl, C. (1978). *Americans and German scholarship, 1770–1870.* New Haven, CT: Yale University Press.

Donabedian, A. (1988). The quality of care. How can it be assessed? *JAMA, 260*(12), 1743–1748.

Edwardson, S.R. (2010). Doctor of philosophy and doctor of nursing practice as complementary degrees. *Journal of Professional Nursing, 26*(3), 137–140.

Fee, E., & Garofalo, M.E. (2010). Florence Nightingale and the Crimean War. *American Journal of Public Health, 100*(9), 159.

Geitz, H., Heideking, J., & Herbst, J. (Eds.), (1995). *German influences on education in the United States to 1917.* Cambridge, United Kingdom: Press Syndicate of the University of Cambridge.

Grove, S.K., Burns, N., & Gray, J.R. (2013). *The practice of nursing research: Appraisal, synthesis, and generation of evidence* (7th ed.). St. Louis, MO: Elsevier/Saunders.

Harris, J.L. (2014). Turning health policy into practice: Implications for advanced practice registered nurses. In A.Goudreau, & M.C. Smolenski (Eds.). *Health policy and advanced practice nursing: Impact and implications,* pp 13–28. New York, NY: Springer Publishing Company.

Harris, Q. (2011). *7 important principles of total quality management.* Retrieved from http://managementhelp.org/quality/total-quality-management.htm

Health Resources and Services Administration (HRSA). (2011). *Quality Improvement.* Retrieved from http://www.hrsa.gov/quality/ toolbox/508pdfs/quality improvement.pdf

Institute of Medicine. (2001). *Crossing the quality chasm: A new health system for the 21st century.* Washington, DC: National Academies Press. Retrieved from http://books.nap.edu/openbook.php?record_id=10027

Institute of Medicine. (2011). *The future of nursing: Leading change, advancing health.* Washington DC: National Academies Press. Retrieved from https://www.iom.edu/~/media/Files/Report%20Files/2010/The-Future-of-Nursing/Future%20of%20 Nursing%202010%20Recommendations.pdf

Institute of Translational Health Sciences (ITHS). (2015). *Learn about ITHS.* Retrieved from https://www.iths.org/sites/www.iths.org/files/files/intranet/Learn-About-ITHS_031015.pdf

Khoury, M.J., Gwinn, M., Yoon, P.W., Dowling, N., Moore, C.A., & Bradley, L. (2007). The continuum of translation research in genomic medicine: How can we accelerate the appropriate integration of human genome discoveries into health care and disease prevention? *Genetics in Medicine, 6*(10), 665–674.

Kirkpatrick, J., & Weaver, T. (2013). The doctor of nursing practice capstone project: Consensus or confusion? *Journal of Nursing Education, 52*(8), 435–441.

Magyary, D., Whitney, J.D., & Brown, M.A. (2006). Advancing practice inquiry: Research foundations of the practice doctorate in nursing. *Nursing Outlook, 54*(3), 139–151.

Melnyk, B.M. (2013). Distinguishing the preparation and roles of doctor of philosophy and doctor of nursing practice graduates: National implications for academic curricula and health care systems. *Journal of Nursing Education, 52*(8), 442–448.

Moran, K., Burson, R., & Conrad, D. (2014). *The doctor of nursing practice scholarly project: A framework for success.* Burlington, MA: Jones & Bartlett Learning.

National Academies Press (NAP). (2005). *Advancing the nation's health needs.* Washington DC: National Academies Press.

National Organization of Nurse Practitioner Faculties Statement. (2013). *Titling of the doctor of nursing practice project.* Retrieved from http://c.ymcdn.com/sites/www.nonpf.org/resource/resmgr/dnp/dnpprojectstitlingpaperjune2.pdf

Newman, M.A. (1975). The professional doctorate in nursing: A position paper. *Nursing Outlook, 23,* 704.

Nowacek, R. (2011). *What makes writing so important?* Milwaukee, WI: Marquette University. Retrieved from http://www.marquette.edu/wac/WhatMakesWritingSo Important.shtml

Nursing informatics. (2013). Retrieved from http://explorehealthcareers.org/en/Career/91/Nursing Informatics

Palmer, I.S. (1977). Florence Nightingale: Reformer, reactionary, researcher. *Nursing Research, 26*(2), 84–89.

Parse, R.R. (1994). Scholarship: Three essential processes. *Nursing Science Quarterly, 7*(4), 143.

Polit, D.F., & Beck, C.T. (2012). *Nursing research: Generating and assessing evidence for nursing practice* (8th ed.). Philadelphia, PA: Wolters Kluwer/Lippincott Williams & Wilkins.

Reavy, K., Hobbs, J., Hereford, M., & Crosby, K. (2012). A new clinic model for refugee health care: Adaptation of cultural safety. *Rural and Remote Health, 12*(1), 1826.

Sampselle, C.M. (2010). The Michigan Center for Health Intervention (MICHIN): Facilitating translational science. *Research and Theory for Nursing Practice: An International Journal, 24*(1), 6–8.

Titler, M.G. (2008). The evidence for evidence-based practice implementation. In R.G. Hughes (Ed.). *Patient safety and quality: An evidence-based handbook for nurses.* Rockville, MD: Agency for Healthcare Research and Quality.

Titler, M.G. (2010). Translation science and context. *Research and Theory for Nursing Practice: An International Journal, (24)*1, 35–55. Townsend, R.B. (2006). How long to the PhD? *Perspectives on History: The Newsmagazine of the American Historical Association.* Retrieved from https://www.historians.org/publications-and-directories/perspectives-on-history/february-2006/how-long-to-the-phd

Titler, M.G., & Everett, L.Q. (2001). Translating research into practice: Considerations for critical care investigators. *Critical Care Nursing Clinics of North America, 13*(4), 587–604.

Udlis, K.A., & Mancuso, J.M. (2012). Doctor of nursing practice programs across the United States: A benchmark of information. Part I: program characteristics. *Journal of Professional Nursing, 28*(5), 265–273.

Wholey, J.S., Hatry, H.P., & Newcomer, K.T. (Eds.) (2010). *Handbook of practical program evaluation* (3rd ed). San Francisco, CA: Jossey-Bass.

Woods, N.F., & Magyary, D.L. (2010). Translational research: Why nursing's interdisciplinary collaboration is essential. *Research and Theory for Nursing Practice, 24*(1), 9–24.

Woolf. S.H. (2008). The meaning of translational research and why it matters. *JAMA, 292*(2), 211–213.

IF YOU WANT TO READ MORE...

Policy Design

Desouza, K.C., & Lin, Y. (2011). Towards evidence-driven policy design: Complex adaptive systems and computational modeling. *The Innovation Journal: The Public Sector Innovation Journal, 16*(1), Article 7. Retrieved from http://www.innovation.cc/scholarly-style/desouza_lin_policy_informatics_v16i1a7.pdf

Program Evaluation

Wholey, J.S., Hatry, H.P., & Newcomer, K.T. (Eds.). (2010). *Handbook of practical program evaluation* (3rd ed.). San Francisco, CA: Jossey-Bass.

Quality Improvement

HRSA. (2011). *Introduction and overview.* Retrieved from *http://www.hrsa.gov/quality/toolbox/508pdfs/introductionandoverview.pdf*

2

Underpinnings of the DNP Project

Successful change is more likely to take place in contexts with leaders who inspire and act within a supportive organization.

SANDSTROM, BORGLIN, NILSSON, & WILLMAN, 2011

OUTCOME OBJECTIVES

- Reflect on the meaning and direction of scholarly activity within the practice scope of the DNP.
- Correlate Boyer's concepts of scholarship with American Association of Colleges of Nursing essentials of scholarly activity.
- Describe the importance of context of your project within the framework of patient-centered care.
- Explore leadership roles for the DNP scholar.
- Discuss the correlations between patient-centered care and population health.
- Analyze the underpinnings of the DNP project related to rigor and outcome.

TERMS

Authentic leadership	Patient-centered care	Transformation
Collaboration	Population	Transformational
Direct patient-	Population health	leadership
centered care	Scholarship	Translation
Indirect patient care	Social justice	Organization
Leadership	Systemic leadership	
Management	model	

Underpinnings provide a basis for conceptualizing and understanding the foundations that buttress the DNP project. Taken individually, each foundational underpinning provides a different aspect of strength. Viewed holistically, the underpinnings convey a solid foundation for growth and evolution of the DNP project. This chapter provides information regarding underpinnings for the purpose of giving meaning to roles and opportunities realized from creation and implementation of a DNP project. Each underpinning is correlated with at least one of the essentials from *The Essentials of Doctoral Education for Advanced Nursing Practice* published by the American Association of Colleges of Nursing (AACN, 2006). This important document can be accessed from http://www.aacn.nche.edu/publications/position/DNPEssentials.pdf. Underpinnings discussed in this chapter include scholarship, patient-centered care, leadership, population health, and social justice. Each underpinning connects to the project, thus predicating that the project represents a demonstration of meaningful knowledge and use.

SCHOLARSHIP

Scholarship is a primary underpinning of the DNP project because it emphasizes students' learning and assists faculty's focus for teaching, guiding, and mentoring. The AACN (2006) Essential III (p 11) frames scholarship within Boyer's (1990) model. Boyer advocated for scholarship to be less restrictive and more inclusive of different ways of knowing and learning. Boyer advocated for encompassing discovery, integration of ideas, teaching, and application as scholarly activities. Essential VIII focuses on the multiple choices for context and specialization open to advanced practice DNP nurses' scholarly directions. A more focused educational journey enhances depth of knowing, learning, and competence in "highly complex areas of practice" (AACN, 2006, p 16). The DNP project assists the DNP student to integrate, teach, or apply best evidence in a specialty area of his or her choice.

What is the meaning of scholarship? The conceptualization of scholarship varied throughout history to meet the norms and mandates of the times. For our current era and needs, Dr. Ernest Boyer (1990), a national leader in education and former president of the Carnegie Institution, wrote *Scholarship Reconsidered: Priorities of the Professoriate.* This seminal publication updated and broadened the concept of scholarship for higher education by emphasizing the equal importance of discovery, integration of ideas, teaching, and application. Boyer noted that scholarship is not a linear model of research, publication, and teaching, but an interconnected method of creating and using knowledge.

The *scholarship of discovery* is most similar to the current understanding of original research and implies a systematic investigation that contributes to the body of knowledge about a specific topic. The scholarship of discovery is considered basic science that contributes interesting new knowledge to draw on "when the time for intelligent use arrives" (Boyer, 1990, p 18). Indeed, the scholarship of discovery describes Phase I in the Translational Science Model, and research publications in peer-reviewed journals provide usable evidence in designing, implementing, and leading change in the practice setting.

The *scholarship of integration* speaks to the importance of giving meaning and understanding to information from multiple scholarly sources. The AACN (2006) wrote that "scholars give meaning to isolated facts and make connections across disciplines through the scholarship of integration" (p 11). In nursing, the scholarship of integration is about connectedness of nursing knowledge with other disciplines' knowledge. Information from interdisciplinary sources places knowledge into a larger context, thereby gaining interpretive ways of solving problems. Scholarly integration is "serious, disciplined work that seeks to interpret, draw together, and bring new insight to bear on original research" (Boyer, 1990, p 19). The scholarship of integration implies that when searching for best available evidence to address practice issues, you are encouraged to increase the interdisciplinary breadth and depth of your literature search. The scholarship of integration may also suggest Phases III and IV of the Translational Science Model wherein dissemination and population randomized controlled trials are conducted. Communication leading to collaboration for and integration of research and new ideas are possible. See Chapter 16 for an in-depth discussion on postgraduation collaborative science within the framework of translational science.

The *scholarship of application* addresses the responsible execution of knowledge to solve problems. Boyer (1990) emphasizes, however, that scholarship of application is much more than finding and applying knowledge. Increased meaning and understanding through scholarly integration enhance scholarly application. "In activities such as these, theory and practice vitally interact and one renews the other" (p 23). The discipline of nursing embraces the scholarship of application. The AACN (2006) wrote that the scholarship of application is "referred to as the scholarship of practice in nursing" (p 11). The scholarships of integration and application, therefore, embody Phase II of the Translational Science Model. Integration addresses evidence-based practice and synthesis of best knowledge leading to practice-based recommendations that can be applied or implemented to a specific advanced nursing context. This is the purview of the DNP project.

The *scholarship of teaching* is the fourth concept in Boyer's (1990) reconceptualization of scholarship. He states that "teaching is a dynamic endeavor involving all the analogies, metaphors, and images that build bridges between the teacher's understanding and the student's learning" (p 23). Teaching and learning grounded in interpretation, utilization, and implementation of knowledge are integral to the multiple roles and contexts of a DNP. Although Boyer's narrative was directed at the professoriate in academia, his concepts of teaching are applicable to clinical practice and introduction of change. Enticing students, peers, and patients to be continuous learners and encouraging them to recognize that all of us are both teachers and learners are important lessons for practice. The scholarship of teaching applies to faculty members who guide you through the learning process of your project, as well as the specific context of advanced practice nurses who aspire to be teachers, either in the practice setting or within the academic realm of higher education.

Boyer's classic contribution to expanding the meaning of scholarship is a pertinent underpinning of a DNP project. Boyer wrote: "In our complicated, vulnerable world, the discovery of new knowledge is absolutely crucial" (p 17). Indeed, without the rigor of research and application of evidence, the quality and safety of practice in a healthcare setting are exposed. New knowledge can be viewed as cyclical and bidirectional when knowledge is applied and used, followed by collaborations both interprofessional and intraprofessional to validate and discover more new knowledge.

PATIENT-CENTERED CARE

Whereas scholarship is framed in Boyer's model, practice is framed in patient-centered care, a concept first presented by the Institute of Medicine (IOM, 2001). The IOM's *Crossing the Quality Chasm: A New Health System for the 21st Century* resulted in major rethinking about the delivery of health care. Six outcome goal attributes specific to core needs of health care were presented:

safe, effective, patient-centered, timely, efficient, and equitable. Patient-centered health care was described as "care that is respectful of and responsive to individual patient preferences, needs, and values, and ensuring that patient values guide all clinical decisions" (IOM, 2001, p 3). Patient-centered care is based on quality and safety. Patient-centered care is actualized through personal, professional, and organizational relationships (Epstein & Street, 2011). Most hospitals have incorporated the patient-centered care model within their institutions' missions and models; patient-centered care is now accepted as the ideal (Cleary, 2012).

Ten general principles to inform redesign, change, and meet outcome goals are included in the following list. Interpretation of the general principles encourages change or improvement based on technology and evidence-based knowledge. The following list describes the 10 principles or general rules to achieve quality in health care. The entire IOM report can be read online, as provided in the Reference list.

1. *Care is based on continuous healing relationships.* The intent is that patients receive care when they need it, not just during a scheduled face-to-face appointment. Alternative routes for continuous access to care involve technology such as cell phones and the Internet.

2. *Care is customized according to patients' needs and values.* Sigma Theta Tau International defined evidence-based nursing as "an integration of the best evidence available, nursing expertise, and the values and preferences of the individuals, families, and communities who are served" (DiCenso, Provost, & Titler, 2004, p 69). Use of technology and evidence to increase patient-centered care is, therefore, recognized throughout the suggested principles or rules.

3. *The patient is the source of control.*

4. *Knowledge is shared, and information flows freely.*

5. *Decision is evidence based.*

6. *Safety is a system property.*

7. *Transparency is necessary.*

8. *Needs are anticipated.*

9. *Waste is continuously decreased.*

10. *Cooperation among clinicians is a priority.*

Two of the eight AACN (2006) Essentials focus on using evidence in practice and information technology as a means of meeting patients' needs, thus aligning with the IOM (2001) report that includes patient-centered care as a desired outcome. The IOM report specifically recommends four areas for improvement in structures and processes to meet the desired outcome goals: (1) applying evidence to healthcare delivery, (2) using information technology, (3) aligning payment policies with quality improvement, and (4) preparing the workforce. These interventions are good starting points in consideration of general areas of focus for your DNP project.

The AACN (2006) Essential I titled *Scientific Underpinnings for Practice* focuses on principles and laws to understand "the wholeness or health of human beings recognizing that they are in a continuous interaction with their environments" (p 9). Using the term *scientific* in the context of nursing practice emphasizes the importance placed on evidence and, by association, evidence-based practice. Essential IV, *Information Systems/Technology and Patient Care Technology for the Improvement and Transformation of Health Care,* focuses on the importance of technology in patient care, education, and administration. The influence of the IOM (2001) report on the AACN Essentials report demonstrates the importance of all aspects that we currently apply to patient-centered health care.

Outcomes from numerous research studies support the finding that patient-centered care makes a positive difference. For example, research findings discovered that improvements in patients' experiences of care increased the public's perceptions of value for services including increased quality and safety of health care and decreased cost. Provider satisfaction also increased. To summarize, patient-centered care has been noted to positively affect business metrics (Australian Commission on Safety and Quality in Health Care, 2010).

Within the patient-centered care model, there are advanced nursing practices and roles that are described as *direct patient care* and *indirect* patient care. *Direct patient-centered care* focuses on clinical interactions between a nurse practitioner and a patient regarding the patient's needs and perceptions. Information related directly to patient care includes physical, mental and emotional assessments. Patient information is collected through communication and interactions with a practitioner. The intent of direct patient-centered care is to empower patients to become active learners and participants in their health care (Grey, 2013).

Indirect patient-centered care is increasingly focused on administration, management, policy, information technology, and education (Grey, 2013; Melnyk, 2013). Although many advanced practice roles that employ indirect patient care have moved beyond the bedside, the patient remains the center of focus.

Skill sets for indirect patient-centered care include principles of practice management, strategies for balancing productivity with quality of care, assessment of practice policies and procedures, proficiency in quality improvement strategies, and systems thinking related to the organization, culture, and financial structures (AONE, 2015).

All DNP projects relate to patient-centered care, whether the process is direct or indirect. Examples of DNP projects centered on sustainability and improvement of quality patient care include financial incentives, program operations, and policy improvements to instill new norms. Information technology projects also contribute to patient-centered care with projects that address access to health-related information and personal healthcare records, workflow issues, computer literacy for patients, or improved patient-provider communication.

POPULATION HEALTH

The resurgence of a population health model was realized because of the importance of lifestyle and culture in health-related issues. It is a movement away from the traditional medical model (Radzyminski, 2007). The Institute of Medicine's (2002) report titled *The Future of the Public's Health in the 21st Century* discussed movement to more actively and effectively create partnerships to involve diverse communities in health actions. The AACN's (2006) Essential VII, *Clinical Prevention and Population Health for Improving the Nation's Health,* focuses on decreasing unhealthy lifestyle behaviors through clinical prevention and population health activities. The AACN wrote that *Healthy People 2010* encouraged clinical education for nursing and other health professionals to include curricular content of core competencies in "health promotion and disease prevention" (p 15).

Since the introduction of the Affordable Care Act in 2010, the term *population health* has been increasingly used by healthcare professionals and corporations. The term has slightly different meanings for researchers, practitioners, policy makers, and public health officials. Yet a common theme shared by all professionals implies that *population health* creates "a potent opportunity for health care delivery systems, public health agencies, community-based organizations, and many other entities to work together to improve health outcomes in the communities they serve" (Bialek, Moran, & Kirshy, 2015, p 1). An example is improved collaboration across boundaries or borders between hospitals and public or community health. The health of a population is influenced by socioeconomics, physical environments, lifestyle choices, coping skills, human biology, early childhood development, and access to healthcare services. The focus of population health is on "interrelated conditions and factors that influence the health of populations over the life course, identifies systematic variations in their patterns of occurrence, and applies the resulting knowledge to develop and implement policies and actions to improve the health and well-being of those populations" (Bialek et al., 2015).

Distinguishing a population from population health is important in understanding the concept. *Population* as a research term is conceptualized as a set of people with an identified or common need that can be measured or examined. The important element is to clearly define the population from which a sample will be drawn (LoBiondo-Wood & Haber, 2010). *Population health* as a practice term refers to people with commonalities. Population health crosses boundaries to increase understanding of a population's health within the healthcare setting or the community and focuses on both wellness and illness (Radzyminski, 2007). Population health examines the influence of everyday life and social interactions, as well as physical and mental illness (Grove, Burns, & Gray, 2013). The World Health Organization (2000) defined population health as not merely absence of disease or infirmity, but a state of total physical, mental, and social well-being. Population health helps practitioners understand trends in a population's health status and the performance of the healthcare system (Radzyminski, 2007).

Opportunities for DNP projects may include behaviors and lifestyles or socioeconomic and cultural factors of populations within a specified environmental context that inhibit or encourage change. A population's attitudes, beliefs, and values regarding motivators or barriers to a specified change could increase understanding of a population's health. Increased understanding of a population's healthcare needs is often correlated with opportunities for social justice.

SOCIAL JUSTICE

Social justice is rooted in societal differences dealing with inequalities of power. The term *social* denotes daily living and development of skills, access to necessary services, and reliance on others in time of need. *Justice* is an ethical principle meaning equal and fair treatment (Oxford Dictionaries, 2013). Social justice is an important value for individuals and for the discipline of nursing (Grace & Wills, 2012). The United Nations (1948) codified the *Universal Declaration of Human Rights*, which declares that each individual is important and has fundamental human rights. *The Code of Ethics* of the American Nurses Association (ANA, 2001) and the AACN's (2006) Essential V, *Health Care Policy for Advocacy in Health Care*, state that the influence of "political activism and a commitment to policy development ... on behalf of the public as well as nursing profession" are influential in multiple areas of ethics, equity, and social justice in the delivery of health care (p 13). In social systems, unfair treatment of others is often perpetuated because of socioeconomics, culture, and race—many of the same issues that inhibit healthy lifestyles and access to health care. The dimensions of unjust treatment are generally interrelated and interactive. Indeed, the combination of unjust effects is greater than that of only one (Grace & Willis, 2012; Powers & Faden, 2006). Dr. Woolf (2008) poignantly points out that "poverty matters as much as proteomics in understanding disease" (p 213).

How does this affect nursing? Paquin (2011) claims that nurses' involvement in social justice is an extension of advocacy. The focus on the unjust in society blends with a population health perspective of advocacy. Interest in understanding social systems assists nursing interventions to address inequities and access to health care for a population. Nursing presence and communication, as suggested in patient-centered care principles, assist in accessing appropriate information to forecast consequences of social actions on health care (Grace & Willis, 2012). Basic concepts of social justice include the following:

- *Personal security* or a sense of safety free from injury, violence, neglect, or abuse

- *Reasoning* abilities to negotiate and personal freedom to question authority

- *Respect* for others, from others, and self-respect or dignity

- *Attachment* or the ability to have feelings of belonging to one's community

- *Self-determination* to live life based on personal values and priorities free from undue outside interference (Powers & Faden, 2006)

"Although we may speak the words of social justice, it is how we act that clearly demonstrates our philosophy" (Drevdahl, Kneipp, Canales, & Dorcy, 2001, p 29). Social justice is more than words; it is about equity.

LEADERSHIP

Leadership is a necessary role for implementation of the DNP project. Your ability to conceptualize new ideas and lead implementation of new programs, policies, or system improvements for a target population is warranted. AACN's Essential II, *Organizational and Systems Leadership for Quality Improvement and Systems Thinking,* is important whether your practice includes direct or indirect care. As a DNP leader, your knowledge and abilities distinguish you "to conceptualize new care delivery models that are based in contemporary nursing science and that are feasible within current organizational, political, cultural, and economic perspectives" (AACN, 2006, p 10).

Leadership is an essential element in all areas of nursing and is the topic of numerous publications. *Graduate-Level QSEN Competencies* identify the need for graduate nurses to "provide leadership by example and promote the importance of providing quality care and outcome measurement" (AACNa, 2012, p 3). The Magnet Recognition Program identifies transformational leadership as the way of thinking to meet the organizational needs of the future (AACNb, 2012). The American Organization of Nurse Executives (AONE) emphasizes the importance of innovative and expert leadership skills in advanced nursing practice. Leadership competencies identified by AONE (2015) include foundational thinking skills, the ability to use systems thinking, success planning, and change management. Finally, the Institute of Medicine's (2010) publication *The Future of Nursing: Leading Change, Advancing Health* emphasizes the important role of nursing leadership in transforming health care in today's changing economy. Foundational competencies for leadership identified by the IOM include the following:

- Knowledge of the care delivery system

- Work in teams

- Effective collaboration within and across disciplines

- Basic tenets of ethical care

- Effective patient advocacy

- Theories of innovation

- Quality and safety improvement (p 224)

A system wherein a nursing leader might work can be defined as a collection of interconnecting parts. The real power of systems, however, is in the way they come together to fulfill a specific purpose. **Systems thinking** is an ongoing evolutionary approach to change and improvement within a large, complex healthcare organization or healthcare system because the focus is on understanding how parts within a whole influence each other (Oxford Dictionaries, 2013). The breadth of potential direct and indirect roles for DNPs within a healthcare system requires leadership and systems thinking to address issues as they arise.

Leadership and **management** are conceptualized differently but work conjointly. Management implies contextual skills rooted in legitimate power for the purposes of supervision of self, population, or organization. Leadership implies a personal skill set that models, motivates, and empowers others to achieve best outcomes (Curtis & O'Connell, 2011). Today's nursing leader-managers must meet increased demands of cost efficiency, monitoring high standards of quality and safety in patient care, stressful work environments, recruiting and retaining high-performing personnel, technology updates, integrating best available evidence, and evaluation of change specific to context, time, and place (Bish, Kenny, & Nay, 2012; Salmela, Eriksson, & Fagerstrom, 2011; Sandstrom, Borglin, Nilsson, & Williams, 2011; Wong & Laschinger, 2012). The varied and important nursing roles identified for leadership in health care demand that "nurses should practice to the full extent of their education and training" (IOM, 2010, p 29). The DNP project provides opportunities for practicing your leadership role or roles.

Leadership Theories Specific to the DNP Project

The DNP curriculum generally includes entire classes related to leadership theories and roles wherein quality resources exist for intensive learning. It is not the intent of this book to supplement leadership curriculum. Rather, the intent is to provide a leadership framework for this book that focuses on the DNP project. Transformational and authentic leadership theories applied within a systemic leadership model have been selected. Together, they provide ideas for structuring, modeling, motivating, and empowering.

Systemic Leadership Model

The *Systemic Leadership Model* is a function of an organizational system, not an individual role, with a focus on interconnectedness of the *whole* system in addition to the individuals and leaders who energize the system. Tate (2013) describes the current emphasis of organization development as being *dialogic*, compared with an older view of organization development, which is considered *diagnostic*. Whether new or old, organization development encompasses humanistic and democratic values. These values are practiced with high levels of participation to balance the many interests represented in the system. A summary of elements in Tate's (2013) overview of systemic leadership includes the following.

- The services of an organization are delivered to customers and markets by systems, not by individuals.

- Leadership is a resource to be managed if it is to reach its full potential.

- An organization should strive for a reputation of being well led as a whole and having good leaders.

- Individual leadership *and* systemic leadership are important and are intertwined.

- A carefully developed system liberates leadership, focuses its energy on the organization's needs, and provides an ethical culture.

- A leader's application of change requires courage to lead as well as obtaining management consent and support.

- Leadership is a relational activity.

- Leaders are more effective if they have a good perspective of how the organization works as a system.

- Issues can be best analyzed, understood, and explained with a multidisciplined understanding of the complexity and dynamics of the system.

- Simple mental models help differentiate the need for leading or managing.

- Leadership is a fit for future challenges when the organization's current paradigm is questioned.

- Leadership should be particularly aware of the culture because it sends powerful messages about leadership values, ethics, and how managers are expected to perform.

- An organization should consider how the power of leadership is distributed for the purpose of achieving improvement.

- Leadership should be accompanied by a sound governance structure (Tate, 2013, pp 35–36).

Transformational Leadership Theory

Transformational Leadership Theory was selected because it is used by the AONE (2011) and is implied in AACN documents (2006). Transformational leaders offer expertise to transform clinical, program, and system cultures to be more conducive to implementation of best evidence. Effective nursing leaders have abilities to meld the application of science and technology with the art of translating evidence into caring actions (Rycroft-Malone, 2012). Authentic leadership theory is presented within the construction of transformational leadership because it adds depth and understanding to the transformational leadership role.

The terms *transformational* and *translational* are often used as modifiers for DNP leadership roles, including the DNP leadership role for scholarly actions. *Transformation* implies metamorphosis or change in appearance, form, or direction (Oxford Dictionary, 2013). The term is used in the IOM (2010) report,

Part II: *A Transformation of the Nursing Profession.* The first three sections of Part II are titled Transforming Practice, Transforming Education, and Transforming Leadership. *Translation* implies changing context without changing meaning or form (Oxford Dictionary, 2013). Translation is best understood as changing or translating a written statement from one language to another without changing the meaning. For the DNP role, translating relevant evidence into the context of practice provides a means for introducing change or improvement but requires transformational leadership for implementation.

The development of *Transformational Leadership Theory* began in 1973 with J.V. Downton's introduction of the term, followed in 1978 by J. M. Burns's conceptualizations of transactional and transformational leadership. Transactional leaders were noted to lead through social exchange, whereas transformational leaders motivated, inspired, and empowered. B.M. Bass is the most published contributor of research validating the theory of transformational leadership. Many of Bass's research studies centered on the military's leadership styles. Included in Bass's publications are the topics of authentic and inauthentic leadership (Bass, 1985; Bass, 1995; Bass & Riggio, 2006).

A review of the theory of transformational leadership identifies transformational leaders as people who empower followers by focusing on positions and objectives of the individuals, the leader, the group, and the larger organization. Transformational leaders move themselves and others to exceed their practice expectations. Transformational leadership uses a style that empowers others to achieve better outcomes, including processes that ensure emotional and intellectual satisfaction (Bass, 1995; Bass & Riggio, 2006; Doody & Doody, 2012).

Bass (1995) identified four conceptual constructs in his theory of transformational leadership:

1. *Idealized influence.* This construct implies confidence, respect, and trust in a charismatic leader who is admired and viewed as a role model for others (Bass, 1995; Curtis & O'Connell, 2011; Doody & Doody, 2012).

2. *Individualized consideration.* Bass (1995) conceptualized "individual consideration as giving personal attention to each individual team member" (p 471). This is a method of motivation leading to empowerment by encouraging and mentoring others to learn and change to advance their careers (Bass, 1995; Curtis & O'Connell, 2011; Doody & Doody, 2012).

3. *Intellectual stimulation.* Transformational leaders encourage and stimulate new ideas based on best evidence. Bass (1995) stated that intellectual stimulation "enabled me to think about old problems in new ways" (p 471). Transformational leaders share knowledge and demonstrate critical thinking and problem-solving skills, thereby increasing the capacity of others to

advance their knowledge in the practice setting (Curtis & O'Connell, 2011; Doody & Doody, 2012).

4. *Inspirational motivation* "inspires loyalty in the organization" (Bass, 1995, p 472). Transformational leaders motivate and create a team spirit for the work to be done. They inspire a shared vision of the organization by communicating high expectations (Curtis & O'Connell, 2011; Doody & Doody, 2012).

Bass's (1995) research found that transformational factors were correlated more closely with the outcomes of effectiveness and satisfaction than with contingent rewards. A transformational leadership style that practices shared accountability, responsibility, and power is empowering to employees and reduces resistance to change. Transformational leadership assists the organization to achieve goals and is consistent with the leadership styles and environments of contemporary health care (Curtis & O'Connell, 2011).

Authentic Leadership Theory

Bass (1995) studied many aspects of transformational leadership including the power and charisma of leaders. However, are charismatic leaders always authentic? Early philosophical conversations between Burns and Bass focused on authentic and inauthentic leadership within the theory of transformational leadership (Bass & Riggio, 2006). Aviolio, who studied with Bass, subsequently wrote about authentic leadership.

The *Theory of Authentic Leadership* relates to the development or making of leaders, whereas the theory of transformational leadership relates to development after the fact or after an identified leader is in place (Aviolio & Gardner, 2005). Advocates of the authentic leadership model practiced by nurse leaders note that job satisfaction and performance improve because authentic leaders emphasize "transparency, balanced processing, self-awareness, and high ethical standards" (Wong & Laschinger, 2012, p 955). Nine constructs are associated with the theory of authentic leadership:

1. Positive psychological capital

2. Positive moral perspectives

3. Leader self-awareness

4. Leader self-regulation

5. Leadership processes and behaviors

6. Follower self-awareness and regulation

7. Follower development

8. Organizational content

9. Veritable sustained performance beyond expectations (Avolio & Gardner, 2005)

To summarize, there is a positive relationship between transformational and authentic leaders and employee motivation. Authentic, transformational leaders have vision. They are innovative and stimulate followers' thinking about change. Leaders are skilled communicators who promote trust within their teams by inspiring self-confidence (Curtis & O'Connell, 2011).

The constructs of authentic leadership theory overlap with transformational leadership theory and the systemic leadership model. The foci are on three structures: leader, follower, and organization. Authentic leaders are confident, optimistic, and resilient. Leaders are transparent in the decision-making process because they draw on moral capacity, efficiency, and courage. Authentic leaders are self-aware of their values, motives, and emotions including self-control and self-analysis. Leaders model positive behaviors (Avolio & Gardner, 2005). Followers of authentic leaders also demonstrate clarity of values, identity, and emotions that contribute to transparent relations between leader and peers. Both follower and leader are shaped in their development through role modeling (Avolio & Gardner, 2005). Finally, context within the system or organization provides opportunity and access to information and resources. The organization can provide nonfinancial incentives that contribute to building human, social, and psychological capital (Avolio & Gardner, 2005).

COLLABORATION

The AACN's (2006) Essential VI, *Interprofessional Collaboration for Improving Patient and Population Health Outcomes,* emphasizes the importance of collaboration. "In order to accomplish the IOM mandate for safe, timely, effective, efficient, equitable, and patient-centered care in a complex environment, healthcare professionals must function as highly collaborative teams" (p 14). Collaboration strengthens the actualization of the essentials. It is an important item to learn and to practice.

Interprofessional, intraprofessional, and transprofessional collaboration and partnership work are characterized as the "new frontier of co-production" (Fenwick & Nerland, 2014, p 6). Collaboration implies ways in which individuals and groups share or recontextualize knowledge across professional boundaries. Collaboration draws energy from others and initiates ideas for practice improvement or change. Collaboration provides synergistic opportunities to enhance population health and patient-centered care (Montero, Lupi, & Jarris, 2015; O'Daniel & Rosenstein, 2008). Put another way, collaboration begins with a good conversation. See Chapter 16 in this text for detailed information regarding interprofessionalism, intraprofessionalism, and transprofessionalism.

An example of a project that characterizes the collaborative underpinning of intraprofessionalism and transprofessionalism is the Million Hearts Initiative (IOM, 2015). The aim of the Million Hearts Initiative is to prevent 1 million heart attacks and strokes by 2017. Million Hearts "brings together communities, health systems, nonprofit organizations, federal agencies, and private-sector partners from across the country to fight heart disease and stroke" (p 3). Among the intended deliverables is to "identify, share, and assist implementation of best practices/strategies to promote population health" (IOM, 2015, p 3). Imagine a DNP project in your specific context that recommends and implements an evidence-based strategy to prevent heart attacks and strokes in your identified population based on the Million Hearts Initiative.

CHAPTER SUMMARY AND AFTERTHOUGHTS

Underpinnings of scholarly inquiry and activity for the role of DNP are multifaceted in meaning and opportunity. Boyer's conceptualization of scholarship encompasses four areas of meaning that apply, in part or in full, to development of the DNP project. Leadership roles practiced in the development and implementation of the DNP project increase understanding of process and assist in successful outcomes. Population health and systems thinking assist in identifying context for the project. Patient-centered care and social justice ground the DNP project in the ethical cloak of nursing while communication and collaboration tie the parts together. The content of the chapter is grounded in AACN (2006) essentials.

CASE STUDY

Jack worked as an adult nurse practitioner in the emergency department (ED) of a large urban medical center. The ED has rooms for emergency care, trauma, and nonemergency health care. Jack works in the nonemergency clinic of the ED where he examines and treats many patients with illnesses that could have been prevented days or weeks before the ED visit. Some of these patients are underinsured, some have Medicaid through the Affordable Care Act, and only a few have a medical home. Jack provides medication prescriptions and education in a caring manner, yet he remains frustrated because the patients he sees are economically and socially marginalized, and he recognizes that these circumstances affect their health.

- Analyze Jack's combined role in patient-centered care, population health, and social justice.

- Using a systems thinking approach, discuss Jack's role within the hospital where he works and the overall healthcare system.

- Discuss potential solutions to the problems Jack identified.

WRITING REMINDERS...

Pay Attention to How the Experts Write

- Read peer-reviewed nursing journals on a regular basis.

- Read for more than content.

- Observe the author's writing skills.

- Observe the sentence structure. Clarity begins by creating well-structured sentences.

- Observe the organization of content. Look for subheadings that organize topics.

- Observe paragraph content and length. Do the sentences in the paragraph connect to each other?

- Your goal in professional writing is to write clearly. Clarity demonstrates your intelligence and logic.

REFERENCES

American Association of Colleges of Nursing (AACN). (2006). *The essentials of doctoral education for advanced nursing practice.* Retrieved from http://www.aacn.nche.edu/publications/position/DNPEssentials. pdf

American Association of Colleges of Nursing (AACN). (2012a). *Graduate-level QSEN competencies: Knowledge, skills and attitudes.* Retrieved from http://www.aacn.nche.edu/faculty/qsen/competencies.pdf

American Association of Colleges of Nursing (AACN). (2012b). *Magnet recognition program model*. Retrieved from http://www.nursecredentialing.org/Magnet/Program Overview/New-Magnet-Model.aspx

American Nurses Association (ANA). (2001). *Code of ethics for nurses with interpretive statements*. Washington, DC: American Nurses Association.

American Organization of Nurse Executives (AONE). (2015). *Nurse executive competencies*. Washington DC: AONE.

Australian Commission on Safety and Quality in Health Care. (2010). *Patient-centred care: Improving quality and safety by focusing care on patients and consumers*. Discussion paper. Retrieved from www.safetyandquality.gov.au/wp-content-uploads/2012/01/PCCC-DiscussPaper.pdf

Avolio, B.J., & Gardner, W.L. (2005). Authentic leadership development: Getting to the root of positive forms of leadership. *The Leadership Quarterly, 16*(3), 315–338.

Bass, B.M. (1985). *Leadership and performance beyond expectations*. New York, NY: The Free Press.

Bass, B.M. (1995). Theory of transformational leadership. *Leadership Quarterly, 6*(4), 463–478.

Bass, B.M., & Riggio, R.E. (2006). *Transformational leadership* (2nd ed.). Mahwah, NJ: Lawrence Erlbaum Associates, Inc., Publishers.

Bialek, R., Moran, J., & Kirshy, M. (2015). *Using a population health driver diagram to support health care and public health collaboration*. Washington, DC: Institute of Medicine. Retrieved from http://nam.edu/perspectives-2015-using-a-population-health-driver-diagram-to-support-health-care-and-public-health-collaboration/

Bish, M., Kenny, A., & Nay, R. (2012). A scoping review identifying contemporary issues in rural nursing leadership. *Journal of Nursing Scholarship, 44*(4), 411–417.

Boyer, E.L. (1990). *Scholarship reconsidered: Priorities of the professoriate*. The Carnegie Foundation. New York, NY: Jossey-Bass.

Cleary, P.D. (2012). *Why is patient-centered health care important?* Retrieved from http://www.scholarsstrategynetwork.org/brief/why-patient-centered-health-care-important

Curtis, E., & O'Connell, R. (2011). Essential leadership skills for motivating and developing staff. *Nursing Management, 18*(5), 32–35.

DiCenso, A., Provost, S., & Titler, M. (2004). Evidence-based nursing: Rationale and resources. *Worldviews on Evidence-Based Nursing, 1*(1), 69–75.

Doody, O., & Doody, C.M. (2012). Transformational leadership in nursing practice. *British Journal of Nursing, 21*(2), 1212–1218.

Drevdahl, D., Kneipp, S.M., Canales, M.K., & Dorcy, K.S. (2001). Reinvesting in social justice: A capital idea for public health nursing? *Advances in Nursing Science, 24*(2), 19–31.

Epstein, R.M., & Street, R.L. (2001). The values and value of patient-centered care. *Annals of Family Medicine, 9*(2), 100–103. Retrieved from http://www.ncbi.nlm.nih.gov/pmc/articles/PMC3056855

Fenwick, T., & Nerland, M. (Eds.). (2014). *Reconceptualising professional learning: Sociomaterial knowledge, practices, and responsibilities*. San Francisco, CA: Jossey-Bass.

Grace, P.J., & Wills, D.G. (2012). Nursing responsibilities and social justice: An analysis in support of disciplinary goals. *Nursing Outlook, 60*(4), 198–207.

Grey, M. (2013). The doctor of nursing practice: Defining the next steps. *Journal of Nursing Education, 52*(8), 462–465.

Grove, S.K., Burns, N., & Gray, J.R. (2013). *The practice of nursing research: Appraisal, synthesis, and generation of evidence* (7th ed.). St. Louis, MO: Elsevier.

Institute of Medicine. (2001). *Crossing the quality chasm: A new health system for the 21st century.* Washington, DC: National Academies Press. Retrieved from http://books.nap.edu/openbook.php?record_id=10027

Institute of Medicine. (2002). *The future of the public's health in the 21st century.* Washington, DC: National Academies Press. Retrieved from http://www.iom.nationalacademies.org/Reports/2002/The-Future-of-the-Publics-Health-in-the-21st-Century.aspx

Institute of Medicine. (2010). *The future of nursing: Leading change, advancing health.* Washington, DC: National Academies Press. Retrieved from http://www.iom.nationalacademies.org/Reports/2010/The-Future-of-Nursing-Leading-Change-Advancing-Health.aspx

Institute of Medicine. (2015). *Collaboration between health care and public health: Workshop in brief.* Washington, DC: National Academies Press. Retrieved from www.nap.edu/catalog.php?record_id=21687

LoBiondo-Wood, G., & Haber, J. (2010). *Nursing research: Methods and critical appraisal for evidence-based practice* (7th ed.). St. Louis, MO: Mosby Elsevier.

Melnyk, B.M. (2013). Distinguishing the preparation and roles of Doctor of Philosophy and Doctor of Nursing Practice graduates: National implications for academic curricula and health care systems. *Journal of Nursing Education, 52*(8), 442–448.

Montero, J.T., Lupi, M.V., & Jarris, P.E. (2015). *Improved population health through more dynamic public health and health care system collaboration.* Institute of Medicine. Retrieved from http://www.nam.edu/perspectives-2015-improved-population-health-through-more-dynamic-public-health-and-health-care-system-collaboration/

O'Daniel, M., & Rosenstein, A.H. (2008). Professional communication and team collaboration. In R. G. Hughes (Ed.). *Patient safety and quality: An evidence-based handbook for nurses.* Rockville, MD: Agency for Healthcare Research and Quality. Retrieved from http://www.ncbi.nlm.nih.gov/books/NBK2637/

Oxford Dictionaries. (2013). Retrieved from http://oxforddictionaries.com

Paquin, S.O. (2011). Social justice advocacy in nursing: What is it? How do we get there? *Creative Nursing, 17*(2), 63–67.

Powers, M., Faden, R. (2006). *Social justice: The moral foundations of public health and health policy.* New York, NY: Oxford University Press.

Radzyminski, S. (2007). The concept of population health within the nursing profession. *Journal of Professional Nursing, 23*(1), 37–46.

Rycroft-Malone, J. (2012). Leadership matters. *Worldviews on Evidence-Based Practice, 127–128.*

Salmela, S., Eriksson, K., & Fagerstrom, L. (2011). Leading change: A three-dimensional model of nurse leaders' main tasks and roles during a change process. *Journal of Advanced Nursing, 68*(2), 423–433.

Sandstrom, B., Borglin, G., Nilsson, & Willman, A. (2011). Promoting the implementation of evidence-based practice: a literature review focusing on the role of nursing leadership. *Worldviews on Evidence-Based Nursing, 8*(4), 212–223.

Tate, W. (2013). *Managing leadership from a systemic perspective.* London: The Centre for Progressive Leadership. Retrieved from http://www.systemicleadershipinstitute.org/wp-content/uploads/2013/01/CPL-white-paper-09-January-2013.pdf

United Nations. (1948). *Universal declaration of human rights.* Retrieved from http://www.un.org/en/universal-declaration-human-rights/index.html

Wong, C.A., & Laschinger, H.K.S. (2012). Authentic leadership, performance, and job satisfaction: The mediating role of empowerment. *Journal of Advanced Nursing,69*(4), 947–959.

Woolf, S.H. (2008). The meaning of translational research and why it matters. *JAMA, 299*(2), 211–213.

World Health Organization (WHO). (2000). *World health reports.* Geneva: World Health Organization.

IF YOU WANT TO READ MORE...

Avolio, B.J., & Gardner W.L. (2005). Authentic leadership development: Getting to the root of positive forms of leadership. *Leadership Quarterly, 16*(3), 315–338.

Bass, B.M. (1995). Theory of transformational leadership. *Leadership Quarterly, 6*(4), 463–478.

Boyer, E.L. (1990). *Scholarship reconsidered: Priorities of the professoriate.* The Carnegie Foundation. New York, NY: Jossey-Bass.

Bunkers, S.S. (2000). The nurse scholar of the 21st century. *Nursing Science Quarterly, 3*(2), 116–123.

Grace, P.J., & Wills, D.G. (2012). Nursing responsibilities and social justice: An analysis in support of disciplinary goals. *Nursing Outlook, 60*(4), 198–207.

Institute of Medicine. (2011). *The future of nursing: Leading change, advancing health.* Washington, DC: National Academies Press. Available electronically, free of charge: http://www.iom.nationalacademies.org/Reports/2010/The-Future-of-Nursing-Leading-Change-Advancing-Health.aspx

Marshall, E.S. (2011). *Transformational leadership in nursing: From expert clinician to influential leader.* New York, NY: Springer Publishing Company.

Inquiry

PURPOSE

The aim of this section is to provide detailed information regarding structure and process in planning and organizing your DNP project from idea to searchable question to evidence-based practice (EBP) recommendations for practice.

Inquiry, the topic of Section II, is about investigation and creativity, from asking a question to making a practice recommendation for change or improvement. EBP provides the most rigorous framework for planning the DNP project. EBP is a rational, critical thinking structure that is linear but iterative. The EBP process begins with development of a searchable question and concludes with creation of EBP recommendations for practice.

Chapter 3 presents conceptual frameworks or models for EBP. The frameworks or models presented in the chapter are from seminal publications authored by nursing leaders. Chapter 4 is about harnessing an idea and turning the idea into a searchable question or statement. This is the beginning of the process that leads to recommendations for practice. Beginnings, however, are difficult, but a good beginning is foundational for a quality DNP project. The chapter begins by analyzing the components of an idea before writing the EBP searchable question or statement using the PICO(T) format. Chapter 5 introduces the reader to the nature of evidence and what constitutes best evidence for a DNP project. Search strategies and organizational plans for finding best evidence are

EBP Process for DNP Project

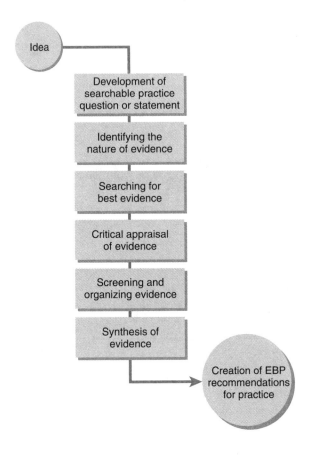

presented in Chapter 6. Organization of findings is essential for orderliness of thought and is best demonstrated with an evidence table. The importance of critiquing evidence leading to establishment of trust in the evidence is the focus of Chapter 7. Analysis or critique of evidence is time consuming, but it is an essential step in creating a rigorous DNP product. Forms are provided to assist learning about critiques. Chapter 8 directs the reader in writing a synthesis of the evidence findings. A well-written synthesis addresses the EBP searchable question and provides the basis for the EBP recommendations for practice.

3

Evidence-Based Practice: Background and Models

A framework is a place to think and strategize.

Author Unknown

OUTCOME OBJECTIVES

- Reflect on the history of research and evidence-based practice (EBP) as it relates to development of EBP models.
- Discuss expected outcomes of EBP models.
- Categorize the commonalities and differences of the processes in the EBP models.
- Discuss the usefulness of an EBP model related to planning your DNP project.

TERMS

Concept	Framework	Research utilization
Evidence-based practice (EBP)	Model	(RU)
		Theory

Evidence-based practice (EBP) is a logical process that guides problem-solving for practice. Making recommendations for improvement or change based on best available evidence provides strength and trust in your practice recommendations. The five EBP models presented in this chapter are similar but with some differences, and they are created by experts in the field. The purpose of reviewing the models is to assist your understanding of the process and problem-solving methods using EBP related to planning your DNP project.

ORIGINS OF EVIDENCE-BASED PRACTICE IN NURSING

Nursing research, research publications, and research utilization (RU) did not substantially grow until the 1960s and 1970s. RU became prominent in the 1970s, thanks in part to Weise's (1979) publication titled *The Problem Solving Model* and Stetler's (1985) model titled *Research Utilization: Defining the Concept.* The models implied direct application to practice of empirical research results. Expectations were that empirical research findings would solve a policy or practice problem. Research was expected to provide "missing knowledge" about the problem and inform decisions. However, users often applied the findings in a context that differed from the one described in the research, thereby altering the linear expectation of the RU model. Additionally, policy and practice changes were often based on a single study (Estabrooks,1999; Melnyk & Fineout-Overholt, 2011) that did not lead to a convincing conclusion. RU models, including the *Problem Solving Model,* failed to clearly guide the use of research in practice. The lack of clarity in process in addition to a lack of adequate nursing research evidence contributed to disillusionment and confusion in implementation of RU (Weiss, 1979).

During the same period, Archie Cochrane, M.D. (1972) published his influential book, *Effectiveness and Efficiency: Random Reflections on Health Services.* Dr. Cochrane was critical of the lack of research evidence to guide healthcare decisions effectively. His concerns led to the establishment of The Cochrane Center, which opened its doors in 1993. As of 2013, more than 5,000 systematic reviews had been published (Cochrane Collaboration, 2013). Dr. Cochrane stressed the use of randomized controlled trials (RCTs) for the systematic reviews because RCTs were considered the most reliable sources of evidence (Grove, Burns, & Gray, 2013; Shah & Chung, 2009). For nursing practice, the development of the Cochrane Collaboration and Library in addition to the focus on RU had limited influence. The reasons were partly the lack of research publications and journals applicable to nursing practice and the narrow interpretation of direct application of RU (Grove et al., 2013). An increase in nursing research journals and a broader view of context for using research in practice subsequently evolved RU into models of EBP.

The concept of EBP was originally presented by medicine. A group of physicians, calling themselves the *Evidence-Based Medicine Working Group*, recognized a need for a new paradigm in medicine wherein "intuition, unsystematic clinical experience, and pathophysiologic rationale" (p 2420) were no longer recognized as best provider practices for patient care (Guyatt, Cairns, Churchill, & Tugwell, 1992). The group recommended that medical students be taught the importance of finding, evaluating, and using evidence in their practices. Dr. David Sackett was a member of the Evidence-Based Medicine Working Group and is given credit for the first definition of EBP: "evidence-based medicine is the conscientious, explicit, and judicious use of current best evidence in making decisions about the care of individual patients" ((Sackett, Rosenberg, Gray, Haynes, & Richardson, 1996, p 71).

Definitions adapted for nursing's use of EBP included a statement by Dr. Marita Titler, who wrote that EBP is "the conscientious and judicious use of current best evidence in conjunction with clinical expertise and patient values to guide health care decisions" (Titler, 2008). Sigma Theta Tau International defined evidence-based nursing as "an integration of the best evidence available, nursing expertise, and the values and preferences of the individuals, families, and communities who are served" (DiCenso, Provost, & Titler, 2004, p 69).

Although EBP was initially adopted by nursing in the early 1990s, wide acceptance of the EBP process was lacking. EBP incorporated some concepts from RU, but it broadened the meaning of *current best evidence* beyond quantitative research and systematic reviews of research to include findings from qualitative research, quality improvement reports, policies, theoretical publications, and organizational data. Today, evidence also includes expert opinion and patients' preferences or values (Melnyk & Fineout-Overholt, 2005; Polit & Beck, 2012).

The importance of EBP is recognized in all aspects of nursing from education to clinical practice to healthcare organizations and systems. EBP increases understanding of who nurses are, what nurses do, and how nurses affect patient care, outcomes, and cost effectiveness (Fineout-Overholt, Levin, & Melnyk, 2004/2005). Undergraduate and graduate curricula, organizational policies and standards, and Magnet recognition are examples of EBP's integration into all practice settings of nursing. Making practice decisions based on current best evidence is a sound and important principle. EBP models assist in explaining the EBP process.

EVIDENCE-BASED PRACTICE MODELS

EBP models provide blueprints to understand and visualize a road map or process to address practice issues. Indeed, the purpose of an EBP model is to provide a structure or organization with rationale as a guide for construction of the EBP process (Green, 2000). A model assists the DNP in the process of connecting concepts, theory, or knowledge with process. EBP models connect concepts with linear and iterative planning and organizing and are considered guides for strategizing about the DNP project. EBP models systematically present ideas to enhance clarity and understanding of process (Burns & Grove, 2011; Rycroft-Malone, 2013; Schaffer, Sandau, & Diedrick, 2012).

Sometimes a model is referred to as a framework. As the quotation at the beginning of this chapter states, "a framework is a place to think and strategize." EBP models provide a place for you to think and strategize about moving from *idea* to *recommendations for practice*. Keep in mind that the EBP models are intended to frame the EBP process for best project outcomes. The intent of an EBP model is *not* to frame the content of your topic.

Five EBP models were selected for this section. As you read them, consider the similarities and differences in how each model adds to or interprets the EBP experience. The EBP models include: the Stetler Model (Melnyk, & Fineout-Overholt, 2011; Stetler, 2001; Stetler & Marram, 1976), the Iowa Model of Evidence-Based Practice (Titler, Kleiber, Steelman, & Goode, 2001), the Rosswurm and Larrabee Model for Change to Evidence-Based Practice (Rosswurm & Larrabee, 1999), the ARCC Model: Advancing Research and Clinical Practice Through Close Collaboration (Melnyk & Fineout-Overholt, 2011, and the Johns Hopkins Nursing Evidence-Based Practice Model (Newhouse, Dearholt, Poe, Pugh, & White, 2007). A brief overview of the models is hereafter presented.

Stetler Model of Research Utilization to Facilitate Evidence-Based Practice

Cheryl Stetler (2001) was an early champion for promoting RU in the practice setting. Her early works on RU provided the conceptual basis for the Stetler-Marram Model of Evidence-Based Practice (Stetler & Marram, 1976). The early model was a prescriptive approach emphasizing steps in critical thinking and decision making, but it was also designed as a process for safe and effective use of research findings (Stetler, 2001). Stetler's early works evolved over time into the current model that integrates RU concepts with the EBP process. Critical thinking and problem-solving are emphasized. The current Stetler Model is presented as an algorithm under five headings. Put another way, the Stetler Model is presented as a five-step decision-making process. The model emphasizes critical thinking and practical application (Stetler, 2001) (Fig. 3.1). The five steps in the Stetler Model (2001) are as follows:

1. *Preparation* emphasizes the purpose of consulting relevant evidence sources as well as consideration of important contextual elements.

2. *Validation* assesses credibility and use of evidence.

3. *Comparative evaluation or decision making* emphasizes synthesis of findings and making recommendations for use that contribute to logical decision making and organization of a plan.

4. *Translation or application* identifies the evidence that will be used and the context of its use.

5. *Evaluation* clarifies formative and expected outcomes, then articulates types of evaluation (Stetler, 2001).

The Stetler Model emphasizes decision making during planning. Organizing is described in the first three phases of the model. An emphasis on *applicability* and *feasibility* to determine whether the study is a fit for the practice context and identification of stakeholders lies within step three. Information from steps four and five relate to contextual translation of evidence and evaluation (Stetler, 2001).

Iowa Model of Evidence-Based Practice

Nursing leaders from University of Iowa Hospitals and Clinics were also early leaders of EBP. Led by Dr. Marita Titler, the Iowa Model was first published in 1994 as an RU tool and was updated in 2001 to reflect integration of RU with EBP. Changes incorporated in 2001 included new terminology, new feedback loops, and utilization of evidence other than research. Expert opinion and patient values or preferences,were considered evidence when research evidence was lacking (Titler et al., 2001).

The Iowa Model provides a decision-making process for the planning stage of a DNP project (Fig. 3.2). The model has been used successfully in multiple settings. It is popular with practitioners because it reflects considerations from all parts of a healthcare organization, including patient, provider, and infrastructure (Melnyk & Fineout-Overholt, 2005). Useful elements from the Iowa Model include problem-focused and knowledge-focused triggers to assist in development and prioritization of project and research ideas. The Iowa Model

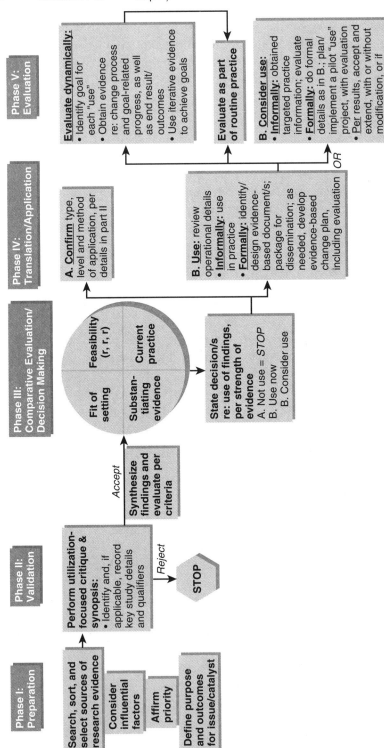

FIGURE 3.1 The Stetler Model of Research Utilization to Facilitate Evidence-Based Practice

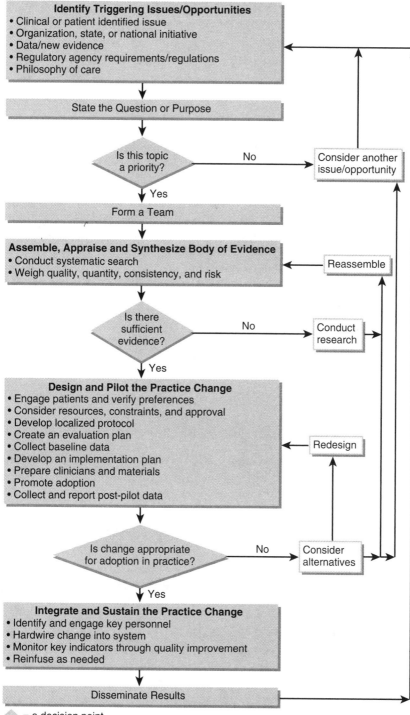

Identify Triggering Issues/Opportunities
- Clinical or patient identified issue
- Organization, state, or national initiative
- Data/new evidence
- Regulatory agency requirements/regulations
- Philosophy of care

State the Question or Purpose

Is this topic a priority? — No → Consider another issue/opportunity

Yes

Form a Team

Assemble, Appraise and Synthesize Body of Evidence ← Reassemble
- Conduct systematic search
- Weigh quality, quantity, consistency, and risk

Is there sufficient evidence? — No → Conduct research

Yes

Design and Pilot the Practice Change ← Redesign
- Engage patients and verify preferences
- Consider resources, constraints, and approval
- Develop localized protocol
- Create an evaluation plan
- Collect baseline data
- Develop an implementation plan
- Prepare clinicians and materials
- Promote adoption
- Collect and report post-pilot data

Is change appropriate for adoption in practice? — No → Consider alternatives

Yes

Integrate and Sustain the Practice Change
- Identify and engage key personnel
- Hardwire change into system
- Monitor key indicators through quality improvement
- Reinfuse as needed

Disseminate Results

◆ = a decision point

Used with permission from University of Iowa Hospitals and Clinics, Revised June 2015. To request permission or to reproduce, go to http://www.uihealthcare.org/nursing-research-and-evidence-based-practice/

FIGURE 3.2 The Iowa Model of Evidence-Based Practice. *(Reprinted with permission from the University of Iowa Hospitals and Clinics and Marita G. Titler, PhD, RN, FAAN. Copyright 1998. For permission to use or reproduce the model, please contact the University of Iowa Hospitals and Clinics at 319-384-9098.)*

has been a leader in EBP because of its extensive application and clarity (Titler et al., 2001).

Rosswurm and Larrabee Model

A model for change to EBP was developed in 1999 by Rosswurm and Larrabee (Fig. 3.3). The focus is on changing the clinical culture from status quo to incorporation of an EBP process. The Rosswurm and Larrabee Model was constructed from theoretical and research literature, RU, and change theory. Usefulness of the model was tested during its implementation stage of mentoring clinical nurses in the EBP process (Rosswurm & Larrabee, 1999).

The Rosswurm and Larrabee Model is a six-step process that focuses on critical thinking in making clinical decisions about quality and cost effectiveness of care in primary care settings. The six steps in the Rosswurm and Larrabee Model include the following:

1. Assess need for change in practice

2. Link problem, intervention, and outcomes

3. Synthesize best evidence

4. Design practice change

5. Implement and evaluate change in practice (Rosswurm & Larrabee, 1999)

Nursing Interventions Classifications (NIC) and Nursing Outcomes Classifications (NOC) are connected with an identified problem in step two. Steps three and four synthesize the evidence and propose designing a practice change. Step five relates to implementation and evaluation using appropriate evaluation methods. Following a contextual implementation of findings, change and sustainability occur in step six (Rosswurm & Larrabee, 1999).

ARCC Model: Advancing Research and Clinical Practice Through Close Collaboration

The Advancing Research and Clinical Practice Through Close Collaboration (ARCC) Model (1999) was a strategic planning initiative created by faculties from the School of Nursing and the School of Medicine and Dentistry at the University of Rochester in New York. Headed by Bernadette Melnyk, the goal was to enhance the use of research in the acute care clinical setting, thereby changing to an organizational culture of EBP. Mentorship was identified as a key component in successful integration of research into the practice setting and subsequently became a key component of the ARCC Model. Intended

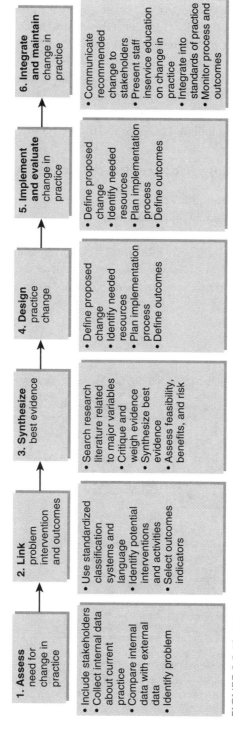

FIGURE 3.3 The Rosswurm and Larrabee Model for Change to Evidence-Based Practice

1. Assess need for change in practice

- Include stakeholders
- Collect internal data about current practice
- Compare internal data with external data
- Identify problem

2. Link problem intervention and outcomes

- Use standardized classification systems and language
- Identify potential interventions and activities
- Select outcomes indicators

3. Synthesize best evidence

- Search research literature related to major variables
- Critique and weigh evidence
- Synthesize best evidence
- Assess feasibility, benefits, and risk

4. Design practice change

- Define proposed change
- Identify needed resources
- Plan implementation process
- Define outcomes

5. Implement and evaluate change in practice

- Define proposed change
- Identify needed resources
- Plan implementation process
- Define outcomes

6. Integrate and maintain change in practice

- Communicate recommended change to stakeholders
- Present staff inservice education on change in practice
- Integrate into standards of practice
- Monitor process and outcomes

audiences for the ARCC Model are advanced practice nurses and staff nurses. Contextual emphasis of the ARCC Model is the clinical setting. Evaluation fine-tuned the construction of the model and led to its practical use in growing clinically based EBP. Review of the ARCC Model reflects an educational approach regarding integrating EBP with the clinical setting and contributing to an EBP nursing culture (Fineout-Overholt, Levin, & Melnyk, 2004/2005; Melnyk & Fineout-Overholt, 2011; Melnyk, Fineout-Overholt, Giggleman, & Cruz, 2010; Wallen, Mitchell, & Hastings, 2010) (Fig. 3.4).

Johns Hopkins Nursing Evidence-Based Practice Model

The Johns Hopkins Model (2007) was developed in conjunction with the Johns Hopkins University Hospital and the Johns Hopkins University School of Nursing. The conceptual model is grounded in three domains of professional nursing: practice, research, and education (White & Dudley-Brown, 2012). Depiction of the model presents each major concept as a point on a triangle. The structure is subsequently acted on by internal and external factors. Internal

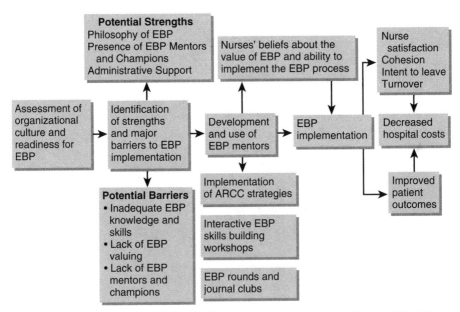

Source: Melnyk, B.M., & Fineout-Overholt, E. (2011). *Evidence-based practice in nursing and healthcare: a guide to best practice.* Philadelphia, PA: Walters Kluwer/Lippincott Williams & Williams.

FIGURE 3.4 The Advancing Research and Clinical Practice Through Close Collaboration (ARCC) Model. EBP, evidence-based practice. *(From Melnyk, B.M., & Fineout-Overholt, E. (2011). Evidence-based practice in nursing and healthcare: A guide to best practice. Philadelphia, PA: Walters Kluwer/Lippincott Williams & Williams.)*

factors are the organizational structures and cultures. External factors act on and with the EBP core in decision making for nursing practice (Newhouse et al., 2007). The acronym PET (practice, evidence, translation) guides the EBP process. The Johns Hopkins Model is useful for working nurses and students in learning and implementing the EBP process (Newhouse et al., 2007).

CHAPTER SUMMARY AND AFTERTHOUGHTS

EBP models or frameworks provide a means for thinking about the planning and organization of the DNP project. Common elements among the identified EBP models include the following:

1. Identification of a practice problem or idea

2. Creation of a searchable question

3. Search for current and relevant best evidence

4. Analysis and synthesis of evidence findings

5. Creation of EBP guidelines or recommendations for practice

Planning and organizing (i.e., structuring) the DNP project are best achieved by selecting and adapting a specific EBP model or by selecting elements from more than one model. An EBP model provides a rigorous decision-making process for making recommendations for practice. Chapter 9 in Section III provides the planning and organizational tools for actualizing (i.e., implementation and evaluation) of the practice recommendations.

CASE STUDY

Colleen has worked as a cardiac intensive care unit nurse since graduating with her baccalaureate degree in nursing 10 years ago. She is currently enrolled in an adult-geriatric acute care DNP program and looks forward to practicing in a rural setting where she and her family would like to move. For her DNP project, Colleen is focusing on cost-effective treatment of elevated blood pressure in older rural residents, many of whom are economically challenged and at great distances from hospitals.

- *Evaluate Colleen's needs in making a decision regarding the best evidence-based framework or model for structuring her DNP project.*

- *Describe an evidence-based practice framework or model that best meets the needs for successful planning of Colleen's project.*

WRITING REMINDERS...

"The fundamental purpose of scientific discourse is not the mere presentation of information and thought but rather it is actual communication. It does not matter how pleased an author might be to have converted all the right data into sentences and paragraphs; it matters only whether a large majority of the reading audience accurately perceives what the author had in mind" (Gopen & Swan, 1990, p 550).

Tips for Writing Clearly

- Before you write:

  - Think about the intent of your message. What do you want the reader to remember?

  - Focus on your intended audience. Whom do you want to read your publication?

  - Create an outline (see Chapter 4, Writing Reminders).

- Clarity in writing paragraphs:

  - Develop only one concept per paragraph.

  - The first sentence in a paragraph is a statement of the purpose for the paragraph.

- Clarity in writing sentences:

  - Use active voice, not passive voice (see Chapter 8, Writing Reminders).

  - Use the subject-verb sentence structure. Beginning a sentence with a prepositional phrase should be avoided or used only for emphasis.

  - Use action verbs; avoid "wordy verbs."

  - Use sparingly: *There is...*, *There are...*, *It is...*

  - Use pronouns sparingly.

- Use terms familiar to your readers. Avoid terms or names that have meaning only for your institution or region. Strive to reach the wider audience.

- "Put wordy phrases on a diet."

Adapted from Williams J. (1989) *Style:Ten lessons in clarity and grace* (3rd ed.). Glenview, IL: Scott Foresman. In University of Wisconsin Writing Center. (2013). *How to write clear, concise, and direct sentences*. Retrieved from http://writing.wisc.edu/Handbook/Clear,_Concise,_and_Direct_Sentences.pdf
Additional information on clarity in writing is available from Purdue Online Writing Lab (Purdue OWL). *Improving sentence clarity*. Retrieved from https://owl.english.purdue.edu/owl/resource/600/01/

REFERENCES

Burns, N., & Grove, S.K. (2011). *Understanding nursing research: Building an evidence-based practice*. Maryland Heights, MO: Elsevier Saunders.

Cochrane, A.L. (1972). *Effectiveness and efficiency: Random reflections on health services*. London, UK: Royal Society of Medicine Press.

Cochrane Collaboration. (2013). *About us*. Retrieved from http://www.cochrane.org/about-us

DiCenso, A., Provost, S., & Titler, M. (2004). Evidence-based nursing: Rationale and resources. *Worldviews on Evidence-Based Nursing, 1*(1), 69-75.

Estabrooks, C.A. (1999). The conceptual structure of research utilization. *Research in Nursing and Health, 22,* 203-216.

Fineout-Overholt, E., Levin, R.F., & Melnyk, B.M. (2004/2005). Strategies for advancing evidence-based practice in clinical settings. *Journal of the New York State Nurses Association, Fall/Winter,* 28-32.

Gopen, G.D., & Swan, J.A. (1990). The science of scientific writing. *American Scientist, 78,* 550-558.

Green, J. (2000). The role of theory in evidence-based health promotion practice. *Health Education Practice, 15*(2), 125-129.

Grove, S.K., Burns, N., & Gray, J.R. (2013). *The practice of nursing research: Appraisal, synthesis, and generation of evidence* (7th ed.). St. Louis, MO: Elsevier.

Guyatt, G., Cairns, J., Churchill, D., & Tugwell, P. (1992). Evidence-based medicine: A new approach to teaching the practice of medicine. *JAMA, 268*(17), 2420-2425.

Melnyk, B.M., & Fineout-Overholt, E. (2011). *Evidence-based practice in nursing and healthcare: A guide to best practice*. Philadelphia, PA: Walters Kluwer/Lippincott Williams & Williams.

Melnyk, B.M., Fineout-Overholt, E., Giggleman, M., & Cruz, R. (2010). Correlates among cognitive beliefs, EBP implementation, organization, culture, cohesion, and job satisfaction in evidence-based practice mentors from a community hospital system. *Nursing Outlook 58*(6), 301-308.

Newhouse, R.P., Dearholt, S.L., Poe, S.S., Pugh, L.C., & White, K.M. (2007). *Johns Hopkins nursing evidence-based practice model and guidelines.* Indianapolis, IN: Sigma Theta Tau International.

Polit, D.F., & Beck, C.T. (2012). *Nursing research: Generating and assessing evidence for nursing practice* (9th ed.). Philadelphia, PA: Wolters Kluwer/Lippincott Williams & Wilkins.

Rosswurm, M.A., & Larrabee, J.H. (1999). A model for change to evidence-based practice. *Image: The Journal of Nursing Scholarship, 31*(4), 317-322.

Rycroft-Malone, J. (2013). Reflecting back, looking forward: 10 years of *Worldviews on Evidence-Based Nursing. Worldviews on Evidence-Based Nursing, 10*(2), 67-68.

Sackett, D.L., Rosenberg, W.C., Gray, J.A.M., Haynes, R.B., & Richardson, W.S. (1996). Evidence-based medicine: What it is and what it isn't. *BMJ, 312,* 71-72.

Schaffer, M.A., Sanda, .E., & Diedrick, L. (2012). Evidence-based practice models for organizational change: Overview and practical applications. *Journal of Advanced Nursing, 69*(5), 1197-1209.

Shah, H.M., & Chung, K.C. (2009). Archie Cochrane and his vision for evidence-based medicine. *Plastic and Reconstructive Surgery, 124*(3), 982-988.

Stetler, C.B. (1985). Research utilization: Defining the concept. *Journal of Nursing Scholarship, 17*(2), 40-44.

Stetler, C.B. (2001). Updating the Stetler Model of Research Utilization to facilitate evidence-based practice. *Nursing Outlook, 49*(6), 272-279.

Stetler, C.B., & Marram, G. (1976). Evaluating findings for applicability in practice. *Nursing Outlook, 24,* 559-563.

Titler, M.G. (2008). The evidence for evidence-based practice implementation. In R.G. Hughes (Ed.), *Patient safety and quality: An evidence-based handbook for nurses.* Rockville, MD: AHRQ. Retrieved from http://www.ncbi.nlm.nih.gov/books/NBK2659/

Titler, M.G., Kleiber, C., Steelman, V. & Goode, C.J. (2001). The Iowa model of evidence-based practice to promote quality care. *Critical Care Nursing Clinics of North America, 13*(4), 497-509.

Wallen, G.R., Mitchell, S.A., & Hastings, C. (2010). Implementing evidence-based practice: Effectiveness of a structured multifaceted mentorship programme. *Journal of Advanced Nursing, 68*(12), 2761-2771. Retrieved from http://www.ncbi.nlm.nih.gov/pmc/articles/PMC2981621/#!po=1.92308

Weiss, C.H. (1979). The many meanings of research utilization. *Public Administration Review, 39*(5), 426-431.

White, K.M., & Dudley-Brown, S. (2012). *Translation of evidence into nursing and health care practice.* New York, NY: Springer Publishing Company.

IF YOU WANT TO READ MORE...

Fineout-Overholt E., Melnyk, B.M., & Schultz, A. (2005). Transforming health care from the inside out: Advancing evidence-based practice in the 21st century. *Journal of Professional Nursing, 21*(6), 335-344.

Newhouse, R.P., Dearholt, S.L., Poe, S.S., Pugh, L.C., & White, K.M. (2007). *Johns Hopkins Nursing evidence-based practice model and guidelines.* Indianapolis, IN: Sigma Theta Tau International.

Rosswurm, M.A., & Larrabee, J.H. (1999). A model for change to evidence-based practice. *Image: The Journal of Nursing Scholarship, 31*(4), 317-322.

Stetler, C.B. (1985). Research utilization: Defining the concept. *Image: The Journal of Nursing Scholarship, 17*(2), 40-44.

Stetler, C.B. (2001). Updating the Stetler model of research utilization to facilitate evidence-based practice. *Nursing Outlook, 49*(6), 272-279.

Titler, M.G., Steelman, V.J., Budreau, G., Buckwalter, K.C., & Goode, C.J. (2001). The Iowa model of evidence-based practice to promote quality care. *Critical Care Nursing Clinics of North America, 13*(4), 497-509.

4

From Idea to Searchable Question

As leaders, probably the most important role we can play is asking the right question.

TIM BROWN, 2013, p 48

OUTCOME OBJECTIVES

- Justify the importance of ideas.
- Analyze how effective questions are developed and written.
- Describe similarities and differences between a practice question and a research question.
- Develop a searchable evidence-based practice question.

TERMS

Background questions	Ideas	Population health
Context	Idea triggers	Problems
Foreground questions	Issues	Search terms
Foundational concepts	Population	Stakeholder(s)

Getting started is the hardest part of any project. Critical thinking and reflection about the background and significance of a project are required before turning an idea into a well-formed question. The purpose of this chapter is to provide logical tools to assist turning an idea that may have been initially perceived as too broad or too narrow into a searchable, answerable question.

FRAMING AN IDEA

Where do ideas come from? The Iowa Model of Evidence-Based Practice (Titler, Kleiber, Steelman, & Goode, 2001) proposes problem-focused and knowledge-focused triggers as catalysts for ideas. Problem-focused triggers are aligned with clinical practice such as data from risk management, process improvement, benchmarking, financial, and clinical problem identification. Knowledge-focused triggers arise from established sources of written evidence such as new publications, national and organizational standards and guidelines, philosophies of care, or questions from an institutional standards committee (Polit & Beck, 2012; Titler et al., 2001).

Interprofessional and intraprofessional communication and collaboration in identifying practice problems and issues also contribute to framing an idea (AACN, 2006; Interprofessional Education Collaborative Expert Panel, 2011). For example, communication with staff nurses often establishes questions about issues relating to patient-centered care. On the other hand, a *top-down* approach may originate with administrators who attempt to stimulate a culture of evidence-based practice (EBP) as part of the Magnet Recognition Program (Polit & Beck, 2012).

Another idea source is human curiosity. "It is the process of imagining that generates new ideas and new ways of being in the world" (Bunkers, 2000, p 119). Ideas are described as ways to express objective knowledge, with knowledge implying a place of reason (Blackburn, 1994). However, places of reason are constantly evolving as practice changes occur and the current knowledge base is redefined. Social and situational circumstances affect change, as do context and the nature of a problem when bringing forward new and evolving ideas (Bronowski, 1978; Bunkers, 2000; Roy & Jones, 2007).

ANALYZING THE IDEA WITH BACKGROUND QUESTIONS

Analysis of an idea begins the process for critically thinking and reflecting about an idea's complexity related to practice issues. Structure for critical reasoning of the foundational concepts of the practice idea is termed *background questions*.

Put another way, time spent reflecting on answers to background questions conceptualizes the foreground practice idea and subsequent EBP question. Explicit background information enhances the quality and clarity of an EBP searchable and answerable question (Fineout-Overholt & Johnston, 2005; Paul & Elder, 2002; Paul & Elder, 2007). To summarize, "a good question is powerful" (Killen, 2010, p 251).

Sackett, Straus, Richardson, Rosenberg, and Haynes (2000) defined background questions as the "full range of biologic, psychologic, and sociologic aspects of human illness" (p 16). DNPs who practice direct patient care as pediatric, adult, or family nurse practitioners follow methods similar to the medical model regarding diagnosis and treatment, but with additions of nursing philosophy regarding holistic patient-centered care. Nursing leaders in management, education, or information technology focus indirectly on different populations or systems, but the outcome goal is the same: reflective background questions to critically think about issues related to patient-centered care (Fineout-Overholt & Johnston, 2005; Melnyk & Fineout-Overholt, 2011; Polit & Beck, 2012; SUNY, 2003). Examples of background questions specific to an EBP question are presented in Box 4.1.

Narrative explanations and rationale for background questions are provided in the following sections.

BOX 4.1 Background Questions to Assist in Idea Creation

1. What is your desired DNP role? Describe it.

2. What is the population or system of interest?

3. Describe the context or the practice setting.

4. Describe the background of the practice issue or problem.

5. Describe the current status of the practice issue or problem.

6. Discuss the significance of the issue or problem.

7. Are community, institutional, or unit policies and/or procedures currently available regarding the issue or problem? Are the documents current?

8. Describe your perception: what you want to know, change, or improve.

1. **What Is Your Desired DNP Role? Describe It.**

   Being a DNP student brings opportunities for implementing and/or evaluating practice ideas, issues, or problems. In the development of the idea for the EBP question, consider the DNP role you desire. Are your personal expectations to function as a DNP in your current work setting? Do you anticipate acquiring skills to work in a different setting? Are you motivated to be an entrepreneur and implement a new healthcare program or create a new patient care device? Do you plan to become involved with socially just causes? Think about and describe your desired role perceptions and goals.

2. **What Is the Population or System of Interest?**

   The concept of population or system from a statistical perspective implies an accessible aggregate of people or elements with common properties or characteristics from which a sample representation can be made (Grove, Burns, & Gray, 2013; LoBiondo-Wood & Haber, 2010; Polit & Beck, 2012). A population health perspective includes an approach that describes physical, mental, cultural, and socioeconomic properties of the population of interest. Descriptions of the population or system of interest align with a qualitative, holistic approach to patient care. Ideas emanating from a population health perspective may reflect relationships, behaviors, lifestyles, and social and environmental factors such as culture, history, employment, education, and housing. Issues may also focus on assessment of the healthcare system. Other ideas embraced by practice include a population's knowledge, attitudes, beliefs, and values that motivate change, reward adoption, or resources that hinder change (Radzyminski, 2007). The importance of detail and clarity in describing the population of interest is a salient point.

3. **Describe the Context of the Practice Setting.**

   Understanding and describing the context in which an EBP plan is to be implemented or evaluated are essential because they guide the clinical question from the perception of end users. A clear description of context also informs stakeholders of potential impact and outcomes (Titler, 2010). Context implies organizational setting, culture, and values, in addition to depth and breadth of the environment and social systems. When evaluating the context of your project, consider the depth and breadth of the environment and the social systems. Other contextual elements to consider include the following: (1) organizational type and size; (2) administration; (3) communication and decision-making structures; (4) policies, procedures, documentation, and data capture systems; and (5) openness to new knowledge and ideas. Contextual understanding indicates perception of the culture, human relationships, and the organizational approach (Titler, 2010;

Zaccagnini & White, 2014). Introduction of new ideas, policy, or change is more successful when integrated into existing strategies in a known culture (Rycroft-Malone, 2004; Rycroft-Malone, 2008).

4. Describe the Background of the Practice Issue or Problem.

Whereas a problem implies a topic in search of a solution, an issue suggests a topic for discussion. Problems and issues contextually arise when members of the discipline perceive a need for more information to make a decision. As you develop your EBP idea, reflect on when and why the problem or issue gained your attention. What social and other situational factors influenced the evolution of the problem's definition? (Rodgers, 2007).

5. Describe the Current Status of the Practice Issue or Problem.

Connecting the history of a practice problem or issue to the current status and conditions of here and now focuses attention on change over time identified from experience and observation. Analysis of the current status increases understanding and may contribute alternative thoughts (Rodgers, 2007). Policies and performance measures are examples of documents that direct the current status of practice. Ideas generated from observations and nursing journals specific to your practice may generate a dialogue regarding outdated performance measures or resources.

6. What Is the Significance of the Issue or Problem?

Significance implies making sense and providing rationale about risk and cost of an identified issue or problem. The significance of a problem is an important element for conversations with stakeholders. Answer this question with clarity, detail, relevance, breadth, and logic (Paul & Elder, 2002).

7. Are Institutional or Unit Policies and/or Procedures Currently Available Regarding the Issue or Problem? Are the Documents Current?

Policies provide guidelines and establish boundaries for best practices. Indeed, written policies contribute to the norms and values that influence the culture and context of the practice setting (Kokemuller, 2014). Policy and procedure documents are valuable assets in comprehending the current context for analyzing the problem. Frequent policy reviews and/or updates are important because of cost and safety risks.

8. Describe Your Perceptions of What You Want to Know, Improve, or Change Regarding the Identified Issue or Problem.

Expected outcomes generally envision an action or reaction to your identified problem or issue. Visualizing important outcomes helps you sharpen the focus of your EBP because it describes where you want to end up. Perceptions of outcomes based on an EBP question differ from perceptions of outcomes based on implementation and evaluation. Implementation outcomes and evaluations related to cost, patient outcomes, policy change, or new program are presented in Section III.

WRITING A SEARCHABLE AND ANSWERABLE QUESTION

Ideas generated from background questions lead to foreground questions or EBP questions that are the basis for searching for best evidence. EBP questions should be well-structured presentations of what is problematic, what needs to be fixed, or what is not well understood. The searchable and answerable question needs to be written clearly and with adequate detail. Indeed, a relevant clinical question is another important part of the EBP process because it puts critical thinking into the real world (Fineout-Overholt & Johnson, 2005; Paul & Elder, 2002; Polit & Beck, 2012; Schardt, Adams, Owens, Keitz, & Fontelo, 2007). Several formulas exist to assist the writer in developing searchable and answerable questions. The PICO-T format is the most recognizable.

PICO-T (defined in Table 4.1) is an acronym for a questioning strategy used with EBP projects, generally intervention or comparison projects, and it contributes to ease in finding evidence and relevance of findings. It is the most widely recognized acronym and has its origins in the medical model of diagnosis and intervention. The PICO-T acronym is also finding increased use in well-written problem statements or questions to guide the literature search that precedes framing of a hypothesis or research statement. Good tools for writing a quality question that is searchable and answerable enhance the quality of the entire EBP process (Health Evidence, 2016; Melnyk & Fineout-Overholt, 2011; Polit & Beck, 2012; Riva, Malik, Burnie, Endicot, & Busse, 2012; Schardt et al., 2007).

Alternative forms of the PICO-T format exist for other projects. PIOT is an acronym for nonintervention, knowledge, quality improvement projects or research studies (Stillwell, Fineout-Overholt, Melnyk, & Williamson, 2010). PICo and PS are other acronyms for nonintervention and descriptive approaches, but they do not require an outcome statement as noted in PIOT (Cooke, Smith, & Booth, 2012). Outcome statements are optional in descriptive, nonintervention, quality improvement projects. The choice of acronym for use in developing your EBP question belongs to you, the user of the tool, based on perceived needs in development of your EBP question. Table 4.2 provides acronyms and definitions as guidelines for writing EBP questions for descriptive, nonintervention projects.

TABLE 4.1 PICO-T Format for Evidence-Based Practice Questions Regarding Intervention or Comparison

P = Population or system; problem or issue, patient situation **I** = Intervention, exposure, test, treatment **C** = Comparison (e.g., current practice, alternative treatment, no treatment), intervention, control group, prognosis, risk factor **O** = Projected outcome relevant to issue or problem of identified population, risk of disease, or accuracy of diagnosis **T** = Time it takes for an intervention to demonstrate an outcome (optional) (Health Evidence, 2010; Melnyk & Fineout-Overholt, 2011; Polit & Beck, 2012; Riva et al., 2012; Woods, n.d.)	In _____ (P), how does _____ (I) compared with _____ (C) affect _____ (O) within _____ (T)? (Stillwell et al., 2010, p 60)	In newly arrived, pregnant refugee women currently living in the northwest United States (P), how do group prenatal care and education (I) compared with individual prenatal care and education (C) affect the patient's experience (O) of the birthing process? (T)

PICO-T is generally used with intervention or comparison projects and research studies.

Additional examples specific for EBP questions used in quality improvement and policy development or revision are presented in Table 4.3.

IDENTIFYING SEARCH TERMS

Your well-written, well-focused search question yields the key words that drive the search for best evidence. A well-focused question contributes to a relevant search that is efficient and organized. Search terms are generally population, problem or issue, intervention, or comparison nouns identified from the EBP question (Fineout-Overholt & Johnston, 2005; Schardt et al., 2007; Stillwell et al., 2010). Effective use of search terms to find best evidence for a searchable and answerable EBP question can be found in Chapter 5.

TABLE 4.2 Examples of Evidence-Based Practice Nonintervention, Descriptive Questions

Strategy	Template	Example
P = Population, system, problem **I** = Issue **O** = Outcome **T** = Time period (optional)	How do ___ (P) with (I) perceive (O) during (T)? (Stillwell et al., 2010, p. 60)	How do nurses who care for pregnant refugee women (P) diagnosed with anemia (I) perceive the effectiveness of patient nutritional education (O) during patient prenatal visits (T)?
P = Characteristics of population or system **I** = Issue/Interest related to event, activity, experience, process **Co** = Context/setting or distinct characteristics	How do (P) introduce (I) in (Co)? (Cooke et al., 2012)	How do large, urban healthcare systems (P) introduce new software for healthcare charting (I) in outpatient clinics?
P = Characteristics of population or system **S** = Phenomenon or situation related to circumstances, conditions, experiences	How do (P) experience/ live with (S)? (Health Evidence, 2009)	In women receiving chemotherapy for breast cancer and returning to work, (P), what modifications are made by the employer (S)?

PICO, PICo, and PS are generally used with nonintervention or descriptive projects or research studies.

PLANNING FOR SUCCESS

Ideas are the first step in opening the conversation about your DNP project. It is prudent that the second step focus on forming your DNP project team, your leadership responsibilities, and stakeholder identification. Begin early in this EBP phase.

Forming a Team

Forming a team early in the process of doing a DNP project or a professional practice project is important. Similarities and differences exist, however, between team roles and responsibilities with the interprofessional practice team and the intradisciplinary DNP project team (AACN, 2015; Titler et al., 2001).

TABLE 4.3	Examples of Evidence-Based Practice Questions for Quality Improvement, Policy Revision, Process, and Context
Quality improvement	What are the benefits of implementing information technology to improve the consistency of nursing documentation (HRSA, 2011)?
Policy creation or revision	Does the new electronic health record (EHR) policy and procedure improve the quality and safety of patient care compared with the previous information technology (HRSA, 2011)?
Process	Is effective workflow of nursing care demonstrated by new information technology for medication delivery and documentation? (HRSA, 2011)
Context	What are the contextual factors that influence people with depression to seek or not seek medical care (Kent & McCormack, 2011)?

From HRSA, 2011; Kirkpatrick & Weaver, 2013; Magyara, Whitney, & Brown, 2006.

The purpose of a DNP project is to individually learn and demonstrate planning, implementation, evaluation, and leadership. When building your DNP project team, AACN (2015) recommends that your project team consist of "a student or group of students, a doctorally prepared faculty member [who is your advisor and will submit your final grade] and a practice mentor who may be from outside the university. In some instances, additional experts/mentors/partners/facilitators can be formal or informal collaborators and may provide intermittent or limited support throughout the project stages as needed" (p 5).

The following excerpt from the AACN (2015) white paper describes the intent of the student's responsibility if a team project is a selection for the individual DNP project.

Guidelines for the entire project as well as for individual contributions to the project and a rubric used for each individual's evaluation should be developed and shared with students prior to the initiation of the project. Each member of the group must meet all expectations of planning, implementation, and evaluation of the project, and be evaluated accordingly. Each student must have a leadership role in at least one component of the project and be held accountable for a deliverable. The following serve as illustrative projects:

1. *The student serves as a vital member of an interprofessional team, implementing and evaluating a component of a larger project.*
2. *Students work on the same project, for example improving hand washing, across multiple units within the same organization or across multiple organizations.*

3. *Students focus on different aspects of improving diabetic outcomes of care by meeting criteria for guidelines for diabetes care such as eye exams, time frames for HgA$_{1c}$ screening, and foot care.*

4. *Students analyze and implement changes in state immunization policies to improve access to immunizations and increase immunization rates" (AACN, 2015, pp 4–5).*

Similarities between a student DNP project team and an interprofessional or intraprofessional practice team begin by creating a learning environment where collaboration and communication are goal focused for best outcomes. A team brings people together and provides opportunity for asking good questions. Brownowski (1978) noted that interprofessional teams are "both an individual and a social activity, for even great minds cannot work in isolation" (p 117). The composition of an interprofesional practice team or DNP project team should be thoughtful and deliberate. Personalities need to fit together to achieve high output and low ego. Teams should strive for organizational creativity wherein pieces of information come together and problems are solved. Variety in teams, especially interprofessional, brings a different perspective and may enable team members to look at the clinical issue or problem from a different angle. Whether your team is interprofessional or intradisciplinary, always model good team behavior, think creatively, communicate respectfully, and learn from each other (Napier et al., 2013).

Leadership

Consider the roles you need for your DNP project team. Your academic adviser or other identified nursing faculty member should be the first formal member of your team because of university requirements for doctoral programs. A knowledge expert for your specific topic is also a wise choice as a formal team member. The team leader for your committee should be you. Research studies increasingly find that the role of leadership is a critical factor for a successful EBP process (Rycroft-Malone, 2012). Therefore, all phases of your DNP project provide opportunities for experiential learning regarding the leadership role.

A leader in DNP projects is described as a transformational leader who inspires confidence, respect, and trust, which are correlated with effective outcomes (Bass, 1995; Curtis & O'Connell, 2011). Clarity of roles within the group or team increases adaptation through interdependence, integrity, and relational growth and also contributes to achievement of identified common goals (Boston College, 2013; Roy, 1988). You are encouraged to lead through motivation, inspiration, and efficient and effective communication to create an adaptive team that empowers team members for best outcomes.

Stakeholders

Stakeholders may be formal or informal members of your DNP project team. Stakeholders have significant interest in your project and the project's evaluation because they may be directly or indirectly affected as a result of their official roles in management or other leadership positions in a healthcare organization. You are encouraged to involve stakeholders early in the development of your project because they can positively or negatively influence implementation and adoption of your EBP recommendations. Negative influences or barriers may revolve around organizational access, lack of adequate resources, cost of implementation, lack of evidence, or negative attitudes. On the other hand, opportunities that exist through supportive stakeholders include quality evidence, communication, and organization. Stakeholders can open doors for the success of your project. Building a positive relationship with supportive stakeholders by keeping them informed is important for the success of your project (LoBiondo-Wood & Haber, 2010; Zaccagnini & White, 2014).

Identification and selection of a relevant stakeholder for your project may be assisted by asking yourself the following questions:

- Who is the intended audience for your project?

- What is the desired setting or system for your project?

- Who is interested in your project, the expected outcome, and evaluation? Who might champion your project?

- How are decisions made in the practice area where your EBP project may be implemented? Who is involved in decision making and can influence implementation of your project?

- What types of cooperation do you need from the stakeholder? (LoBiondo-Wood & Haber, 2012, p 394)

CHAPTER SUMMARY AND AFTERTHOUGHTS

Ideas are concepts, problems, or issues derived from experiences in the practice setting and/or knowledge gained from professional publications and/or internal documents. Time spent with your EBP team in communicating, collaborating, and analyzing the idea contributes to increased understanding of the issue or problem and leads to creation of a searchable and answerable question. A detailed, clearly written question or statement is the greatest asset when searching for evidence that is meaningful for the DNP project (Titler, 2010).

CASE STUDY

Eric is a doctorally prepared nurse practitioner. He works at the men's state correctional institution in the role of medical director. In the prison population, chronic pain and drug-seeking behaviors are common diagnoses. Recently, Eric formed and now leads an evidence-based practice (EBP) team composed of a nurse, a pharmacist, a social worker, and a prison guard. The goals of the team are to (1) evaluate the use of long-term pain medication in the prison population and (2) evaluate the current treatment of pain based on best evidence.

- *Evaluate the composition of Eric's EBP team. Should representatives from other disciplines be included on the team?*

- *Appraise the benefits of working in teams.*

- *Identify background questions that will assist in writing a searchable question or statement.*

- *Write a searchable, answerable EBP question.*

- *Identify search terms from your EBP question or statement.*

WRITING REMINDERS...

Active Voice or Passive Voice

- A sentence written with *active voice* means that the subject of the sentence performs the action.

- A sentence with *passive voice* means the subject receives the action.

Examples of active and passive voice.

Active: The DNP implemented a new pain protocol for returning veterans.

Passive: It was decided that returning veterans should receive a new pain protocol.

Active: The nurse medicated the patient.

Passive: The patient was medicated by the nurse.

(University of Wisconsin, 2014.)

A tradition of using passive voice occurred nearly a century ago. In the 1920s, the accepted form of medical and scientific writing was objective, impersonal, and passive. Passive writing, however, often lacks clarity because of the overuse of modifiers, prepositional phrases beginning with *by*, future verb tense *to be*, and an overuse of the pronoun *it* in place of *I* or *we*. Passive voice often conveys evasiveness. You are encouraged to use an active voice in your writing because the sentences are more clear and concise. However, passive voice is still accepted in some journals when the focus of the article is on the recipient of the action (UNC, 2012).

REFERENCES

American Association of Colleges of Nursing (AACN). (2006). *Position statement on nursing research*. Washington, DC: AACN. Retrieved from http://www.aacn.nche.edu/publications/position/nursing-research

American Association of Colleges of Nursing (AACN). (2006). *The essentials for doctoral education for advanced nursing practice*. Washington, DC: AACN. Retrieved from http://www.aacn.nche.edu/publications/position/DNPEssentials. pdf

American Association of Colleges of Nursing (AACN). (August 2015). *The doctor of nursing practice: Current issues and clarifying recommendations*. Retrieved from http://www.aacn.nche.edu/aacn-publications/white-papers/DNP-Implementation-TF-Report-8-15.pdf

Bass, B.M. (1995). Theory of transformational leadership. *Leadership Quarterly, 6*(4), 463–478.

Blackburn, S. (1994). *The Oxford dictionary of philosophy*. NY: Oxford University Press.

Boston College. (2013). *The Roy Adaptation Model*. Retrieved from https://www.bc.edu/schools/son/faculty/featured/theorist/Roy_Adaptation_Model.html

Bronowski, J. (1978). *The origins of knowledge and imagination*. London: Yale University Press.

Bunkers, S.S. (2000). The nurse scholar of the21st century. *Nursing Science Quarterly, 13*, 116–123.

Cooke, A., Smith, D., & Booth, A. (2012). Beyond PICO: The SPIDER tool for qualitative evidence synthesis. *Qualitative Health Research, 22*(10), 1435–1443. Retrieved from http://www.ncbi.nlm.nih.gov/pubmed/22829486

Curtis, E., & O'Connell, R. (2012). Essential leadership skills for motivating and developing staff. *Nursing Management, 18*(5), 32–35.

Fineout-Overholt, E., & Johnston, L. (2005). Teaching EBP: Asking searchable, answerable clinical questions. *Worldviews on Evidence-Based Nursing, 2*(3), 157–160.

Grove, S.K., Burns,N., & Gray,J. (2013). *The practice of nursing research* (7th ed.). St. Louis, MO: Elsevier Saunders.

Health Evidence. (2013). Evidence-informed decision making (EIDM) checklist. *Practice Tools*. Ontario, Canada: McMaster University. Retrieved from http://www.healthevidence.org/practice-tools.aspx

Health Evidence. (2016). Developing an efficient search strategy using PICO. *Practice Tools*. Ontario, Canada: McMaster University. Retrieved from http://www.healthevidence.org/practice-tools.aspx#PT1

Health Resources and Services Administration (HRSA). (2011). Quality improvement (QI) and the importance of QI. In *Quality Improvement*. Retrieved from http://www.hrsa.gov/quality/toolbox/508pdfs/qualityimprovement.pdf

Interprofessional Education Collaborative Expert Panel. (2011). *Core competencies for interprofessional collaborative practice: Report of an expert panel*. Washington, DC: Interprofessional Education Collaborative.

Kent, B., & McCormack, B. (Eds.). (2010). *Clinical context for evidence-based nursing practice*. Hoboken, NJ: Wiley-Blackwell.

Killen, P.O. (2010) Building questioning strategies or why am I asking these questions and where are they taking us? *Teaching Theology and Religion, 13*(3), 251–253.

Kirkpatrick, J.M., & Weaver, T. (2013). The doctor of nursing practice capstone project: Consensus or confusion? *Journal of Nursing Education, 52*(8), 435–441.

Kokemuller, N. (2014). What is the purpose of a workplace policy? *Chron.com*. Retrieved from http://smallbusiness.chron.com/purpose-workplace-policy-41601.html

LoBiondo-Wood, G., & Haber, J. (2010). *Nursing research: Methods and critical appraisal for evidence-based practice* (7th ed.). New York, NY: Mosby Elsevier.

Magyara, D., Whitney, J.D., & Brown, M.A. (2006). Advancing practice inquiry: Research foundations of the practice doctorate in nursing. *Nursing Outlook, 54*(3), 139–151.

Melnyk, B.M., & Fineout-Overholt, E. (2011). *Evidence-based practice in nursing and healthcare: A guide to best practice*. New York, NY: Lippincott Williams & Wilkins.

Napier, N.K., Cooper, J., Hoflund, M., Kemper, D., Loken, B., Petersen, C., Raney, G., & Schert, J.M. (2013). *Wise beyond your field*. Boise, ID: CCI Press.

Oxford Dictionaries. (2013). Retrieved from http://www.oxforddictionaries.com

Paul, R., & Elder, L. (2002). *Critical thinking: Tools for taking charge of your professional and personal life*. Saddle River, NJ: Prentice Hall.

Paul, R., & Elder, L. (2007). Critical thinking: The art of Socratic questioning. *Journal of Developmental Education, 31*(1), 36–37.

Polit, D., & Beck, C.T. (2012). *Nursing research: Generating and assessing evidence for nursing*. Philadelphia, PA: Wolters Kluwer/Lippincott Williams & Wilkins.

Radzyminski, S. (2007). The concept of population health within the nursing profession. *Journal of Professional Nursing, 23*(1), 37–46.

Riva, J.J., Malik, K.M.P., Burnie, S.J., Endicot, A.R., & Busse, J.W. (2012). What is your research question? An introduction to the PICOT format for clinicians. *Journal of the Canadian Chiropractic Association, 56*(3), 167–171.

Rodgers, B.L. (2007). Knowledge as problem solving. In C. Roy & D.A. Jones (Eds.). *Nursing knowledge development and clinical practice*. New York, NY: Springer Publishing Company, pp 107–117.

Roy, C. (1988). An explication of the philosophical assumptions of the Roy Adaptation Model. *Nursing Science Quarterly, 1*(1), 26–34.

Roy, C., & Jones, D.A. (Eds.). (2007). *Nursing knowledge development and clinical practice.* New York, NY: Springer Publishing Company.

Rycroft-Malone, J. (2008). Evidence-informed practice: From individual to context. *Journal of Nursing Management, 16*(4), 404–408.

Rycroft-Malone, J. (2012). Leadership matters. *World Views on Evidence-Based Practice, 9*(3), 127–128.

Rycroft-Malone, J., Harvey, G., Seers K., Kitson, A., McCormack, B., & Titchen, A. (2004). An exploration of the factors that influence the implementation of evidence into practice. *Journal of Clinical Nursing, 13*(8), 913–924.

Sackett, D.L., Straus, S.E., Richardson, W.S., Rosenberg, W., & Haynes, R.B. (2000). *Evidence-based medicine: How to practice and teach EBM.* Edinburgh: Churchill Livingstone.

Schardt, C., Adams, M.B., Owens, T., Keitz, S., & Fontelo, P. (2007). Utilization of the PICO framework to improve searching PubMed for clinical questions. *BMC Medical Informatics and Decision Making, 7,* 16. Retrieved from http://www.ncbi.nlm.nih.gov/pmc/articles/PMC1904193/

Stillwell, S.B., Fineout-Overholt, E., Melnyk, B.M., & Williamson, K.M. (2010). Asking the clinical question: A key step in evidence-based practice. *American Journal of Nursing, 110*(3), 58–61.

SUNY, Medical Research Library of Brooklyn. (2003). *Background/foreground questions.* Retrieved from http://library.downstate.edu/EBM2/foreground.htm

Titler, M.G. (2010). Translation science and context. *Research Theory for Nursing Practice: An International Journal, 24*(1), 35–55.

Titler, M.G., Kleiber, C., Steelman, V.J, & Goode, C.J. (2001). The Iowa model of evidence-based practice to promote quality care. *Critical Care Nursing Clinics of North America, 13*(4), 497–509.

University of North Carolina. (2012). Passive voice. *The Writing Center.* Retrieved from https://writingcenter.unc.edu/files/2012/09/Passive-Voice-The-Writing-Center.pdf

University of Wisconsin. (2014). Use the active voice. *The Writer's Handbook.* Retrieved from https://writing.wisc.edu/Handbook/CCS_activevoice.html

Woods, N.F. (2009). *Clinical scholarship and practice inquiry: Contributions of DNP- and PhD-prepared nurses to evidence-based practice* (PowerPoint). Retrieved from http://www.cumc.columbia.edu/nursing/research/pdf/ORR/Woods_Presentation.pdf

Zaccagnini, M.E., & White, K.W. (2014). *The Doctor of Nursing Practice essentials: A new model for advanced practice nursing.* Sudbury, MA: Jones & Bartlett.

IF YOU WANT TO READ MORE...

Faculty of Health, School of Nursing and Midwifery, University of Newcastle. (2009). *Clinical reasoning: Instructor resources.* Australia: University of Newcastle. Retrieved from   http://www.utas.edu.au/data/assets/pdf_file/0003/263487/Clinical-Reasoning-Instructor-Resources.pdf

Fineout-Overholt, E., & Johnston, L. (2005). Teaching EBP: Asking searchable, answerable clinical questions. *Worldviews on Evidence-Based Nursing, 2*(3), 157–160.

Health Resources and Services Administration (HRSA). (2011). Quality improvement (QI) and the importance of QI. In *Quality Improvement*. Retrieved from http://www.hrsa.gov/quality/toolbox/methodology/qualityimprovement/

5

The Nature of Evidence

Whilst few would disagree with the notion of delivering patient-centered care based on information about what works, there remain significant challenges about what evidence is, and thus how practitioners use it in decision-making in the reality of clinical contexts.

RYCROFT-MALONE (2004), p 82

OUTCOME OBJECTIVES

- Discuss the nature of evidence.
- Describe attributes of best evidence.
- Differentiate sources of research evidence, conceptual evidence, and contextual evidence.
- Correlate empirical reasoning, conceptual reasoning, and contextual reasoning with practice.

TERMS

Best evidence	Contextual evidence	Gray literature
Cochrane review	Contextual reasoning	Integrative review
Conceptual evidence	Empirical reasoning	Meta-analysis
and reasoning	Evidence	Metasynthesis

Continued

TERMS—cont'd

Policy	Research evidence	Rule of law
Quality	Randomized controlled	Search terms
improvement	trial (RCT)	Systematic review

Evidence is a central component of evidence-based practice (EBP) for patient-centered care. Evidence influences the following: use of safe patient practices; institutional policies; patient, student, and staff education; use of medical equipment and devices; and effective, efficient management of patient data. In other words, patient-centered care grounded in a culture of creating, using, and evaluating best evidence is a desired outcome to which DNP scholars are expected to contribute. But what is the nature of evidence? What constitutes best evidence? Reaction to these questions is found in research, philosophical, theoretical, clinical, and practical sources of evidence, in addition to contextual sources of evidence. This chapter develops the concepts of evidence and the nature of best evidence.

WHAT IS EVIDENCE?

The term *evidence* is grounded in the ideas of experience and observation, thus lending support to a definition meaning obvious, factual, testimonial, or informational (Rycroft-Malone, Seers, & McCormack, 2004). From a legal perspective, evidence is used to convince a judge or jury regarding *facts* of a case. Facts consist of witness testimony, expert opinions, public documents and records, objects, photographs, or depositions (Hill & Hill, 2013; Kitson, 2002). From a research perspective, evidence is perceived as having a rigorous methodology and contributing new knowledge to a specific domain of study. Terms repeatedly used to describe research evidence include *observation, verifiable,* and *subject to scrutiny* (Rycroft-Malone et al., 2004). From an EBP perspective, *evidence* is used for answering questions, making practice improvements, or validating current actions with the intended outcome being quality and safety of patient-centered care. Definitions of EBP expand the term *evidence* to include "nursing expertise, and the values and preferences of the individuals, families, and communities who are served" (DiCenso et al., 2004, p 69). The term *evidence,* whether through the eyes of the law, research, or practice, can be viewed as the basis for thinking or reasoning about your EBP question.

In nursing, the meaning of evidence was not actively discussed until the early 1990s. At that time, evidence was assumed to be research evidence, especially evidence from randomized controlled trials (RCTs) (Sackett, Richardson, Rosenberg, & Haynes, 1997). RCTs have historically been called the gold standard for best evidence because RCTs have the highest statistical probability of representing the population of study. RCTs are considered to have rigorous methodologies that control for confounders in intervention research and answer the question of efficacy for diagnosing and treatment of disease. Based on this background, RCTs gained the reputation of being the most valuable form of evidence, but at the expense of other evidence designs and sources that may be useful for nursing practice (Rycroft-Malone et al., 2004). For example, RCTs do not answer the questions of *where* or *why* new discoveries work, yet the domain of nursing is relational and patient centered (Cartwright, 2011; Kitson, 2002). Nonexperimental quantitative research designs and qualitative research designs are examples of research evidence for nursing practice that are not RCTs.

Other sources of evidence include patient preferences and values, as well as expert opinion. Credibility of nonresearch evidence can be established through objective documentation such as narrative charting. The objective recording of subjective patient values or expert opinion is a form of qualitative data collection. This broader concept of evidence for practice therefore contributes to sources of evidence wherein empirical data are collected and used to increase conceptual understanding of an identified EBP issue (Higgs & Jones, 2000; Kitson, 2002; Rycroft-Malone et al., 2004).

Finally, evidence informs beliefs (Joanna Briggs Institute [JBI], 2014a). In other words, evidence contributes to thinking or reasoning about your topic for the purpose of answering your EBP question. Three constructs of reasoning that are reflected in EBP definitions include empirical reasoning, conceptual reasoning, and contextual reasoning. *Empirical reasoning* is the means for understanding qualitative and quantitative research evidence. Empirical reasoning implies using your critique skills to assess the rigor and methodology of research publications, thereby trusting or not trusting the findings of the study (Barnard Library, 2014). *Conceptual reasoning* looks at patterns and connections in research, nonresearch, and clinical situations and identifies underlying issues. Use of theory or nonresearch or opinion publications about trends or situations that can be applied to your EBP question is an example of conceptual reasoning or thinking (Sales, Smith, Curran, & Kochevar, 2006). *Contextual reasoning* implies that "cognitive processes are contextual in the sense that they depend on the environment, or context" (Giunchiglia, 1992, p 1). Contextual reasoning grounds your thoughts in the realities of your practice setting. The empirical, conceptual, and contextual constructs of reasoning work together to guide your search and identify best evidence that fits the context to answer your EBP question.

To summarize, RCTs alone do not necessarily translate well into practice. Adding different philosophical and theoretical foundations from nonexperimental quantitative research designs and qualitative research designs contributes to different realities of nursing. The integration of evidence based on multiple worldviews offers a clearer understanding of the components that influence patient-centered care (Phillips, 1996; Romyn, Boschma, & Warnock, 2003). Evidence is built from experience, relationships, proof and rationality, core concepts of law, theory, observations, and rigorous scrutiny to detail and data (Rycroft-Malone, 2004). Understanding the many blended forms that compose the basic nature of evidence assists your knowledge base and reasoning in planning your DNP project (Wilkinson, Rycroft-Malone, Davies, & McCormack, 2012).

WHAT CONSTITUTES BEST EVIDENCE FOR PRACTICE?

Evidence is used to increase understanding of a problem or issue, population, or system, but it depends on the DNP conducting or leading the literature search to determine best fit for the evidence (Grove, Burns, & Gray, 2013; Polit & Beck, 2012). Best evidence implies retrieval of research and nonresearch literature relevant to the reader's contextual needs.

Confidence and trust of evidence, irrespective of design or source, are paramount when making practice decisions. Trust in published research findings is based on confidence of rigorous methodology and high ethical standards. Confidence is gained by critically analyzing the methodology, thereby creating confidence in the findings. Clarity and detail in writing also contribute to the reader's confidence in the researcher's abilities and therefore the publication. Recognition of usefulness from other types of evidence such as patient preferences, theory, and expert opinion also depends on trust and confidence. A critique of each piece of evidence, whether research or nonresearch, is important in the process of identifying best evidence wherein the findings can be trusted and practice decisions made (Polit & Beck, 2012).

Rigor, a term implying credibility, accuracy, validity, and reliability, is a hallmark of research methodology (Polit & Beck, 2012). Rigor should also be applied to patient communication about values and preferences for care by objectively recording details of the patient-provider conversation or observation in the patient's chart. Patient charts subsequently become sources of data for making practice decisions. Expert consultation or opinion is another source of data for making decisions. Conversations should be objectively recorded in your personal field notes. Personal notes become sources of qualitative evidence that can be used to increase contextual understanding of a problem.

To summarize, "the emphasis on best evidence in EBP implies that evidence about a clinical problem or issue has been gathered, evaluated, and synthesized so that conclusions can be drawn about the most effective practices" (Polit & Beck, 2012, p 20).

Evidence Hierarchies

Evidence hierarchies comprise a way to rank the strength of evidence. There are several evidence hierarchies, but no consensus about what constitutes best evidence for ranking purposes. According to Polit and Beck (2012), EBP evidence hierarchies are not universally appropriate, "a point that is not always made sufficiently clear" (p 28). Hierarchal rankings of evidence contribute information to level or rank a study design initially. However, leveling is not a substitute for critical appraisal and empirical reasoning (JBI, 2014b).

Research designs that minimize risk of bias through randomization and control groups are given the highest level or ranking in hierarchies. Quantitative experimental designs demonstrate the least risk of bias, whereas quantitative nonexperimental and qualitative study designs are considered at greater risk of bias and are given lower rankings (JBI, 2014b).

Experimental research, however, is not always possible in the practice setting because of ethical issues, financial costs, flexibility, or difficulty in recruiting participants. Reliance on evidence hierarchies of experimental research therefore may limit findings of best available evidence. Quasiexperimental, nonexperimental, and qualitative designs offer practical alternatives (JBI, 2014a; Mantzoukas, 2008). There are no valid leveling hierarchies for qualitative designs because qualitative methodology and findings are embedded rather than distinct. Themes evolve through data analysis. The richness of the philosophic traditions of qualitative studies is intended to discover the depth of the phenomenon of interest and types of qualitative designs. Strength and trust of a qualitative research publication become choices of the reader and do not rely on relevance of ranking (JBI, 2014b).

In summary, current evidence-based nursing definitions recommend integration of rigorous practice knowledge, patient preferences, and expert opinion with rigorous research studies (Mantzoukas, 2008). Evidence hierarchies based on study design are tools for establishing initial strength of large experimental studies, but they should be used in conjunction with other critical thinking tools. Factors influencing decisions and recommendations suggest assessment of quality of evidence, balance of desirable and undesirable consequences, values and preferences, and cost (Falck-Ytter & Schünemann, 2009; JBI, 2014b).

Types of Evidence

Multiple types of evidence exist for EBP. RCTs have large sample sizes, a comparison and control group, and multiple sites for gathering data. Other types of research evidence may be socially and historically constructed and are generally designed using nonexperimental quantitative methods or qualitative methods. Nonresearch sources of evidence also contribute important evidence from nursing practice and are increasingly being respected and used. Examples include benchmarking data, pathophysiological information (including secondary sources such as textbooks), chart reviews, quality improvement (QI) projects, risk-management data, data on patient preferences, clinical expertise, and information from content experts (Polit & Beck, 2012). Nonresearch sources of evidence should include rationale based on critical thinking or reasoning, but, more importantly, demonstrations of observational or experiential evidence (Kitson, 2002). This section looks briefly at many categories of evidence that may be retrieved for addressing a problem or issue. Table 5.1 presents an overview of *research evidence, conceptual evidence,* and *contextual evidence,* as well as gray literature, to emphasize the integrative importance of research, conceptual, and contextual reasoning in problem solving.

Research Evidence

Research implies evidence that comes through observation or experimentation. *Research* is a broad and important category of empirical evidence. Research is a methodical process to investigate ideas and contribute to nursing's body of knowledge. The following are descriptions of research designs.

Quantitative research designs use numbers to collect data and statistically analyze the results. True *experimental research designs* such as large *RCTs* are used primarily to address efficacy of new products, devices, treatments, and medications. Methodology of a true experimental design includes an intervention or a comparison, a control group, and randomization, thereby decreasing confounding variables as well as risk of bias (LoBiondo-Wood & Haber, 2010; Polit & Beck, 2012). RCTs are often *blinded,* meaning that study subjects or patients and healthcare workers involved in the study have no information about the intervention and, therefore, do not influence findings either intentionally or unintentionally (JBI, 2014a).

Quasiexperimental research designs generally lack randomization, but they have intervention and control (LoBiondo-Wood & Haber, 2010; Polit & Beck, 2012).

Continued

TABLE 5.1 Categories of Evidence

Research Evidence	Conceptual Evidence	Contextual Evidence	Gray Literature
Definition	*Definition*	*Definition*	*Definition*
Observational and experimental methodological processes that contribute to the body of knowledge (Polit & Beck, 2013).	Contributes to increased understanding of patterns and connections in addressing practice issues. Accessed when research evidence is lacking and explanations or strategies are needed to enhance understanding of the issue or problem (Leeman & Sandelowski, 2012; McHugh & Lake, 2010).	Based the on premise that increased understanding of local context is related to yielding a desired outcome (Horner, Blitz, & Ross, 2014).	Print and electronic sources created on all levels of government, academics, businesses, and healthcare systems and not controlled by commercial publishers (New York Academy of Medicine, 2013).
Examples	*Examples*	*Examples*	*Examples*
Quantitative research designs rely on statistical analyses to describe findings. • Experimental (intervention or comparison; control group; randomization; e.g., RCT) • Quasiexperimental (lacks randomization but has intervention or comparison, and control) • Nonexperimental, also referred to as quantitative descriptive (no randomization, intervention or comparison, and control)	*Theory* is abstract thought integrating concepts that describe, explain, and predict. An example is Maslow's Hierarchy of Needs. *Concept* is an abstract idea with similar meaning to the qualitative research term *phenomenon.* *Philosophy,* also an abstract thought, explores the principles of being and knowledge.	*Quality improvement reports* are specific to a healthcare organization or system for the purpose of improving delivery and process of patient-centered care. *Policies* increase understanding of political, social, and safety principles that underlie action and give structure to institutions and employee roles.	• Conference papers and proceedings • Technical reports • Market research reports • Unpublished dissertations • Raw data such as census reports • Websites • Blogs

TABLE 5.1 Categories of Evidence—cont'd

Research Evidence	Conceptual Evidence	Contextual Evidence	Gray Literature
Qualitative research designs are influenced by philosophical traditions and analyze a composite of realities to identify themes. • Common designs include case study, community-based participatory research, grounded theory, ethnography, critical theory, phenomenology.		*Rule of Law* refers to an end state in which all individuals and institutions, public and private, and the state itself are held accountable to the law because it has supreme power. Examples include CHIP, Medicare, and individual state Nurse Practice Acts.	
Mixed methods research designs integrate quantitative and qualitative methods throughout the study to enhance overall understanding of an issue.		*Patient values and preferences* inform and increase understanding of the complexity of illness behavior pertinent to patient-centered care.	
Meta-analysis statistically integrates results from several studies to increase the magnitude of difference between variables.		*Electronic health records* produce large volumes of data that inform systems, organization, policies, and change. Analytics of data stimulate discussions for practice improvement, validate EBP, assess risks and benefits, assist in prioritization of actions, and measure cost effectiveness.	
Metasynthesis integrates and compares themes and understanding from qualitative studies.			

Systematic review is a rigorous, comprehensive synthesis of primary research studies regarding a specific practice topic produced by Cochrane Library and Joanna Briggs Institute.

Integrative review combines quantitative and qualitative research publications, theoretical and philosophical publications, and other sources of evidence to inform nursing research with ideas, contribute to theory development, and contextualize findings for practice and policy.

Clinical practice guidelines synthesize best available evidence and make recommendations for clinicians and practice.

Expert opinion retrieved from published opinion articles or directly from conversations with clinical experts should follow a qualitative research process to establish confirmability of evidence.

Economic evidence specific to the institution or system evaluates and compares health-care effects, process, or devices with costs.

CHIP, Children's Health Insurance Program; EBP, evidence-based practice; RCT, randomized controlled trial.

Quantitative descriptive and observational research designs are nonexperimental and do not have control, intervention, or randomization (LoBiondo-Wood & Haber, 2010; Polit & Beck, 2012).

Qualitative research designs "emphasize the inherent complexity of humans, their ability to shape and create their own experiences, and the idea that truth is a composite of realities" (Polit & Beck, 2012, p 14). Qualitative designs are influenced by philosophical traditions. Common names of qualitative designs include case study, community-based participatory research, critical theory, ethnography, grounded theory, and phenomenology. Qualitative methodology collects data with words and analyzes data through theme identification. The richness of stories and lived experiences add depth to qualitative research (JBI, 2014a).

A *mixed methods* research design integrates quantitative and qualitative methods in the study. The research question or statement should support a mixed methods approach throughout the study. Data collection strategies focus on enhancing an overall understanding of the issue through qualitative and quantitative data collection strategies that complement each other (Polit & Beck, 2012). Numerical demographic data for a qualitative study do not imply mixed methods but describe the study's sample.

A *meta-analysis* is a quantitative process that statistically pools or integrates results from several studies, thereby increasing the effect size or magnitude of the difference among the variables. These findings contribute to increased confidence in the study's results and provide a high level of evidence for efficacy of an intervention (DerSimonian & Laird, 1986; Grove et al., 2013; Polit & Beck, 2012; Russo, 2007).

A *metasynthesis* is an interpretive translation from integrating or comparing findings from qualitative studies (Grove et al., 2013; Polit & Beck, 2012). The intent is to "deepen understanding of the contextual dimensions of health care" (Walsh & Downe, 2005, p 204).

A *systematic review* is a rigorous, comprehensive analysis and synthesis of primary research that focuses on human health care and health policy. The purpose is to "investigate the effects of interventions for prevention, treatment, and rehabilitation" (Cochrane Library, 2016b). The Cochrane Library also looks at the accuracy of a diagnostic test for a specific disease condition in a specific patient population. Cochrane Library and JBI are internationally recognized as meeting highest standards for EBP (Cochrane Library, 2016a; Cochrane Library, 2016b; DiCenso et al., 2004; Grove et al., 2013; Polit & Beck, 2012). Both the Cochrane Collection and the JBI follow stringent guidelines for retrieving and assessing publications. The intent is to ensure that decisions made in health care are based on quality and timely research evidence (Cochrane Library, 2016a; JBI, 2014b).

Databases in the Cochrane Library include the Cochrane Database of Systematic Reviews (CDSR), the Cochrane Central Register of Controlled Trials (CENTRAL), the Cochrane Methodology Register (CMR), the Database of Abstracts of Reviews of Effects (DARE), and the Health Technology Assessment Database (HTA), NSH Economic Evaluation Database (EED) (Cochrane Library, 2016a).

To summarize, systematic reviews of research publications identify, appraise, and synthesize evidence to answer a specific clinical question (Cochrane Library, 2016a; Melnyk & Fineout-Overholt, 2011; Whittemore & Knafl, 2005). Systematic reviews include a detailed, comprehensive process that is created before searching. The result is a rigorous search process that contributes to decreased risk of bias (Ulman, 2011). Some publications include both meta-analysis and systematic review processes. Clarity in distinguishing the systematic review methodology from the meta-analysis methodology must be rigorously exhibited and explained in such publications.

Systematic reviews are often interpreted with the same meaning as *integrative reviews* because of the expanded definition of EBP, the increasing importance of qualitative practice research, and the limitations of research publications that have meaning for practice. Indeed, a literature review has been conceptualized as an integrative review, systematic review, meta-analysis, or metasynthesis. Understanding the subtle differences contributes to clarity in communication and application of evidence. An integrative review, as the title implies, integrates quantitative and qualitative research publications, theoretical and philosophical publications, and other sources of evidence. Findings from integrative reviews inform nursing research and DNP projects with ideas, contextualize findings for practice and policy, and contribute to theory development (Whittemore & Knafl, 2005).

The purpose for *practice guidelines* and *practice measures* is to contribute evidence-based practice recommendations that influence clinical decision making (Polit & Beck, 2012). Recommendations for practice guidelines are "necessity driven" (Sackett, Straus, Richardson, Rosenberg, & Haynes, 2000), and the process for creation of practice recommendations is similar to a systematic review. Sources for clinical practice guidelines and/or measures include the following.

The National Guideline Clearinghouse (AHRQ, 2016) is a public resource that can be accessed at http://www.guideline.gov. A free login may be required. The National Guideline Clearinghouse, established by AHRQ in the early 1990s, is composed of recognized researchers and expert clinicians from multiple healthcare disciplines. Topics are identified, best evidence searched for, a synthesis of the findings completed, and guidelines for practice recommendations developed. After feedback by consultants, revisions are made, and guidelines distributed through publications and repositories (Grove et al., 2013). This structured process is similar to expectations of the EBP process that is part of the DNP project.

The National Quality Measures Clearinghouse (NQMC) is also a public resource and can be accessed at http://www.qualitymeasures.ahrq.gov/content.aspx?id=49267. A free login may be required. NQMC is a database and web page of measures and measure sets that are analyzed for creation of information useful for clinical decision making. NQMC adapted Donabedian's model of structure, process, and outcomes as a framework with a focus on outcome measurements (ANRQ, 2016).

The National Database of Nursing Quality Indicators (NDNQI) collects nursing data on identified indicators that relate to patient-centered quality and care. The NDNQI, established by the American Nurses Association (ANA) in 1998, assists nurses in patient care and QI projects. The NDNQI collects data at the nursing unit level in multiple hospitals throughout the United States. The foci of data collection are patient outcomes and quality nursing care. Quality indicator topics for data collection are identified by ANA. Quarterly and annual reports on structure, process, and outcome (the Donabedian Model, 2005) are distributed to ANA member hospitals (ANA, 2013; Donabedian, 2005). Following the 2015 sale of NDNQI to Press Ganey, ANA continues its leadership position in identifying quality indicator topics that affect nursing quality and care (ANA, 2016).

Conceptual Evidence

Conceptual evidence is nonresearch evidence that contributes to increased understanding of patterns and connections in addressing practice issues or problems. Conceptual evidence is accessed when research evidence is lacking and when explanations or strategies are needed to better understand the practice issue or problem. For example, *theories and conceptual models* provide frameworks for thinking about, connecting, and explaining phenomena (Zaccagnini & White, 2014). *Philosophy* explores abstract thought as it relates to principles of being and knowing (Burns & Grove, 2011). Theories, concepts, and philosophies are the foundations of frameworks wherein writers think and strategize.

A *theory* is abstract thought integrating concepts that describe, explain, and predict (Burns & Grove, 2011). "Theory construction is a creative and intellectual enterprise that can be undertaken by anyone who is insightful, has a firm grounding in existing evidence, and has the ability to knit together evidence into an intelligible pattern" (Polit & Beck, 2012, p 130). Theory explains what we do (Zaccagnini & White, 2014). *Conceptual models, frameworks,* or *schemas* are terms used interchangeably. A concept is an abstract idea with a meaning similar to that of the qualitative research term *phenomenon*. A *schema* is a visual representation of connections among concepts, whereas a *framework* is generally a narrative explanation of conceptual relations (Polit & Beck, 2012). *Philosophy* is similarly abstract thought, but it explores the truth and principles of being and knowledge (Burns & Grove, 2011). Theory and, by association, models and philosophies "guide and generate ideas for research; research assesses the worth of the theory and provides a foundation for new theories" (Polit & Beck, 2012, p 131).

Contextual Evidence

Contextual evidence is an important element in a practice project because of its relationship to increased understanding of direct and indirect patient-centered care in your institution. The evidence from QI reports, patient records, policies, delivery systems, and the sociopolitical environment are contextually fundamental to patient-centered care, yet they may be proprietary to the institution. These unpublished sources of evidence, however, may be important to your DNP project. Communication with stakeholders and Institutional Review Board approval will assist in gaining access, as needed, to some sources of evidence as well as provide for protection of patients (Leeman & Sandelowski, 2012; McHugh & Lake, 2010; Rycroft-Malone, 2008).

QI reports are sources of evidence that have historically not been published, but they are increasingly appearing in professional journals (Orgrinc, 2008). QI reports are associated with specific healthcare organizations and systems for the purpose of improving delivery and process of patient-centered care (Batalden & Davidoff, 2007; Riley et al., 2010). QI is a cyclical, continuous process that is built on the three dimensions of the Donabedian model: *structure, process,* and *outcome.* Continuous QI (CQI) focuses on process and emphasizes organization and systems. Total quality management (TQM) focuses on organizational management to meet or consistently exceed customer requirements (Health Resources and Services Administration [HRSA], n.d., a and b).

Policies are other examples of nonpublished proprietary evidence. Policies are important pieces of evidence to increase understanding of political, social, and safety principles that underlie action and give structure to institutions and employee roles (Bardach, 2009; Carver, n.d.). Policies inform the future by establishing targets or goals for the short and medium terms. Policies assist decision making, planning, and action expected of roles among different groups. Policies inform people and help build consensus (World Health Organization [WHO], 2013). Nursing is guided by public and institutional health policies. Whether policies originate at the unit, institution, state, or federal levels, healthcare policies affect patient care. Policies therefore become important pieces of evidence for a DNP project because they increase understanding of how care is delivered and received in the specific context of your project. Retrieval of important policies can increase understanding of your topic or issue and enhance understanding of the context in which you are working.

The Rule of Law

Kitson (2002) noted that nonresearch evidence is critical reasoning grounded in observation and experience. Laws are based on concepts of lived experience for the purpose of governing. *The rule of law* refers to an end state in which all individuals and institutions, public and private, and the state itself are held accountable to the law because it has supreme power (United Nations, n.d.; World Justice Project, 2016). In the United States, the laws that affect nursing and may contribute evidence to your project include the Children's Health Insurance Program (CHIP), Medicaid, Medicare, and the Patient Protection and Affordable Care Act (PPACA) (innovations.cms.gov). State Boards of Nursing oversee the Nurse Practice Act for individual states (NCSBN, 2016). The rule of law provides parameters for healthcare practice and may be a source of evidence for your EBP question.

Patient values and preferences are increasingly important in EBP because understanding the complexity of illness behavior is pertinent to patient-centered care. Engaging the patient as an active partner in his or her care is empowering for the patient. Communication from the patient regarding his or her lived experiences may also provide qualitative evidence to be used in the DNP project (Birkel, Hall, Lane, Cohan, & Miller, 2003; Romyn, 2003). Preferences are formed from values that arise from culture, family, and religion. Preference perceptions are interpretations of personal lived experiences through the lens of values, lived experiences, and knowledge. Nursing conversations with patients yield information about preferences and values that are important pieces of evidence to be entered as narrative into the patient's nursing chart. The action of charting turns patient values and preferences into data points. The importance of timeliness in narrative charting of patient preferences cannot be underestimated.

Electronic health records (EHRs) produce large volumes of data every day. Analytics from these large volumes of data inform systems, organization, policies, and change. Data stimulate discussions for practice improvement, validate EBPs, assess risks and benefits, assist in prioritization of actions, and measure cost effectiveness. EHRs are important sources of data and should not be overlooked (Harris, 2014). Retrospective chart reviews of EHRs provide primary sources of evidence for clinical practice projects. Data collected from chart reviews have potential to contribute evidence of similar or same preferences and values related to a specific patient population and context.

Expert opinion is another source of evidence. Expert opinion can complement empirical evidence or can stand alone as evidence in the absence of research. Expert opinion can be retrieved from published opinion articles or directly from clinical experts. Your conversation with a clinical expert should follow a qualitative research process to establish confirmability of the evidence. Confirmability, a characteristic of qualitative research methodology, establishes that the evidence collected from a conversation with an expert reflects the objective voice of the expert and not the perspectives of the DNP who is interviewing or questioning. Expert opinion should be explicitly clear for readers (Guba & Lincoln, 1994; JBI, 2014a; LoBiondo-Wood & Haber, 2010; Polit & Beck, 2012).

Economic Evidence

Economic evidence is increasingly important for nurse practitioners and nurse managers for evaluating or comparing healthcare effects and costs. Economic evaluation reports may examine the following:

- Cost minimization, the least expensive process for care is the preferred method.

- Cost-effectiveness results are presented as a ratio of incremental cost to incremental effect. Programs with different types of outcomes, however, cannot be compared.

- Cost-utility analysis measures quality of life adjusted over years.

- Cost-benefit analyses are measured in monetary terms. However, it is difficult to measure the value of life to assess best outcomes (JBI, 2014a). Costs are measured either directly or indirectly and are difficult to measure.

Gray Literature

Relevance and practicality of DNP projects may require information and validation from unpublished evidence sources. Excluding such nonpublished findings is perceived as publication bias, implying that published research studies may overrepresent findings that are statistically significant at the expense of reports where findings were negative (Polit & Beck, 2012). Unpublished information also includes conference presentations that are conceptually practical. Relevant unpublished literature is termed *gray literature* and is defined as "that which is produced on all levels of government, academics, business, and industry in print and electronic formats, but which is not controlled by commercial publishers" (New York Academy of Medicine, 2013).

Examples of gray literature range from conference papers and proceedings to technical reports from governments, business, or academic institutions, market research reports, unpublished dissertations, and raw data such as census reports, economic reports, research, or blogs. Gray literature also includes technological publishing on websites (Huffine, 2010; JBI, 2014a). Gray literature should not be viewed as competition with commercially published literature, but rather as a complementary method of communication that may reach a wider audience (JBI, 2014a). On the other hand, rigorous assessment of gray literature is important for establishing trust in the findings for potential use as evidence in your DNP project.

CHAPTER SUMMARY AND AFTERTHOUGHTS

Understanding the nature of evidence lays the groundwork for finding and applying best evidence in your practice setting. Reasoning about the fit, concept, and science of evidence provides a broad base for meeting the practice goal of indirect and direct patient-centered care.

CASE STUDY

Andrew was deployed to Afghanistan from 2008 to 2009 as an Army flight medic (medevac). On his return to the United States, he returned to school for a master's degree and subsequently certified as a nurse practitioner. Andrew currently works in a limb loss clinic at the Veterans Affairs (VA) Hospital. The patients he sees have complex issues. Most of his patients have some form of post-traumatic stress disorder (PTSD), and many have traumatic brain injury. In addition to the social and family problems that are secondary to PTSD, chronic pain is a common complaint. Andrew thinks that if the patient's pain can be controlled, the patient can gain more control over his or her mental and social issues.

Andrew is currently enrolled in a post-master's DNP program. His topic has been reviewed by his DNP project team. A nurse practitioner at the VA Hospital has been identified and has agreed to work with Andrew as a content expert. Andrew is meeting with his academic adviser and DNP project team next week to present his search question and discuss search strategies.

* *Compose an EBP question based on Andrew's identified issue, population, and context.*

* *Identify search terms from Andrew's EBP question.*

* *What are the best types of evidence for Andrew's project?*

WRITING REMINDERS...

Technical Writing and Scientific Writing: What's the Difference?

Technical writing, scientific writing, and state-of-the-science papers are similar in meaning, yet different. As a nursing scholar, clarity in using terminology is important.

- Technical writing is intended to put complex information into language that is easily understood by others who use the information. Technical writing is mainly associated with information technology, but it is increasingly connected to explaining internal procedures, design products, or implementation of processes and services or for defining policies. Examples of technical writing include instructions, policies, project documents, proposals, training materials, and Web-based training (TechWhirl, 2013).

- Examples of scientific writing include peer-reviewed journal publications, grant proposals, literature review publications, and science articles. The goal of scientific writing is to present detailed ideas clearly so the reader can easily understand the methodology in a research publication or the logical process leading to conclusions. Key elements of scientific writing include precision, clarity, and objectivity (Regents Online Collaborative Campus [RODP], 2010).

- A state-of-the-science-paper is a scholarly synthesis of publications regarding a specific topic. State-of-the-science scholarly papers (1) answer a question or address an issue, (2) synthesize results of a thorough literature search, (3) identify controversial areas in the literature, and (4) create questions for further study (University of North Carolina [UNC], 2004).

REFERENCES

Agency for Healthcare Research and Quality (AHRQ). (2016a). *National guideline clearinghouse.* Retrieved from http://www.guideline.gov

Agency for Healthcare Research and Quality (AHRQ). (2016b). *National quality measures clearinghouse.* Retrieved from http://www.qualitymeasures.ahrq.gov/browse/by-topic .aspx

American Nurses Association (ANA). (January 5, 2016). *The American nurse.* Retrieved from http://www.theamericannurse.org/index.php/2014/09/02/ndnqi-changes -hands/

Bardach, E. (2009). *A practical guide for policy analysis: The eightfold path to more effective problem solving* (3rd ed.). Washington, DC: CQ Press.

Barnard Library. (2014). *What is empirical reasoning?* Retrieved from https://erl.barnard.edu

Batalden, P.B., & Davidoff, F. (2007). What is "quality improvement" and how can it transform healthcare? *Quality and Safety in Health Care, 18*(1), 2–3. Retrieved from http://www.ncbi.nlm.nih.gov/pmc/articles/PMC2464920/

Birkel, R., Hall, L., Lane, T., Cohan, K., & Miller, J. (2003). Consumers and families as partners in implementing evidence-based practice. *Psychiatric Clinics of North America, 26*(4), 867–881.

Burns, N., & Grove, S.K. (2011). *Understanding nursing research: Building an evidence-based practice* (5th ed.). Maryland Heights, MO: Elsevier Saunders.

Cartwright, N. (2011). A philosopher's view of the long road from RCTs to effectiveness. *Lancet, 377*(9755), 1400–1401.

Carver, J. (n.d.). *Basic principles of policy governance.* Retrieved from http://www.dccs.org/uploaded/About_DC/Board/Basic_Principles_of_Policy_Governance.pdf

Cochrane Library. (2016a). *About the Cochrane Library.* Retrieved from: http://www.cochranelibrary.com/about/about-the-cochrane-library.html

Cochrane Library. (2016b). *What is Cochrane evidence and how can it help you?* Retrieved from http://www.cochrane.org/what-is-cochrane-evidence

DerSimonian, R., & Laird, N. (1986) Meta-analysis in clinical trials. *Controlled Clinical Trials, 7,* 177–188.

DiCenso, A., Prevost, S., Benefield, L., Bingle, J., Ciliska, D., Driever, M., Lock, S., & Titler, M. (2004). Evidence-based nursing: rationale and resources. *Worldviews on Evidence-Based Practice, 1*(1), 69–75.

Donabedian, A. (2005). Evaluating the quality of medical care. *Millbank Quarterly, 83*(4), 691–729.

Falck-Ytter, Y., & Schünemann, H. (2009). *Rating the evidence: Using GRADE to develop clinical practice guidelines.* PowerPoint from AHRQ 2009 Conference. Retrieved from http://archive.ahrq.gov/news/events/conference/2009/falck-ytter-schunemann/index.html

Giunchiglia, F. (1992). *Contextual reasoning.* Retrieved from http://citeseerx.ist.psu.edu/viewdoc/download?doi=10.1.1.85.1580&rep=rep1&type=pdf

Grove, S.K., Burns, N., & Gray, J.R. (2013). *The practice of nursing research: Appraisal, synthesis, and generation of Evidence* (7th ed.). St. Louis, MO: Elsevier Saunders.

Guba, E.G., & Lincoln, Y.S. (1994). Comparing paradigms in qualitative research. In N.K. Denzin, & Y.S. Lincoln (Eds.). *Handbook of qualitative research,* Thousand Oaks, CA: Sage Publications, pp 105–117.

Harris, J.L. (2014). Turning health policy into practice: implications for advanced practice registered nurses. In A. Goudreau, & M.C. Smolenski (Eds.). *Health policy and advanced practice nursing: Impact and implications.* Philadelphia, PA: Lippincott Williams & Wilkins, pp 13–28.

Health Resources and Services Administration (HRSA). (n.d.). *Who are the key stakeholders for the project?* Retrieved from http://www.hrsa.gov/healthit/toolbox/RuralHealthIT-toolbox/GettingStarted/stakeholders.html

Health Resources and Services Administration (HRSA). (2011). *Quality improvement.* Retrieved from http://www.hrsa.gov/quality/toolbox/508pdfs/qualityimprovement.pdf

Higgs, J., & Jones, M. (2000) Will evidence-based practice take the reasoning out of practice? In J. Higgs, & M. Jones (Eds.). *Clinical reasoning in the health professionals* (2nd ed.). Oxford, United Kingdom: Butterworth Heinemann, pp. 307–315.

Higgs, J., & Titchen, A. (2000). Knowledge and reasoning. In J. Higgs, & M. Jones (Eds.). *Clinical reasoning in the health professions* (2nd ed.). Oxford, United Kingdom: Butterworth Heinemann, pp 23–32.

Hill, G., & Hill, K. (2013). Search legal terms and definitions. *Law.com.* Retrieved from http://dictionary.law.com/Default.aspx?selected=671

Horner, R., Blitz, C., & Ross, S.W. (2014). The importance of contextual fit when implementing evidence-based interventions; executive summary. *ASPE Issue Brief, (September),* 1–16. Retrieved from http://aspe.hhs.gov/hsp/14/IWW/ib_Contextual.pdf

Huffine, R. (2010). *Value of grey literature to scholarly research in the digital age.* Retrieved from http://www.slideshare.net/richardhuffine/2010-richardhuffine

Joanna Briggs Institute (JBI). (2014a). *Joanna Briggs Reviewers' Manual.* University of Adelaide. Retrieved from http://joannabriggs.org/assets/docs/sumari/Reviewers-Manual-2014.pdf

Joanna Briggs Institute. (JBI) (2014b).Levels of evidence and grades of recommendation. *The JBI Approach.* University of Adelaide. Retrieved from http://www.joannabriggs.org/jbi-approach.html#tabbed-nav=Levels-of-Evidence

Kitson, K. (2002). Recognizing relationships: Reflections on evidence-based practice. *Nursing Inquiry, 9*(3), 179–186.

Leeman, J., & Sandelowski, M. (2012). Practice-based evidence and quality inquiry. *Journal of Nursing Scholarship, 44*(2), 171–179.

LoBiondo-Wood, G., & Haber, J. (2010). *Nursing research: Methods and critical appraisal for evidence-based practice* (7th ed.). St. Louis, MO: Elsevier Mosby.

McHugh, M.D., & Lake, E.T. (2010). Understanding clinical expertise: nurse education, experience, and the hospital context. *Research in Nursing and Health, 33*(4), 276–287. Retrieved from http://www.ncbi.nlm.nih.gov/pmc/articles/PMC2998339/

Mantzoukas, S. (2008). A review of evidence-based practice, nursing research and reflection: leveling the hierarchy. *Journal of Clinical Nursing, 17*(2), 214–223.

Melnyk, B.M., & Fineout-Overholt, E. (2011). *Evidence-based practice in nursing and healthcare: A guide to best practice* (2nd ed.). Philadelphia, PA: Wolters Kluwer Health/Lippincott Williams & Wilkins.

National Council of State Boards of Nursing (NCSBN). (2016). Nurse practice acts guide and govern nursing practice. *Nurse Practice Act, Rules & Regulations.* Retrieved from https://www.ncsbn.org/nurse-practice-act.htm

New York Academy of Medicine. (2013). *What is grey literature?* Retrieved from http://www.greylit.org/about

Orgrinc, G., Mooney, S.E., Estrada, C., & Watts, B. (2008). The SQUIRE (Standards for Quality Improvement Reporting Excellence) guidelines for quality improvement reporting: Explanation and elaboration. *Quality and Safety Health Care, 1*(Suppl I), 13–32.

Phillips, J.R. (1996). What constitutes nursing science? *Nursing Science Quarterly, 9*(2), 48–49.

Polit, D.F., & Beck, C.T. (2012). *Nursing research: Generating and assessing evidence for nursing practice* (9th ed.). Philadelphia, PA: Wolters Kluwer/Lippincott Williams & Wilkins.

Regents Online Collaborative Campus (RODP). (2010). *Scholarly synthesis*. Retrieved from http://www.rodp.org/sites/default/files/syllabi/NURS_5990.pdf

Riley, W.J., Moran, J.W., Corso, L.C., Beitsch, L.M., Bialek, R., & Cofsky, A. (2010). Defining quality improvement in public health. *Journal of Public Health Management Practice, 16*(1), 5–7.

Romyn, D.M., Boschma, G., & Warnock, F. (2003). The notion of evidence in evidence-based practice by the Nursing Philosophy Working Group. *Journal of Professional Nursing, 19*(4), 184–188.

Russo, M.W. (2007). How to review a meta-analysis. *Gastroenterology & Hepatology, 3*(8), 637–642. Retrieved from http://www.ncbi.nlm.nih.gov/pmc/articles/PMC3099299

Rycroft-Malone, J. (2004). The PARIHS framework: A framework for guiding the implementation of evidence-based practice. *Journal of Nursing Care Quality, 19*(4), 297–304.

Rycroft-Malone, J. (2008). Evidence-informed practice: From individual to context. *Journal of Nursing Management, 16,* 404–408.

Rycroft-Malone, J., Seers, K., & McCormack, B. (2004). What counts as evidence in evidence-based practice? *Journal of Advanced Nursing, 47,* 81–90.

Sackett, D.L., Richardson, W.S., Rosenberg, W., & Haynes, R.B. (1997) *Evidence based medicine: How to practice and teach EBM.* Edinburgh, United Kingdom: Churchill Livingstone.

Sackett, D.L., Straus, S.E., Richardson, W.S., Rosenberg, W., & Haynes, R.B. (2000). *Evidence-based medicine: How to practice and teach EBM* (2nd ed.). Edinburgh: Churshill Livingstone.

Sales, A., Smith, J., Curran, G., & Kochevar, L. (2006). Models, strategies, and tools: Theory in implementing evidence-based findings into health are practice. *Journal of General Internal medicine, 21*(Suppl 2), S43–S49.

TechWhirl. (2013). What is technical writing? Retrieved from http://techwhirl.com/what-is- technical-writing/

Ulman, L.S. (2011). Systematic reviews and meta-analysis. *Journal of the Canadian Academy of Child and Adolescent Psychiatry, 20*(1), 57–59.

United Nations. (n.d.). *United Nations and the Rule of Law.* Retrieved from http://www.un.org/en/ruleoflaw/

University of North Carolina (UNC). (2004). *Guidelines from state of the science clinical paper.* Retrieved from http://nursing.unc.edu/files/2012/11/ccm3_037585.pdf

Walsh, D., & Downe, S. (2005). Meta-synthesis method for qualitative research: A literature review. *Journal of Advanced Nursing, 50*(2), 204–211.

Whittemore, R., & Knafl, K. (2005). The integrative review: Updated methodology. *Journal of Advanced Nursing, 52*(5), 547–553.

Wilkinson, J.E., Rycroft-Malone, J., Davies, H.T.O., & McCormack, B. (2012). A creative approach to the development of an agenda for knowledge utilization: Outputs from the 11th International Knowledge Utilization Colloquium. *Worldviews on Evidence-Based Practice.* 9(4), 195–199.

World Health Organization. (2013). *Health policy.* Retrieved from http://www.who.int/topics/health_policy/en/

World Justice Project. (2016). *What is the rule of law?* Retrieved from http://worldjusticeproject.org/what-rule-law

Zaccagnini, M.E., & White, K.W. (2014). *The doctor of nursing practice essentials: A new model for advanced practice nursing.* Burlington, MA: Jones & Bartlett Learning.

IF YOU WANT TO READ MORE...

Joanna Briggs Institute (JBI). (2014). *Joanna Briggs reviewers' manual.* University of Adelaide. Retrieved from http://joannabriggs.org/assets/docs/sumari/ReviewersManual-2014.pdf

Moher, D., Liberati, A., Tetzlaff, J., & Altman, D.F. (2009). Preferred reporting items for systematic reviews and meta-analyses: the PRISMA statement. *BMJ, 339,* 2535.

PRISMA. (2015). *Transparent reporting or systematic reviews and meta-analyses.* Retrieved from http://www.prisma-statement.org/Extensions/Default.aspx

National Information Center on Health Services Research and Health Care Technology (NICHSR). (2011). *Core health policy library recommendations, 2011.* Retrieved from http://www.nlm.nih.gov/nichsr/corelib/corehp-2011.html

PubMed Tutorial: Retrieved from http://www.nlm.nih.gov/bsd/disted/pubmedtutorial

Rycroft-Malone, J., Seers, K., & McCormack, B. (2004). What counts as evidence in evidence- based practice. *Journal of Advanced Nursing, 47,* 81–90.

Whittemore, R., & Knafl, K. (2005). The integrative review: Updated methodology. *Journal of Advanced Nursing, 52*(5), 546–553.

6

Searching and Organizing

The ultimate authority must always rest with the individual's own reason and critical analysis.

DALAI LAMA

OUTCOME OBJECTIVES

- Discuss the importance of a well-designed search strategy.
- Cite effective and efficient strategies in searching for best evidence.
- Analyze the importance of managing findings from evidence searches.
- Discuss the iterative process of searching and managing evidence findings.

TERMS

Booleans

Evidence table

Inclusion and
    exclusion criteria

Limiters and expanders

Organizing or managing

Search strategy

Screening

Searching

The idiom "cast your net wide" applies to the principle of inclusiveness in searching the widest range possible specific to your evidence-based practice (EBP) topic (Joanna Briggs Institute [JBIb], 2014). There is such an abundance of information that it can quite easily become overwhelming, and it is logical to ask oneself what to do with all that evidence, information, and input. The usefulness and credibility of the literature search rest in the comprehensiveness of searching for evidence and finding evidence for best fit with your project. Searching and managing evidence findings require systematic and consistent methods. Clarity of these processes promotes confidence in the evidence-based decisions that you make.

SEARCH STRATEGY

A search strategy should be thoughtfully planned and organized. Development of a search strategy *before* conducting the search saves time and energy later in the process. A detailed search strategy helps you avoid duplication or omission of references, stay focused, manage search terms and databases, and find relevant evidence. Early in the process, experts recommend a consultation with a research librarian at your university. Time spent developing a good search strategy affects the quality of the search (Grove, Burns, & Gray, 2013; Polit & Beck, 2012; Timmins & McCabe, 2005). Box 6.1 presents important

---

BOX 6.1 Elements of a Search Strategy

- Identify *search terms* or phrases from the EBP question.
- Describe *inclusion and exclusion criteria* related to the EBP issue.
  - Use of *Booleans*
- Describe *limiters and expanders,* such as
  - Publication dates
  - Language
- Identify *library databases* to be searched for evidence.
- Identify *Internet sources* to be searched for evidence.
- Identify *other sources* to be searched for evidence.

EBP, evidence-based practice.
Sources: JBIa, 2014; LoBiondo-Wood & Haber, 2010.

information regarding a strategy to search for relevant evidence. Italicized terms are described in the following text.

Search terms are the key concepts or variables identified from your EBP question. Search terms guide your literature search (Tensen, 2010). *Inclusion and exclusion criteria* are also important in the search strategy because they are based on your involvement and understanding of the practice issue, population, and context. Inclusion and exclusion criteria therefore should be established before searching begins. Inclusion and exclusion criteria help you find evidence that will assist your decision making regarding the publication's fittingness. Use of Booleans is effective in fine-tuning search terms and phrases (JBIb, 2014; LoBiondo-Wood & Haber, 2010; Melnyk & Fineout-Overholt, 2011).

Booleans are terms that make searches more exact. Booleans are credited to James Boole, a 19th century mathematician, who developed a model of logical sequencing for searching library catalogs. Booleans are useful in searching library databases and Internet websites (Library of Congress, 2008). The following is a list of Boolean terms and symbols useful in searching library databases and online. Note that Boolean terms are all capital letters.

- " " Words inside the quotation marks are searched as a phrase.
  - Example: "best evidence"
- OR is an expander because more than one term is searched, meaning that literature findings with one and/or both terms will be included in the search.
  - Example: "evidence-based nursing" OR "evidence-based medicine"
- AND decreases the number of publications that may be found.
  - Example: research AND theory
- AND NOT is a limiter that is generally used after the first search and to look for specific words or phrases.
  - Example: "qualitative research" AND "theory" AND NOT "philosophy"
- ( ) Parentheses indicate "nesting" and are used to identify groupings of terms connected by Booleans.
  - Example: "evidence-based nursing" AND evidence-based medicine" AND ("quantitative research" OR "qualitative research") (Barker, n.d.)

Booleans are valuable tools to broaden or narrow the focus of keywords and phrases. Other *limiters and expanders* include dates and languages. These are the two most commonly selected limiters. Limiting the search by date is useful when the topic is a recent intervention or innovation. However, date limitations should be used with caution because a potentially relevant or salient publication may be excluded. Restricting a search by language holds similar problems.

The global reach of relevant publications and knowledge should not be limited by language (JBIb, 2014). Other common limiters include peer review and publication type (e.g., research publication, theory, opinion). Common expanders include *apply related terms* and *search within full text articles*. Expanders and limiters for searching are programmed into database search engines.

Identification of databases and websites is the last step of your strategic search plan before beginning the search. The next section describes databases, websites, and other resources useful in the evidence search.

Resources for searching include library databases, websites, and other sources. These resources are efficiently organized to find evidence about your identified topic. Box 6.2 presents a compilation of resources that may be useful in your search for best evidence to meet your project needs. The lists are not inclusive

Text continued on page 105

BOX 6.2 Databases, Websites, and Other Resources for Searching

Library Databases

- *Allied and Complementary Medicine Database (AMED)* provides resources for nurse practitioners, researchers, and clinicians to learn more about alternative treatments (AMED, 2014).

- *BIOSIS* life sciences databases provide resources about biodiversity, biotechnology, drug discovery, gene therapy, and other topics, with cross-references for gene, disease, and organism names (Biosis, 2014).

- *CINAHL, Cumulative Index to Nursing and Allied Health Literature,* provides full text access to more than 70 journals and publications from the National League for Nursing and the American Nurses Association (ANA). Topics include research, biomedicine, 17 allied health disciplines, and consumer health. CINAHL also provides access to nursing dissertations, proceedings from selected conferences, clinical innovations, and research instruments and studies, including clinical trials (CINAHL, 2014).

- *Embase* is a comprehensive international biomedical database (Embase, 2014).

- The *Education Resource Information Center (ERIC)* is an online library of education research and information. It is sponsored by the Institute of Sciences (IES) of the U.S. Department of Education (ERIC, 2014).

BOX 6.2 Databases, Websites, and Other Resources for Searching—cont'd

- *MEDLINE* databases are created by the U.S. National Library of Medicine (NLM). MEDLINE uses Medical Subject Headings (MeSH) that consist of sets of terms in a hierarchical structure (MEDLINE, 2014).

- *Ovid* is a database for medical information services that is commonly used in hospital libraries (Ovid, 2014).

- *ProQuest Central* is a cross-disciplinary research tool (ProQuest, 2014).

- *ProQuest Government Periodicals Index* (1988 to present). This index links to periodicals published by agencies and departments of the U.S. government (ProQuest, 2014).

- *PsycINFO* is sponsored by the American Psychological Association (APA, 2014).

- *PubMed* is a free service provided by the NLM and is part of the National Institutes of Health (NIH, 2013). It provides biomedical literature from MEDLINE, life science journals, and online books (NCBI, 2014).

- *Sociological Abstracts* is an international database for sociology, social and behavioral sciences (ProQuest, 2014).

Systematic Review Websites

- *Campbell Collaboration* (2014)

- *Cochrane Libraries* (2014)

- *Joanna Briggs Institute* (JBI, 2014a)

Nursing Quality Indicator Databases Used to Monitor Quality of Care

- *Collaborative Alliance for Nursing Outcomes (CALNOC)* (www.calnoc.org)

- *Core Health Policy Library Recommendations, 2011* (http://www.nlm.nih.gov/nichsr/corelib/corehp-2011.html) is a useful resource for locating publications related to policies.

Continued

BOX 6.2 Databases, Websites, and Other Resources for Searching—cont'd

- *National Database of Nursing Quality Indicators (NDNQI).* NDNQI is a national, nursing quality measurement program that provides unit-level performance comparison reports. All data are reported at the nursing unit level. Nursing-sensitive indicators report on structure, process, and outcomes of nursing care. More than 1,500 U.S. hospitals participate. NDNQI is associated with ANA's National Center for Nursing Quality. There is a cost to access this database (access through http://www.nursingworld.org/Research-Toolkit/NDNQI).

- *National Quality Forum (NQF)* reviews and recommends standardized healthcare performance measures, also called quality measures. These tools are used to evaluate delivery of healthcare services. NQF is a not-for-profit membership organization (http://www.qualityforum.org/who_we_are.aspx).

- *National Quality Measures Clearinghouse (NQMC)* is an evidence-based quality measures and measure set resource. It is a public resource overseen by the Agency for Healthcare Research and Quality (AHRQ). (http://www.qualitymeasures.ahrq.gov/browse/nqf-endorsed.aspx)

Theses and Dissertations

- ProQuest Dissertations and Theses Database (PQDT): (http://www.proquest.com/products-services/proquest-dissertations-theses-full-text.html)

U.S. Government Websites

- AHRQ   (http://www.ahrq.gov/research/findings/index.html): summary of research findings and full research reports

- Centers for Medicare and Medicaid Services (December, 2015). Research, statistics, data & systems. *CMS.gov.* Retrieved from https://www.cms.gov/Research-Statistics-Data-and-Systems/Statistics-Trends-and-Reports/CMSProgramStatistics/index.html

- National Guideline Clearinghouse (http://www.guideline.gov/browse/by-topic.aspx): guidelines categorized by topic

BOX 6.2 Databases, Websites, and Other Resources for Searching—cont'd

- National Institute on Alcohol Abuse and Alcoholism (http://www. niaaa.nih.gov): lead agency for research on alcohol abuse, alcoholism, and other health and developmental effects of alcohol abuse

- NIH (http://www.nih.gov): the U.S. medical research library

- Partners in Information Access for the Public Health Workforce (http:// phpartners.org/guide.html): public health organizations and health sciences library

- Patient Protection and Affordable Care Act (PPACA) (http://www.hhs. gov/healthcare/rights/law/index.html): website for the Affordable Care Act

- United States Health Information Knowledgebase (USHIK; http:// ushik.ahrq.gov): a repository of healthcare-related data, metadata, and standards

International Websites

- *Bandolier*: Evidence Based Thinking About Health Care (http://www. medicine.ox.ac.uk/bandolier)

- *Canadian Health Network* (http://www.canadianhealthcarenetwork.ca)

- *Department of Health* (www.dh.gov.uk)

- *Health In Site* (http://www.healthinsite.gov.au)

- *National Electronic Library for Health* (http://www.bmj.com/ content/319/7223/1476)

- *National Institute for Health and Care Excellence (NICE)* (www.library.nhs. uk)

- *Office of National Statistics* (www.statistics.gov.uk)

- *World Health Organization (http://www.who.int/gho/database/en/* Global health observatory data repository)

- **The York Research Database** (https://pure.york.ac.uk/portal/en/ (http://www.york.ac.uk/inst/crd/projects/euronheed.htm

Continued

BOX 6.2 Databases, Websites, and Other Resources for
Searching—cont'd

Open Access Sites

- *BMJ* open access to *Clinical Evidence* database (www.clinicalevidence. com)

- *BMJ* open access to *Evidence-Based Nursing* journal (www. evidencebasednursing.com)

- *BMF* open access to *Evidence Based Medicine* journal (ebm.bmj.com)

- Wiley open access to *Worldviews on Evidence-Based Practice* journal (http:// onlinelibrary.wiley.com/journal/10.1111/(ISSN)1741-6787/earlyview)

National Nursing Organizations

- *American Association of Critical-Care Nurses* (www.aacn.org)

- *ANA publications* (http://www.nursingworld.org/HomepageCategory/ ANAPublications)

- *Robert Woods Johnson Foundation.* (http://www.rwjf.org/en/how-we-work/rel/tools-and-resources.html)

Economic Evaluation Websites

- Connaissance et Décision en Economie de la Santé (CODECS; http:// asp.bdsp.ehesp.fr/Webs/Scripts/Show.bs?bqRef=218)

- Cost-Effectiveness Analysis (CEA) Registry (https://research.tufts-nemc.org/cear4/Home.aspx)

- Health Economic Evaluations Database (HEED)/HTAi vortal (http:// www.htai.org/vortal/?q=node/227)

- Health Technology Assessment (HTA) database (http://www.cochrane. org/editorial-and-publishing-policy-resource/health-technology -assessment-database-hta)

- National Health Service Economic Evaluation Database (NHS EED; http://www.cochrane.org/editorial-and-publishing-policy-resource/ nhs-economic-evaluation-database)

- Pediatric Economic Database Evaluation (PEDE; http://pede.ccb. sickkids.ca/pede) because there are hundreds of databases and websites covering multiple disciplines. However, remember the importance of identifying databases, websites, and other evidence sources for the purpose of establishing trust in the references that influence your recommendations for practice.

Example: Search Strategy Statement

The following excerpt from Wollery et al. (2008) is an example of a search strategy written for a synthesis report. This is a reminder that the processes of searching and selecting best evidence to answer your question must be thoroughly documented because the search strategy statement becomes part of the synthesis of evidence report.

In consultation with a medical librarian, the researchers conducted computerized searches of a variety of databases in July 2006 to identify meta-analyses, systematic reviews, research studies, and practice guidelines for interventions related to the prevention and management of constipation. The search was limited to English language publications. Databases searched included Wiley's Cochrane Database of Systematic Reviews, Ovid's MEDLINE (1966 to July 2006), the National Guideline Clearinghouse, the National Cancer Institute's PDQ, the National Comprehensive Cancer Network, and the Cumulative Index to Nursing and Allied Health Literature (CINAHL) (1982 to July 2006). In addition, a search for critically appraised topics was conducted in Ovid's Clinical Evidence and in the American College of Physicians' Information and Education Resource. Search terms included constipation, defecation, fecal incontinence, bowel function, colonic transit, stool impaction, colonic inertia, *and* cancer, neoplasms, oncology. *Additional search terms included specific pharmacologic (e.g., laxatives, polyethylene glycol [PEG], senna) and nonpharmacologic (e.g., diet changes, biofeedback) interventions related to constipation. Abstracts of the literature search were reviewed to determine whether articles met the inclusion criteria. Articles were retrieved and critiqued if they included constipation as an outcome variable or contained guidelines for the prevention and management of constipation. Additional data sources were identified from manual searches in article bibliographies. Published references before October 2006 were retrieved (Woolery et al., 2008, p 318).*

SEARCHING

A *standard approach* to searching for evidence uses inductive thinking with databases serving as the primary source for finding evidence, whether the databases are accessed through a university library or through the Internet. There is also a *network approach* to finding evidence that includes searching reference lists from pertinent publications, conference presentations, similar current events, or professional journals with a focused theme (Timmins & McCabe, 2005). Be thorough and aggressive in your search, and retrieve as much relevant evidence as possible. Search until your evidence findings are repetitive or saturated. This is a qualitative data gathering principle that is effective in evidence searching (Polit & Beck, 2012).

The *title* is your first introduction to a publication. A well-written title should identify the population and variables or key terms of the publication. If the identified population and terms are similar to your EBP question, make a decision whether or not to retrieve the article or read the abstract for additional information about the article's relevance to your need. The purpose of an *abstract* is to assist your decision in retrieving relevant evidence for your scholarly needs. The abstract is approximately 150 words and is completed after the article is written. Abstracts are "dense with information but also readable, well-organized, brief, and self-contained" (APA, 2001, p 12). Reading an abstract generally guides your decision whether to download the full text.

In your first search of the literature, choose a variety of publications related to your EBP question. Few articles, if any, will directly answer your question, but many will have parts that address key concepts of your topic. Select relevant information from the found publications because your EBP question generally fits into a broader scope. To summarize, look for themes similar to your EBP question, population, and context. Above all, keep good search notes about your search process, and consult the research librarian at your university (Driscoll & Brizee, 2010).

SCREENING

Searching and screening occur concurrently. Screening the findings of the search implies a first assessment of suitability of evidence for use in answering your EBP question (Oxford Dictionary, 2014). The first screening is about separating relevant articles from nonrelevant articles. Relevant articles are publications or other sources of evidence that appear appropriate for your project based on your first introduction to the title and abstract. A full-text of a relevant finding can then be downloaded for critical appraisal.

ORGANIZING

There is much emphasis on keeping organized notes during your searching. Indeed, the importance of keeping notes cannot be overestimated (Polit &

Beck, 2012; Timmins & McCabe, 2005). Evidence tables are essential for organizing and accessing evidence discovered during your search. Tables can be created at no cost with Microsoft Word or Excel. Reference management software can also be purchased. Common software programs include Bookends, EndNote, Reference Manager, and RefWorks. Evidence tables are working documents to record information from searching and critiquing each piece of evidence. See Chapter 7 for an example of an evidence table.

VALIDATING THE SEARCH PROCESS

Validating the quality of your search adds strength to your findings, thereby increasing trust in your recommendations for practice. A section of the PRISMA tool assists in tracking and reporting sets of items found while searching (Moher et al., 2009).

Following are suggestions to assist validation of your search:

1. Total number of identified publications from your database search

2. Total number of identified evidence from other sources

3. Total number of duplicate publications and other evidence removed

4. Total number of publications and other evidence screened and excluded

5. Total number of full text publications and other evidence critically assessed for eligibility in answering your EBP question (keepers)

6. Total number of full text publications and other evidence critically assessed but excluded (Moher et al., 2008)

CHAPTER SUMMARY AND AFTERTHOUGHTS

The quote at the beginning of this chapter from the Dalai Lama focuses on the authority of individual reasoning and critical analysis in selecting best evidence to answer an EBP question. His wise advice resonates in the screening and selection of relevant evidence found in your database searches and institutional documents. It will enhance the value of evidence because of the clarity and interpretation of your thoughts. Chapter 7 describes critical analysis of the identified evidence *keepers* from your search, thereby adding rigor to the identified publications to answer the EBP question.

CASE STUDY QUESTIONS

Refer to the case study in Chapter 5, "The Nature of Evidence." The following questions continue the decision-making process of Andrew's DNP project related to care of chronic pain.

- *Design a search strategy for Andrew.*

- *What databases should Andrew search?*

- *Find a minimum of six research publications that might be helpful for Andrew's project.*

- *What websites should Andrew search?*

- *Find a minimum of six websites that might be helpful for Andrew's project.*

- *Provide rationale why you chose the websites.*

- *Where else should Andrew search to find evidence?*

WRITING REMINDERS...

Titles, Headings, and Subheadings

- Purposes

  - Inform the reader about the content that follows.

  - Keep content organized.

  - Provide a *road map* for quick scanning.

A *title's* function is to assist evidence searchers in identifying publications that meet the evidence-based practice needs of the DNP project. A title therefore should be written with care. Use clear, concise wording. The title should reflect the variables and population of a study, not the findings.

Headings and subheadings show the reader how the publication is organized. Organization begins with equally important parts of the paper identified with a header. Parts subordinate to each header are termed subheadings. Subheadings are useful for readers, but they also contribute to your writing by keeping you focused. A good outline contributes to identification of headings and subheadings.

Chronological order of the five subheadings for APA formatting can be reviewed on the Purdue Owl website (https://owl.english.purdue.edu/owl/resource/560/16/).

Adapted from Pyrczak, & Bruce, 2011; Reimer, 2010; The Writing Center, University of Wisconsin-Madison, 2014; Write, 2015.

REFERENCES

Allied and Complementary Medicine Database (AMED). (2016). *A definitive guide to complementary medicine and alternative treatments.* Retrieved from https://www.ebscohost.com/academic/amed-the-allied-and-complementary-medicine-database

American Psychological Association (APA). (2001). *Publication manual of the American Psychological Association* (6th ed.). Washington, DC: APA.

American Psychological Association (APA). (2014). *PsychINFO.* Retrieved from http://www.apa.org/pubs/databases/psycinfo/index.aspx

Barker, J. (n.d.). *Basic search tips and advanced Boolean explained.* Retrieved from http://www.lib.berkeley.edu/TeachingLib/Guides/Internet/Boolean.pdf

BIOSIS Previews. (2014). Retrieved from http://thomsonreuters.com/biosis-previews/

Campbell Collaboration. (2016). *Campbell systematic reviews.* Retrieved from http://www.campbellcollaboration.org

CINAHL (Cumulative Index to Nursing and Allied Health Literature). (2014). Retrieved from http://www.ebscohost.com/biomedical-libraries/the-cinahl-database

Cochrane Library. (2016). Retrieved from http://www.thecochranelibrary.com/view/0/AboutTheCochraneLibrary.html

Cooke, A., Smith, D., & Boorth, A.. (2012). Beyond PICO: The SPIDER tool for qualitative evidence synthesis. *Qualitative Health Research, 22*(10), 1435–1443.

Driscoll, D.L., & Brizee, A. (2010). What is primary research and how do I get started? *Owl, Purdue Online Writing Lab.* Retrieved from https://owl.english.purdue.edu/owl/resource/559/01/

Embase. (2014). *A biomedical database that speaks your language.* Retrieved from http://www.elsevier.com/online-tools/embase

ERIC (Institute of EDUCATION SCIENCE). (2014). Retrieved from http://eric.ed.gov

Grove, S.K., Burns, N., & Gray, J.R. (2013). *The practice of nursing research: Appraisal, synthesis, and generation of evidence* (7th ed.). St. Louis, MO: Elsevier Saunders.

Joanna Briggs Institute (JBI). (2014a). *Joanna Briggs reviewers' manual.* University of Adelaide. Retrieved from http://joannabriggs.org/assets/docs/sumari/Reviewers-Manual-2014.pdf

Joanna Briggs Institute (JBI) Levels of Evidence and Grades of Recommendation Party. (2014b). Summary of findings tables for Joanna Briggs Institute systematic reviews. Retrieved from joannabriggs.org/assets/docs/sumari/ReviewersManual-2014-Summary-of-Findings-Tables.pdf

Library of Congress Online Catalog. (2016). *Search/browse help—Boolean operators and nesters.* Retrieved from https://catalog.loc.gov/vwebv/ui/en_US/htdocs/help/searchBoolean.html

LoBiondo-Wood, G., & Haber, J. (2010). *Nursing research: Methods and critical appraisal for evidence-based practice* (7th ed.). St. Louis, MO: Mosby Elsevier.

MEDLINE. (2014). *Medline complete.* Retrieved from http://www.ebscohost.com/nursing/products/medline-databases

Melnyk, B, & Fineout-Overholt, E. (2011). *Evidence-based practice in nursing and healthcare: A guide to best practice* (2nd ed.). Philadelphia, PA: Wolters Kluwer Health/Lippincott Williams & Wilkins.

Moher, D., Liberati, A. Tetziaff, J., & Altman, D.G. (2009). Preferred reporting items for systematic reviews and meta-analyses: The PRISMA statement. *PLoS Med 6*(7), e1000097. Retrieved from http://journals.plos.org/plosmedicine/article?id=10.1371/journal.pmed.1000097

National Center for Biotechnology Information (NCBI). (2014). *PubMed.* Retrieved from http://www.ncbi.nlm.nih.gov/pubmed

National Institutes of Health (NIH). (2013). PubMed Tutorial. Retrieved from http://www.nlm.nih.gov/bsd/disted/pubmedtutorial/020_390.html

Ovid. (2014). *Recommended databases in medicine.* Retrieved from http://www.ovid.com

Oxford Dictionary. (2014). Retrieved from http://www.oxforddictionaries.com

Polit, D.F., & Beck, C.T. (2012). *Nursing research: Generating and assessing evidence for nursing practice* (9th ed.). Philadelphia, PA: Wolters Kluwer/Lippincott Williams & Wilkins.

ProQuest. (2014). *About ProQuest.* Retrieved from http://www.proquest.com

Pyrczak, F., & Bruce, R.R. (2011). *Writing empirical research reports* (7th ed.). Glendale, CA: Pryczak Publishing.

Reimer, H. (2010). *Why you should use subheadings.* Retrieved from http://ezinearticles.com/?Why-You-Should-Use-Subheadings&id=4078003

Tensen, B.L. (2010), *Research strategies for the digital age* (3rd ed.). *Boston, MA: Wadsworth.*

Timmins, F., & McCabe, C. (2005). How to conduct an effective literature search. *Nursing Standard, 20*(11), 41–47.

Woolery, M., Bisanz, A., Lyons, H.F., Gaido, L., Yenulevich, M., Fulton, S., & McMillen, S.C. (2008). Putting evidence into practice: Evidence-based interventions for the prevention of management of constipation in patients with cancer. *Clinical Journal of Oncology Nuring, 12*(2), 317–337.

Write. (2015). *How to use headings and subheadings effectively in online content.* Retrieved from http://www.write.com/writing-guides/writing-for-the-web/how-to-use-headings-and-subheadings-effectively-in-online-content

The Writing Center, University of Wisconsin-Madison. (2014). *The writer's handbook: APA documentation guide.* Retrieved from http://writing.wisc.edu/Handbook/DocAPA.html

IF YOU WANT TO READ MORE...

Joanna Briggs Institute. (2014). *Joanna Briggs reviewers' manual.* University of Adelaide. Retrieved from http://joannabriggs.org/assets/docs/sumari/ReviewersManual-2014.pdf

McMaster University. (2014). *Health evidence practice tools.* Retrieved from http://healthevidence.org/practice-tools.aspx#PT3

Moher, D., Liberati, A. Tetziaff, J., & Altman, D.G., The PRISMA group. (2009). *PLoS Med, 6*(7), e1000097.. Retrieved from http://www.plosmedicine.org/article/info%3Adoi%2F10.1371%2Fjournal.pmed.1000097

National Institutes of Health (NIH). (2013). PubMed Tutorial. Retrieved from http://www.nlm.nih.gov/bsd/disted/pubmedtutorial/020_390.html

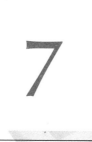

7

Critical Appraisal of Evidence

Make your judgment trustworthy by trusting it.

GRENVILLE KLEISER

OUTCOME OBJECTIVES

- Discuss the purpose of critically appraising evidence for use in the practice setting.
- Identify standards of rigor for best available evidence.
- Differentiate similarities and differences in critically appraising varied sources of evidence.
- Analyze the correlation between establishing trust in published evidence and trust in your recommendations for practice.

TERMS

Analysis	Quality	Systematic review
Critical appraisal	Random bias	Systemic bias
Intentional bias	Relevance	Unintentional bias
Meta-analysis	Rigor	
Metasynthesis	Synthesis	

Confidence and trust in evidence grow with effective skills to evaluate retrievals from your searches. Knowing what to look for as well as understanding the strengths and weaknesses of the evidence increases trust in the findings. Combining trusted findings from research publications with quality improvement (QI) reports, policies, nursing guidelines, and other available documents yield evidence that can be contextually applied for best patient outcomes. This chapter provides critical appraisal tools to assist verification and establishment of trust in evidence findings, thereby increasing the strength of your written synthesis and recommendations for practice.

Critical appraisal tools are also referred to as a critique, evaluation, analysis, or assessment. The purpose, however, remains the same: rigorous, detailed evaluation of evidence. The term *critique* is commonly used and implies an objective analysis of the components of the publication, document, or other evidence. A critique does not mean criticism. A critique requires your full attention to *hear* what the author is saying. Objectivity means to put aside your personal biases; do not attack the author, and refrain from using subjective "I" messages. Your critical appraisal is not about what you would change; the critical appraisal focuses on the strengths and weaknesses of the publication's methodology.

This chapter presents tools and information for critically appraising different types of evidence. The appraisal tools are not intended to be inclusive; rather, the intent is to provide resources and references to enhance choices to best meet your individual needs. Numerous critical appraisal tools are available online and in print, and you are encouraged to access them as needed.

CRITICAL APPRAISAL TOOLS

The process of a critical appraisal is to evaluate published evidence carefully and systematically to establish *quality* and *relevance* (Burls, 2009). *Quality* of research publications relates to methodology and the extent to which a research study has excluded *intentional* and *unintentional bias* (Joanna Briggs Institute [JBI], 2014; Lohr & Carey, 1999). In research studies, bias, whether intentional or unintentional, implies errors in methodology that may affect a study's results. Random, unintentional bias, for example, may include a study participant who consciously or unconsciously strives to present himself or herself in the best light. Systematic bias, on the other hand, consistently distorts and alters findings. For example, a scale in need of calibration consistently provides flawed data. Appraising quality is important for all pieces of evidence, not just research publications. *Relevance* of evidence infers that the evidence is pertinent to answer your evidence-based practice (EBP) question and is applicable to the desired practice setting (Grove, Burns, & Gray, 2013). The outcome goal of a critical appraisal is to establish confidence in the evidence and trustworthiness of the findings for the purpose of making effective recommendations for practice.

Critical appraisals are divided into two sections: *analysis* and *synthesis*. Analysis means to "pull apart" each section of a publication structure for individual appraisal. Synthesis means to combine the parts and to make decisions about the quality and relevance of the publication. Analysis and synthesis are performed for each piece of evidence. The next section provides tools for analyzing and synthesizing different categories of evidence.

RESEARCH PUBLICATIONS

Review of the research process and research designs is encouraged as preparation for critically appraising a research publication. The following textbooks are recommended as references to meet your review needs.

- Grove, S.K., Burns, N., & Gray, J.R. (2013). The Practice of Nursing Research: Appraisal, Synthesis, and Generation of Evidence (7th ed.). St. Louis, MO: Elsevier Saunders.

- LoBiondo-Wood, G., & Haber, J. (2013). Nursing Research: Methods and Critical Appraisal for Evidence-based Practice (8th ed.). St. Louis, MO: Mosby Elsevier.

- Polit, D.F., & Beck, C.T. (2016). Nursing Rresearch: Generating and Assessing Evidence for Nursing Practice (10th ed.). Philadelphia, PA: Wolters Kluwer/ Lippincott Williams & Wilkins.

The critique tool (Box 7.1) is a guide to assist in critically analyzing research publications (Grove et al., 2013; LoBiondo-Wood & Haber, 2010; Polit & Beck, 2012; Pyrczak, 2008).

A *mixed methods research publication* is complex because it integrates both quantitative and qualitative research questions and methodology. Mixed methods research is not demographic data for a qualitative study and is not an open-ended question at the end of a quantitative survey asking whether the respondent would like to write additional information. A mixed methods study integrates qualitative and quantitative data collection and analysis and integrates analytical and interpretive discussion of results. A mixed methods critical appraisal follows the same critique format as a single research study. For a mixed methods critique, however, use both the quantitative and qualitative

Text continued on page 120

BOX 7.1 Critical Appraisal Tool for Research Publications

Complete APA Reference of Publication:

Part I: Analysis

1. Introduction and literature review

• Describe the problem as presented by the authors.

• Is the problem identified in the publication similar to your EBP problem or issue?

• Is current literature cited? If not, is there a reason why older literature is cited?

• What is the framework of the study?

  Conceptual framework

  Theoretical framework

  Physiological framework

  Other (describe)

• Do the authors operationalize the variables from the purpose statement?

• Quote the purpose statement.

2. Methodology

• *Design*

  • Is this study a quantitative or qualitative study?

  • What design is used in this study?

  • *Quantitative*

    Experimental _____

    RCT _____

    Quasiexperimental _____

    Nonxperimental/descriptive _____

    Other (quote the authors' terminology that describes the design)

BOX 7.1 Critical Appraisal Tool for Research Publications—cont'd

- *Qualitative*

  Case study _____

  Community-based participatory research _____

  Ethnography _____

  Grounded theory _____

  Historical _____

  Phenomenological _____

  Qualitative/descriptive _____

  Other (quote the author's terminology that describes the design)

  - Is the design appropriate for the purpose statement or question?
- *Sample and context*
  - How were participants recruited?

    Probability sampling

    Random

    Nonprobability sampling

    Convieniencce

    Purposive

    Quota

    Snowball

    Other (quote the authors' terminology that describes the sample)

  - If study is a large RCT, did the authors complete a power analysis to estimate sample size?
  - Have the authors adequately described the sample participants' demographics? Briefly describe.
  - Is the sample similar to that in your EBP question or statement?

Continued

BOX 7.1 Critical Appraisal Tool for Research Publications—cont'd

- Is the context similar to that in your EBP question? Briefly describe.

- Do the authors state that approval was received from an IRB or ethical board?

- *Quantitative measurement tool*

  - Are the measurement tools adequately described, or is there an example of the actual measurement tool?

  - Do the authors state that the measurement tool has internal consistency to measure the instrument's reliability (e.g., Cronbach's alpha, split-half reliability)?

- *Qualitative measurement tool*

  - Is there a sample of the actual data collection tool?

- *Quantitative data collection*

  - Is more than one method used to collect data on each variable?

  - If more than one researcher or research assistant collected data, is there evidence of interrater reliability?

  - Do authors describe how control and experimental groups were formed if the study is experimental or quasiexperimental?

  - Briefly describe how data were collected.

- *Qualitative data collection*

  - Were data collected through multiple methods to achieve triangulation?

  - If more than one researcher or research assistant collected data, is there evidence of interrater reliability?

  - Was data saturation achieved?

3. Data analysis

- *Quantitative*

  - Are descriptive statistics presented before inferential statistics results?

BOX 7.1 Critical Appraisal Tool for Research Publications—cont'd

- List the statistical tests used to analyze the data.

- Did the authors select appropriate statistical tests to answer the research question or hypothesis? Briefly explain.

- Did the authors note statistical significance? List the statistically significant results.

- *Qualitative*

  - Were themes adequately supported with quotations and/or descriptions of observations?

  - Is theme analysis presented in a logical manner? Explain.

  - List the themes derived from the qualitative data.

4. Discussion of results

  - Are results discussed in relation to current literature, including references first presented in the introduction and literature review section?

  - Were results discussed in relation to the study's framework?

  - Do the authors acknowledge the study's limitations? Briefly describe.

  - Do the authors make specific recommendations for using the findings of the study? Briefly describe.

  - Do the authors make suggestions for future research? Briefly describe.

Part II: Synthesis (Combining the Parts and Making Decisions)

- Based on your critique of the article, is there evidence of bias?

- Based on your critique of the article, can you trust the results of the study?

- What information from this article will help in decision making?

- What additional information do you need to make a decision?

APA, American Psychological Association; EBP, evidence-based practice; IRB, Institutional Review Board; RCT, randomized controlled study.

sections of Box 7.1 (Critical Appraisal Tool for Research). Additional questions to consider in appraising a mixed methods research publication include the following (Polit & Beck, 2012):

- Is the design logically based on the research question or hypothesis?

- Are integration of qualitative and quantitative methodologies demonstrated throughout?

- Do integrated data collection and analyses demonstrate both analytic and interpretive findings?

- Are the authors' inferences and interpretation of results logical?

- Do the authors discuss the study's limitations?

- Based on your critique of the publication, is there evidence of bias?

- Based on your appraisal of the mixed methods publication, do you trust the findings?

Meta-Analysis, Metasynthesis, and Systematic Review Publications

A *meta-analysis* is conducted by systematically searching the literature for single quantitative studies (usually experimental and quasiexperimental) and then statistically combining and analyzing the findings. A meta-analysis process is commonly used for comparative effectiveness reports. The evidence produced from a meta-analysis is considered one of the strongest levels of evidence regarding an intervention's effectiveness. Critical appraisal for a meta-analysis is similar to a research critique wherein the focus is reduction of bias. Bias in a meta-analysis appraisal focuses on effect. The following questions along with the research critical appraisal tool (see Box 7.1) can assist the focus of your critique (Grove et al., 2013; Higgins & Green, 2011, section 1.2.2; Lohr, 2009):

- Is there evidence of a thorough (i.e., complete and adequate) search of the literature?

- Are the studies clinically similar? (Stated another way, studies that are clinically diverse may be meaningless.)

- What is the direction of effect?

- What is the effect size?

- What is the consistency of the effect among identified studies?

- What is the strength of evidence for the effect?

Metasynthesis is a systematic process that integrates findings from similar qualitative studies for an aggregate synthesis of interpretation. This differs from a meta-analysis process that aggregates statistical findings. Researchers disagree about a methodology to integrate qualitative findings from multiple studies. In contrast, qualitative researchers recognize the importance of summarizing qualitative findings to increase the knowledge base, to describe, and to bring fresh insight into nuances and taken-for-granted assumptions. Similar to a meta-analysis, bias within a metasynthesis study can be decreased with a thorough, systematic search for qualitative research publications of a similar clinical problem. Use the qualitative methodology sections from Box 7.1 to assist your analysis. Additionally, consider the following questions in analyzing a metasynthesis (Grove et al., 2013; Walsh & Downe, 2005):

- Does the author describe the strength of the evidence search?

- Are the studies related or clinically similar?

- Does the author describe the quality of the evidence?

- What is the total number of publications?

- Does the author's aim or purpose meet your inclusion criteria?

- Does the author synthesize the findings?

A *systematic review* is the primary knowledge product of the Cochrane Collaboration, the Joanna Briggs Institute, the Campbell Library, and other international institutions for systematic reviews. According to a description from the Cochrane Library (2011), a systematic review is an analysis of published primary studies, whereas a meta-analysis is a statistical combination of results from two or more separate published studies. The main commonality between the systematic review and the meta-analysis is the extensive literature search for best research evidence. Box 7.2 provides questions to assess the strength of a systematic review. Systematic reviews often combine with a meta-analysis methodology by providing a "quantitative estimate of effect (or no difference in effect)" using a confidence interval (CI) (Berkman et al., 2013; Grove et al., 2013; Melnyk & Fineout-Overholt, 2011; Pryczak, 2008).

The PRISMA (Preferred Reporting Items for Systematic Reviews and Meta-Analysis) also provides a checklist to assist authors in reporting meta-analyses and systematic reviews. The stated purpose of PRISMA is transparent reporting of systematic reviews and meta-analyses. PRISMA's checklist can be accessed at http://www.prisma-statement.org. PRISMA may be helpful in assisting your critical appraisal (Moher, 2009).

BOX 7.2 Critical Appraisal Tool for a Systematic Review

Complete APA Reference for Publication:

Part I: Analysis

1. Search question or questions

   • Is the clinical question clearly written?

   • Is the clinical question similar to your clinical question or objective?

   • Quote the clinical question.

2. Search strategy

   • Were search criteria clearly identified?

   • Were inclusion and exclusion criteria clearly stated?

   • What databases were searched? How many records identified?

   • What other sources were searched? How many records were identified?

   • How many records were included? How many records were excluded?

   • How many articles were assessed for eligibility in the systematic review? Was rationale provided?

   • How many articles were excluded for eligibility in the systematic review? Was rationale provided?

3. Synthesis

   • Are evidence findings discussed in relation to the clinical question or objective?

   • Are evidence findings organized by topic and clearly written?

   • Do the authors suggest clinical practice guidelines or recommendations for practice?

   • Were the authors' recommendations for practice supported by the evidence?

BOX 7.2 Critical Appraisal Tool for a Systematic Review—cont'd

Part II: Pulling It All Together

- Based on your critique of the article, is there evidence of bias?

- Based on your critique of the review, can you trust the findings?

- What information from this review will help in your decision making?

- What additional information do you need to make a practice decision?

APA, American Psychological Association.

The Rule of Law

Assessing the contents of a law may be beneficial to increased understanding of your EBP issue and context. In addition, consider retrieving research publications regarding specific lived experiences under a law. This may be helpful if the publication's methodology is rigorous. Retrieving opinion articles or expert opinion on a law is not a valuable investment of your time. The following is a short list of characteristics that should be included in all laws (Quality of Laws, 2008):

- *Spirit of the law* contains the law's purpose and intent.

- *Sanctions* infer strengths by which the law is able to achieve the intended goals.

- *Costs* relate to construction, enforcement, and improvement in the law, if needed.

- *Side effects* such as unintended costs or results are identified over time.

- *Performance* is measured by the sum of the law's benefits minus the sum of burdens.

- *Fallibility* corrects unintended design flaws and outcomes through amendments.

Questions to consider when appraising a law specific to your practice context and issues include the following (Quality of Laws, 2008):

- Is the law clearly written and easy to understand?

- Is the purpose and intent of the law clearly stated? Briefly describe.

- Are the strengths of the law clearly inferred? Briefly describe.

- Are side effects identified? Briefly describe.

- Is the performance measure discussed? Briefly describe.

- Have amendments been added? If so, briefly describe.

- Did you access other sources (e.g., research publications about the law)? Briefly describe.

- In your opinion, is this law helpful for interpreting the context of your EBP question? Briefly describe.

Clinical Practice Guidelines

Published clinical practice guidelines are practice recommendations based on systematic reviews. The purpose of guidelines is to assist clinicians in patient care. Guidelines are suggestions, not rules, because of the variations in context that must be taken into account. Critical appraisal of clinical guidelines is important to recognize credibility and therefore trust in the guideline before implementing and evaluating practice change. AGREE II (Appraisal Guidelines for Research and Evaluation) is an "international tool to assess the quality and reporting of practice guidelines" (Brouwers et al., 2010). You are encouraged to adapt the topics and questions from AGREE II to appraise clinical practice guidelines. The tool is free of charge and can be retrieved from http://www.agreetrust.org/wp-content/uploads/2013/10/AGREE-II-Users-Manual-and-23-item-Instrument_2009_UPDATE_2013.pdf. The organization's home page can be accessed at http://www.agreetrust.org/agree-ii/. Specific critique questions for each topic can be retrieved from the online tool. Critique topics identified in AGREE II include the following:

- Scope and purpose

- Stakeholder involvement

- Rigor of development

- Clarity

- Applicability

- Editorial independence

On completion of the critique, remember to ask yourself the following questions:

- Based on your critique of the clinical guideline report, is there evidence of bias?

- Based on your critique of the clinical guideline report, can you trust the recommendations?

- What information from the clinical guideline report will help in decision making?

- What additional information do you need to make a decision?

Quality Improvement Reports

QI programs systematically collect data, both quantitative and qualitative, on a regular basis for the purpose of making decisions about quality of care provided to patients and improving provider performance, interventions, or efficiency (Health Resources and Services Administration [HRSA], n.d.; Six Sigma, 2014). The American Psychological Association (APA, 2009) identified indicators for measuring QI in programs.

- Quality is measured with empirical evidence and is "psychometrically sound, relevant, actionable, auditable, and feasible" (APA, 2009, p 554).

  - Measures to address quality are reliable, thus implying psychometric properties.

  - Quality indicators are sensitive to change.

  - Quality indicators are relevant or meaningful.

  - Quality indicators are not susceptible to manipulation and are auditable.

  - Sources of data and benchmarks are methods for data collection and reporting.

  - Standards of patient confidentiality (Health Insurance Portability and Accountability Act [HIPAA]) are upheld, and Institutional Review Board (IRB) approval is received.

- Risk is appropriately adjusted. Stated another way, "risk adjustment is the process of adjusting the outcome probabilities for unlike groups so that comparisons can be made" (APA, 2009, p 555). Risk adjustment focuses on (1) service and cost and (2) comparing intervention outcomes.

- Quality measurements focus on providers and patients. Provider measurements relate to interventions and delivery. Patient measurements relate to health, well-being, and function.

- Involvement of stakeholders is indicated for the selection of relevant indicators.

SQUIRE Guidelines (Standards for Quality Improvement Reporting Excellence) is a recommended tool for writing QI reports to increase dissemination and use of findings.. A critical appraisal for QI reports (Box 7.3) was adapted from the SQUIRE guidelines for writing the report (Davidoff, Batalden, Stevens, Ogrinc, & Mooney, 2008; Orgrinc, 2014).

BOX 7.3 Critical Appraisal Tool for Quality Improvement Written Reports

Title of Quality Improvement Report:

Introduction and Literature Review

- Is the intended improvement or intervention clearly described?
- Is the outcome objective or clinical question clearly written?
- Are the study questions precisely stated?

Methods

- Are ethical standards followed (e.g., IRB approval)?
- Are participants and context clearly described?
- Is the proposed intervention appropriate to address the outcome objective or clinical question?
- Are measurement tools and data collection methods appropriate to answer the clinical question?
- Are assessment criteria effective for ensuring data quality and adequacy?
- Are evaluation methods appropriate for collected data? Briefly describe.
- Is there evidence of internal and external validity?

Results

- Are relevant themes or statistically significant results identified?
- Are themes presented about learned characteristics of the setting, structure, patterns of care, or actual intervention? Briefly describe.

BOX 7.3 Critical Appraisal Tool for Quality Improvement Written
Reports—cont'd

• Are statistical data presented about changes in care process and clinical outcomes? Briefly describe.

Discussion

• Are key successes and differences summarized?

• Are the results presented in relation to other evidence?

• Do the authors make recommendations for use of findings?

• Do the authors make recommendations for practice?

Pulling It All Together...

• What information will help in your decision making?

• What additional information do you need to make a decision?

IRB, Institutional Review Board.

Policies

Policies are important pieces of evidence to increase understanding of organizational, political, and social principles that underlie action and give structure to institutions and employee roles (Bardach, 2009; Carver, n.d.). Critical appraisal of a policy (Box 7.4) is generally a review that the policy is clearly written and contributes understanding through the eyes of a practitioner (Bardach, 2009; Melnyk & Fineout-Overholt, 2011).

Patient Preferences or Values and Expert Advice or Consultation

EBP definitions describe patient preferences and expert advice or consultation as significant elements in making decisions about patient-centered care,. yet patient preferences and expert advice are forms of subjective information. How do these elements become more rigorous and trustworthy for use in an EBP

BOX 7.4 Critical Appraisal Tool for Policies

Title of Policy:

Policy #:

- Are important terms clearly conceptualized?

- Is the policy problem clearly described?

- Is the policy problem similar to your EBP issue or problem?

- Are research and best practice publications referenced?

- Is a criterion for efficiency (e.g., cost, benefit, labor) clearly described?

- Are criteria for equity, fairness, and justice clearly described?

- Based on your assessment of the policy, does it increase your understanding of your EBP problem or issue?

- What information will help in decision making?

- What additional information do you need?

EBP, evidence-based practice.

project? The answer lies in where the information is recorded and subsequently retrieved. Patient preferences and expert advice are similar to qualitative data and should be treated as such. Qualitative information becomes usable data when the conversations are documented with as much detail as possible. *Patient preferences* are gleaned through patient-provider or patient-nurse communication and should be narratively charted, thereby contributing usable data for making decisions (Box 7.5). Clarity, timeliness, and detail are important. *Reviews of electronic health records* by DNP scholars can then look for trends in patient preferences and values.

Expert advice or consultation may be an opinion publication or a personal conversation. The information is especially useful for understanding context, culture, and tradition. If possible, the conversations should be recorded and transcribed. If you are unable to record the conversation, details of the communication should be written as soon as possible following the event and kept with your project or field notes (Box 7.6). Use of this qualitative data collection method increases credibility. Written field notes contribute to an audit trail of your project's data collection process. An *opinion article*, such as an editorial,

---

BOX 7.5 Critical Appraisal Tool for Patient Preferences and Expert Advice or Opinion

Topic of Search:

Dates of Electronic Health Record Search:

Patient Preferences:

- Provide a description of the patient; include the date and time of chart entry.

- Was the topic clearly described?

- Were the patient's responses quoted and/or clearly described?

- Were themes (i.e., patient's preferences) clearly summarized?

- Were interventions implemented? Briefly describe.

- Do you trust the contents of the chart?

- Is the information from the chart review helpful in making decisions?

- What additional information do you need?

BOX 7.6 Expert Advice or Consultation

Source of Expert Advice or Consultation:

Date of Event:

- Provide a description of the expert's role, and note the date, time, and context of the communication.

- What was the topic of conversation?

- Was the conversation recorded? If not, when were the field notes written?

- What themes emerged from the conversation?

- Is the information helpful in making decisions?

- What additional information do you need?

gains credibility by examining the author's short biography, if one accompanies the publication, or by reviewing the credibility of the journal or newspaper.

Gray Literature

Examples of gray literature include government publications, white papers, internal documentation, working papers, patents, unpublished dissertations or theses, and conference presentations and proceedings. Gray literature is increasingly useful as evidence because of the speed and ease of access as a result of Internet technology (Huffine, 2010). Strength of gray literature as a primary source can be increased by asking questions about credibility of the information source (e.g., website, sponsor of source, identification and contact of author). Box 7.7 provides a guide to appraising gray literature (Kilborn, 2011; PHCRIS, 2016).

STRENGTH OF EVIDENCE

Consistency of reporting quality and relevance with individual critiques leads to trust of individual pieces of evidence and contributes to overall strength (Berkman et al., 2013). Critiquing the quality and relevance of individual pieces of evidence, however, differs from establishing the overall strength of evidence from all relevant sources. Consistency in establishing strength of evidence occurs before writing the synthesis report and subsequent recommendations for practice. Describing strength of evidence provides stakeholders and decision makers with a sense of how much confidence can be placed in your practice recommendations.

There are variations in rating or grading systems and hierarchies of evidence, but there is no standard formula for how much weight to give individual factors when making clinical decisions (NURSE.com, 2014; Woolf et al., 2012). In other words, no single approach to grading the strength of evidence is accepted by all users. Following are examples of tools that are used to establish strength of evidence. Use them according to your needs to convey clarity of the strength of your overall evidence.

Pyramid-shaped levels of hierarchy are easy to use, and there are several from which to choose. Adaptations of the hierarchal order on the pyramid continue to occur secondary to increasing use and lived experiences of the EBP process. The evidence-based medicine pyramid model suggests the following seven categories of evidence, beginning with the pinnacle as strongest and the base as least strong (Glover, Izzo, Odato, & Wang, 2006). Recall that strength is grounded in methodology and limited bias.

BOX 7.7 Critical Appraisal Tool for Gray Literature

Reference:

- Is the identified author credible (e.g., credentials, professional authority in his or her field)?

- Is the author's contact information provided?

- Is the sponsor of the website, conference, patent, and so forth reputable? Briefly describe.

- Is the sponsoring organization's contact information on the website or conference brochure?

- What is the copyright date of the website information?

- Is the website currently maintained? (Maintenance can be considered current if embedded links are still active.)

- Does the author clearly present a problem?

- Is the context similar to the context of your EBP issue or problem?

- Is the website information clearly written and understandable?

- Are any biases observed in the writing?

- Does the writing have a reference list?

- How many sites or sources contribute similar or same information?

- Based on your assessment, does the website, conference, patent, and so forth contribute credible information for your EBP issue or problem? Do you trust the information?

- What information will help in decision making?

- What additional information do you need?

EBP, evidence-based practice.
Data from Kilborn, 2011; Oncology Nursing Society, n.d.

- Systematic reviews

- Critically appraised topics (evidence synthesis)

- Critically appraised individual articles (article synopses)

- Randomized controlled trials (RCTs)

- Cohort studies

- Case-controlled studies, case series, reports

- Background information, expert opinion (Glover et al., 2006)

Another nursing source for strength of evidence ranks evidence in just three levels plus a multilevel (ML) rank (http://ce.nurse.com/ebp.aspx; NURSE.com, 2014):

- Level A evidence is obtained from an RCT, a systematic review, a meta-analysis, and a clinical practice guideline.

- Level B evidence is obtained from a well-designed control trial without randomization, a clinical cohort study, a case-controlled study, an uncontrolled study, an epidemiological study, and a qualitative or quantitative descriptive study.

- Level C evidence comes from consensus viewpoint and expert opinion and from meta-synthesis.

- Level ML (multilevel) combines clinical practice guidelines and recommendations based on evidence obtained from more than one level of evidence.

A third example of a grading chart that has a solid following in other health disciplines is the Dietary Guideline Advisory Committee (DGAC) Conclusion Grading Chart. Criteria from the chart are useful for systematic reviews and include the following (Greer et al., 2000; U.S. Department of Agriculture [USDA], 2014):

- Quality: scientific rigor and validity, study design, and methodology

- Quantity: number of studies, number of participants

- Consistency: consistency of findings across studies

- Magnitude of effect or impact: importance of studied outcomes, magnitude of effect

- Generalizability: generalizability to population of interest

Each category is leveled as follows: (1) strong, (2) moderate, (3) limited, (4) expert opinion only, or (5) grade not assignable. The DAGC Conclusion Grading Criteria Chart can be retrieved from http://www.nel.gov/topic.cfm?cat=3210

ORGANIZING

Chapter 6 introduced the importance of an *evidence table* in organizing findings from your evidence search (Cooke et al., 2012; Grove et al., 2013; JBI, 2014; Timmins & McCabe, 2005). As you critique each piece of evidence, continue to make entries into your evidence table. Table 7.1 is an example of an evidence table.

CHAPTER SUMMARY AND AFTERTHOUGHTS

Demonstrating the ability to critically appraise various publications and other forms of evidence for the purpose of establishing trust in the findings contributes to your strength and skills as a scholar. Remember to keep ongoing records of each critically appraised piece of evidence. Your *evidence table* is increasingly valuable when establishing strength of the evidence and writing the synthesis of your evidence findings. Your evidence table may be required as an appendix that demonstrates proof of the quality and strength of your evidence.

WRITING REMINDERS...

Analysis and Synthesis

- *Analysis* comes from the Greek word *analyein,* which means "to break up." Analysis applies principles of deductive thinking. Concepts, ideas, problems, or issues are broken into smaller pieces for the purpose of increasing understanding of the whole.

- *Synthesis* comes from the Greek word *syntithenai,* which means "to put together." Synthesis implies integrating and building relationships among the parts to create something new (Oxford Dictionaries, 2013).

Analysis and synthesis are common tools for nurses. Nursing education teaches students to use deductive analysis in head-to-toe assessments and patient histories for the purpose of analyzing the health of the body's systems and then synthesizing the findings for the purpose of focusing on holistic care of the patient. Analyzing research publications, evidence-based practice publications, and other evidence specific to a particular topic is another example of understanding the parts of a problem. Synthesizing all the pieces of best evidence leads to integration of evidence, identifying new relationships, and ultimately finding answers and making suggestions for change (LoBiondo-Wood & Haber, 2010).

TABLE 7.1 Example of an Evidence Table

EBP Question or Statement:

In newly arrived, pregnant refugee women currently living in a western U.S. state (P), how do group prenatal care and education (I) compared with individual prenatal care (C) affect the patient's experience (O) of the birthing process (T)?

Author, Title, Journal, Date: (APA Style)	Database, Website, or Other; Search Terms; Search Dates	Type of Evidence	Population Focus; Setting	Research Design; Data Source; Analysis	PICO-T Variables Identified in Evidence (Fittingness)	Level (Strength) of Evidence	Do You Trust the Quality of Findings Based on Your Critique?
Janevic, T., Savitz, D.A., & Janevic, M., (2011). Maternal education and adverse birth outcomes among immigrant women to the United States from Eastern Europe: a test of the health migrant hypothesis. *Social Science & Medicine, 73*(3).	MEDLINE; group prenatal care; refugees; 2010–2015	Research	Population focus: Pregnant immigrant women from Russia, Ukraine, Poland, former Yugoslavia Republic living in New York City	Design: Quantitative correlational; data source: 253,363 hospital and birth records between 1998 and 2003	Group prenatal care and education; birth outcomes; immigrants	EBM pyramid: strength = 7/7	Yes

Zollo, L., & Tellez, T. (2013); *Provider perspectives on the continuum of care for immigrant and refugee women; a qualitative assessment.* Retrieved from http://newenglandtb.pbworks.com/w/file/fetch/65976922/Perinatal%20PROVIDER%20Perspectives%204.29.pdf	Web search on 12/2013; group prenatal care; refugees; birthing outcomes	Gray literature; PowerPoint from Refugee Health Conference presentation	Population focus: data source: focus group of 39 immigrant and refugee women; 20 perinatal providers; setting: Manchester and Concord, N.H.	Design: qualitative descriptive; data source: immigrant and refugee focus group; provider intervies	Refugee women of childbearing age currently living in United States; prenatal care and education	Not measureable; no measurement tool for strength of gray literature	Yes

EBM, evidence-based medicine.

REFERENCES

Agency for Healthcare Research and Quality (AHRQ, September 2013). *Methods guide for effectiveness and comparative effectiveness reviews.* AHRQ Pub. No. 10(13)-ECH063-EF. Retrieved from http://www.effectivehealthcare.ahrq.gov/ehc/products/60/318/CER-methods-guide-130916.pdf

American Psychological Association. (2009). Criteria for evaluation of quality improvement programs and the use of quality improvement data. *American Psychologist, 64*(6), 551–557.

Bardach, E. (2009). *A practical guide for policy analysis: The eightfold path to more effective problem solving* (3rd ed.). Washington, DC: SAGE.

Berkman, N.D., Lohr, K.N., Ansari, M., McDonagh, M., Balk, E., Whitlock, E., & Chang, S. (2013). Grading the strength of a body of evidence when assessing health care interventions for the Effective Health Care Program of the Agency for Healthcare Research and Quality: An update. *Methods guide for comparative effectiveness reviews.* Publication No. 13(14)-EHC130. Rockville, MD: Agency for Healthcare Research and Quality.

Brouwers, M., Kho, M.D., Browman, G.P., Cluzeau, F., Feder, G., Fervers, B., Hanna, S., & Makarski, J., on behalf of the AGREE Next Steps Consortium. (2010). AGREE II: Advancing guideline development, reporting, and evaluation in healthcare. *Canadian Medical Association Journal, 10*(1503), E839–842.

Burls, A. (2009). *What is critical appraisal?* (2nd ed.). Haywood Group Ltd. Retrieved from http://www.medicine.ox.ac.uk/bandolier/painres/download/whatis/what_is_critical_appraisal.pdf

Carver, J. (n.d.). *Basic principles of policy governance.* Retrieved from http://www.dccs.org/uploaded/About_DC/Board/Basic_Principles_of_Policy_Governance.pdf

Cochrane Library. (2011). *Cochrane Library.* Retrieved from http://www.cochranelibrary.com

Cooke, L., Smith, D., & Booth, A. (2012). Beyond PICO: The SPIDER tool for qualitative evidence synthesis. *Qualitative Health Research, 22.*

Davidoff, F., Batalden, P., Stevens, D., Ogrinc, C., & Mooney, S. (2008). Publication guidelines for quality improvement in health care: Evolution of the SQUIRE project. *Quality and Safety Health Care, 17*(Supplement 1), 13–19.

Glover, J., Izzo, D., Odato, K., & Wang, L. (2006). *Evidence-based clinical practice resources.* Retrieved from http://guides.nyu.edu/managementpyramid

Greer, N., Mosser, G., Logan, G., & Wagstrom Halaas, G. (2000). A practical approach to evidence grading. *The Joint Commission Journal on Quality Improvement, 26,* 700–712.

Grove, S.K., Burns, N., & Gray, J.R. (2013). *The practice of nursing research: Appraisal, synthesis, and generation of evidence* (7th ed.). St. Louis, MO: Elsevier Saunders

Health Resources and Services Administration (HRSA). (n.d.). *Quality improvement.* Retrieved from http://www.hrsa.gov/quality/toolbox/methodology/quality improvement/

Higgins, J.P.T., & Green, S. (2011). *Cochrane handbook for systematic reviews of interventions, (Version 5.1.0)*. Retrieved from http://handbook.cochrane.org

Huffine, R. (2014). *Value of grey literature to scholarly research in the digital age.* Retrieved from http://www.slideshare.net/richardhuffine/2010-richardhuffine

Joanna Briggs Institute (JBI). (2014). *Joanna Briggs Institute reviewers' manual 2014.* University of Adelaide, Australia: Joanna Briggs Institute. Retrieved from http://joannabriggs.org/assets/docs/sumari/ReviewersManual-Methodology-JBI_Umbrella%20Reviews-2014.pdf

Kilborn, J. (2005). *Assessing the credibility of online sources.* Literacy Education Online: St. Cloud University. Retrieved from http://leo.stcloudstate.edu/research/credibility1.html

Kleiser, G. (n.d.). Quotation in *Brainy quote.* Retrieved from http://www.brainyquote.com/quotes/quotes/g/grantlandr118346.html

LoBiondo-Wood, G., & Haber, J. (2013). *Nursing research: Methods and critical appraisal for evidence-based practice* (8th ed.). St. Louis, MO: Mosby Elsevier

Lohr, K.N., & Carey, T.S. (1999). Assessing 'best evidence': Issues in grading the quality of studies for systematic reviews. *The Joint Commission Journal on Quality Improvement, 25*(9), 470–479.

McMaster University. (2014). *Healh evidence: Practice tools.* Retrieved from http://www.healthevidence.org/practice-tools.aspx

Melnyk, B.M., & Fineout-Overholt, E. (2011). *Evidence-based practice in nursing and healthcare: A guide to best practice* (2nd ed.). Philadelphia, PA: Wolters Kluwer Health/Lippincott Williams & Wilkins.

Moher, D., Liberati, A., Tetzlaff, J., & Altman, D.F. (2009). Preferred reporting items for systematic reviews and meta-analyses: The PRISMA statement. *BMJ, 339,* 2535.

NURSE.com. (2014). *Evidence-based practice: Levels of evidence.* Retrieved from http://ce.nurse.com/ebp.aspx

Ogrinc, G. (June 10, 2014). *Publication guidelines for quality improvement: Standards for quality imrprovement reporting excellence (SQUIRE) guidelines.* Retrieved from http://www.academyhealth.org/files/ARM/adjunct/Ogrinc%20Presentation.pdf

Polit, D.F., & Beck, C.T. (2012). *Nursing research: Generating and assessing evidence for nursing practice* (9th ed.). Philadelphia, PA: Wolters Kluwer/Lippincott Williams & Wilkins.

Primary Health Care Research and Information Service. (PHCRIS, 2016). PHCRIS getting started guides. *Introduction to accessing the grey literature.* Retrieved from http://www.phcris.org.au/guides/grey_literature.php

Pyrczak, F. (2008). *Evaluating research in academic journals* (4th ed.). Glendale, CA: Pyrczak Publishing.

Quality of Laws. (2008). *The characteristics of laws.* Retrieved from http://www.qualityoflaws.com/democracy/laws-of-government/characteristics-of-laws.aspx

Six Sigma. (2014). *The purpose of quality improvement in healthcare.* Retrieved from http://www.sixsigmaonline.org/six-sigma-training-certification-information/the-purpose-of- quality-improvement-in-healthcare/

Timmins, F., & McCabe, C. (2005). How to conduct an effective literature search. *Nursing Standard, 20*(11), 41–47.

United States Department of Agriculture (USDA). (2014). *Conclusion grading chart (DGAC, 2010)*. NutritionEvidenceLibrary.gov. Retrieved from http://www.nel.gov/topic.cfm?cat=3210

Walsh, D., & Downe, S. (2005). Meta-synthesis method for qualitative research: A literature review. *Journal of Advanced Nursing, 50*(2), 204–211.

Woolf, S., Schunemann, H.J., Eccles, M.P., Grimshaw, J.M., & Shekelle, P. (2012). Developing clinical practice guidelines: Types of evidence and outcomes; values and economics, synthesis, grading and presentation and deriving recommendations. *Implementation Science, 7*(61). Retrieved from http://www.implementationscience.com/content/7/1/61

IF YOU WANT TO READ MORE...

Bardach, E. (2009). *A practical guide for policy analysis: The eightfold path to more effective problem solving* (3rd ed.). Washington, DC: SAGE.

Kilborn, J. (2005). *Assessing the credibility of online sources*. Literacy Education Online: St. Cloud University. Retrieved from http://leo.stcloudstate.edu/research/credibility1.html

Lohr, K.N. (2009). *Methods guide for comparative effectiveness reviews*. Retrieved from http://effectivhealthcare.ahrq.gov/ehc/products/60/318/2009_0805_grading.pdf

Lohr, K.N., & Carey, T.S. (1999). Assessing "best evidence": Issues in grading the quality of studies for systematic reviews. *The Joint Commission Journal on Quality Improvement, 25*(9), 470–479.

Walsh, D., & Downe, S. (2005). Meta-synthesis method for qualitative research: A literature review. *Journal of Advanced Nursing, 50*(2), 204–211.

8

Synthesizing the Evidence and Making Recommendations for Practice

We can't solve problems by using the same kind of thinking we used when we created them.

ALBERT EINSTEIN

OUTCOME OBJECTIVES

- Discuss the purpose for the synthesis report.
- Examine methods and tools for writing a synthesis report.
- Summarize the usefulness of clinical practice guidelines/recommendations for practice.
- Consider the significance of dissemination at this stage of your DNP project.

TERMS

Clinical practice
　guidelines
Concept

Context
Dissemination
Integrative review

Recommendations for
　practice
Synthesis

How do we use the plethora of evidence from a good evidence search for the purpose of promoting best patient outcomes, providing cost-effective care, and recommending practice change or improvement within the ever-increasing complexity of the healthcare system? The answer is a logical, organized written synthesis that demonstrates quality and strength of evidence in addressing the evidence-based practice (EBP) question. A well-written synthesis report based on best evidence from numerous sources (i.e., integrative review) is intended to increase a reader's trust in the proposed practice recommendations. Indeed, a legacy of evidence begins with rigorous creation of scientific knowledge that informs practice. This is the hallmark of EBP.

Information related to purpose and creation of a well-organized synthesis report comprises the content of this chapter. A synthesis report is a written argument based on best evidence that answers the PICO(T) (**P**opulation or problem; **C**omparison; **O**utcome; **T**ime for intervention to demonstrate outcome) question. The report concludes with recommendations for practice change or improvement.

WHAT IS SYNTHESIS?

Synthesis, according to the philosopher Hegel, is an interpretive method that combines the elements of evidence into a new form. For example, a thesis (proposition) has antithesis (contradiction) that is reconciled by a third proposition (synthesis) (Dictionary.com, 2014). Synthesis is not a summary. Synthesis implies a combination of ideas that make thoughtful connections or relationships and explain why the relationships are important. Synthesizing means comparing different sources of evidence and highlighting similarities, differences, and connections. When a writer synthesizes successfully, he or she presents new ideas based on interpretations of other evidence or arguments. Writing a synthesis report is about critical reading and critical thinking of existing knowledge to answer your EBP question. The result is a persuasive argument for proposing practice guidelines, program recommendations, analyzing policies, or assessing quality improvement as part of your DNP project (Grove et al., 2013; Jamieson, 1999; Polit & Beck, 2012; Walden University, 2014).

WRITING THE SYNTHESIS REPORT

Interpretation of the evidence based on the context for application is the crux of the synthesis report because you, the author and evidence-based expert, have intimate knowledge for making practice recommendations (Grove et al., 2013; Polit & Beck, 2012). Note that the synthesis report becomes the first part of the report that will eventually include the proposal for implementation and evaluation strategies (see Chapter 13). However, the synthesis report with recommendations for practice is also a stand-alone report for the purpose of communicating to stakeholders and DNP faculty at this strategic time of making practice recommendations.

A synthesis report contains the following sections, each building on the previous section for the purpose of a logical argument to address your PICO(T) question or statement.

Title

A *title* is the reader's first introduction to your synthesis report. A title should clearly and briefly describe the population and major concepts or variables of the EBP question. A well-written title catches the reader's attention and invites the reader to investigate the entire paper (Branson, 2004).

Executive Summary

An *executive summary* is written after the synthesis report is completed, yet it becomes the first section of the synthesis report. The executive summary is an important written document for clear, concise dissemination of information to stakeholders. The executive summary is a business tool that has similarities to an abstract in that it summarizes important elements. The length of the executive summary is approximately two pages, compared with an abstract that consists of approximately 250 words. Content of the report includes the EBP question, the search statement and strategy, strength of evidence, synthesis and recommendations for practice (Grove, Burns, & Gray, 2013; JBI, 2014a; Purdue Owl, 2014).

Introduction or Background

The *background* section of the synthesis report introduces and describes the practice or program issue and defines the population of focus and context (Woolf, Schünemann, Eccles, Grimshaw, & Shekelle, 2012). Background questions and answers from the development of your PICO(T) question provide this information. Background information describes the practice issue and context, population of interest, significance of the problem, and the intended audience (See Chapter 4). The background section concludes with your PICO(T) question or problem statement. In addition to background information contextualizing the practice setting, important terms from your PICO(T) question or statement are identified and conceptualized (JBI, 2014a; Moher, Liberati, Tetzlaff, & Altman, 2009).

Search Strategy

Reporting the search strategy is the next section of the synthesis report. The purpose of narrating the search strategy is to help the reader assess the "comprehensiveness and exhaustiveness" (p 68) of the evidence search, including details about *inclusion* and *exclusion criteria,* search terms, databases searched, and expanders and limiters applied to the database search. Information about the search strategy provides details into the author's decision-making process. Information regarding evidence sources also allows the author to demonstrate validity of the synthesis report, thereby enhancing trust in the findings and recommendations for practice (JBI, 2014a).

Synthesizing Results From the Evidence

Recall that you were encouraged to create an evidence table (see Chapters 6 and 7) as a tool for organization of your search findings. The evidence table now assists in synthesizing evidence by topic and commonalities, then organizing under relevant subheadings in the written report (JBI, 2014a; Moher et al., 2009; Patten, 2012).

Tools that may assist in writing your synthesis report include the following. These tools are helpful at this stage of your DNP project and later when your strategy for implementation is proposed (see Chapter 13) prior to real-time implementation.

- The *PRISMA Checklist* is a set of 27 items that can be adapted for reporting and synthesizing evidence findings for a DNP project (Moher et al., 2009). The checklist can be retrieved from http://prisma-statement.org/documents/PRISMA%202009%20checklist.pdf

- The *Health Evidence* practice tools also assist in finding, using, and documenting evidence, then sharing lessons learned (McMaster, 2014). The practice tools can be retrieved from http://www.healthevidence.org/practice-tools.aspx#PT2

Writing the synthesis of evidence section is more than combining information from two or more sources. Combining evidence must be written in a meaningful way that makes an academic argument to answer the EBP question or statement leading to written recommendations for practice improvement or change (Jamieson, 1999). Development of a conceptual model or schema, based on synthesis of evidence, may be a helpful and efficient visual method for presenting linkages of the identified concepts, thereby enhancing the conveyance of your message (Polit & Beck, 2012).

Recommendations for Practice

The last section of a synthesis report gives meaning to the evidence findings and provides written guidelines or recommendations for practice. The terms *evidence-based practice guidelines* and *clinical practice guidelines* are used in publications (American College of Physicians [ACP], 2014; Davis, Goldman, & Palda, 2007; Titler et al., 2001). Synthesis reports for the DNP project are increasingly using the term *recommendations for practice* because of the contextual emphasis for implementation. The terms are similar to the definition by the World Health Organization (WHO, 2012) in *Handbook for Guideline Development:*

> ... *any document containing recommendations about health interventions, whether these are clinical, public health, or policy recommendations. A recommendation provides information about what policy-makers, health-care providers or patients should do. It implies a choice between different interventions that have an impact on health and that have implications for the use of resources (p 1).*

Guidelines or recommendations are linked to cognitive theory because the intent is to change or validate behavior based on best evidence (Timmermans & Berg, 2003). Recommendations for practice are intended to assist providers, recipients of health care, and stakeholders in making informed decisions. Principles that guide quality development of recommendations can be met by ensuring that (1) the recommendations are comprehensively and objectively based on best available evidence and (2) the developmental process is clear for the reader to understand how, why, and for whom the recommendation was developed (WHO, 2012).

Increasing numbers of publications about *writing clinical guidelines* are available, but there is not a standardized method for wording or methodology. The importance of well-written guidelines, however, cannot be overlooked because wording influences the acceptance of recommendations by stakeholders (Woolf et al., 2012).

The National Guideline Clearinghouse encourages guideline statements be written with an active, not passive, voice. GRADE (Grading of

Recommendations Assessment, Development, and Evaluation), supported by the American Medical Association, provides an explanation regarding strength of written guidelines (Woolf et al., 2012). Strength of recommendations is one of the few suggestions based on best evidence for writing practice guidelines (Akl et al., 2007; Schunemann et al., 2003; Woolf et al., 2012).

Other tools to assist in writing practice recommendations are outlined by the JBI (2014b) and the Institute of Medicine (2011). *FAME* is a tool developed by the JBI Levels of Evidence and Grades of Recommendation Working Party (2014b). FAME (feasibility, appropriateness, meaningfulness, effectiveness) provides useful factors to consider when writing a guideline and rationale.

F = Feasibility focuses on the practice context: cost effectiveness, resource availability, and adequate levels of competency and experience.

A = Appropriateness centers on cultural acceptability and transferability.

M = Meaningfulness is associated with positive experiences, not negative experiences.

E = Effectiveness looks at safety versus harm and risk versus benefit.

The Institute of Medicine (IOM, 2011) recommended the following attributes for clinical practice guidelines:

- Validity
- Reliability/reproducibility
- Clinical applicability
- Clinical flexibility
- Clarity
- Multidisciplinary process
- Scheduled reviews
- Documentation

Appraisal of Guidelines for Research and Evaluation (AGREE) provides another guideline development tool. The AGREE II (Brouwers et al., 2013, p 1) is useful to:

- Assess the quality of guidelines
- Provide a methodological strategy for the development of guidelines
- Inform what information and how information ought to be reported in guidelines

Items in the AGREE tool are divided into six sections: (1) scope and purpose, (2) stakeholder involvement, (3) rigor development, (4) clarity of presentation, (5) applicability, and (6) editorial independence. Specific suggestions from each identified AGREE section can be accessed at http://www.agreetrust.org/wp-content/uploads/2013/10/AGREE-II-Users-Manual-and-23-item-Instrument_2009_UPDATE_2013.pdf (Brouwers et al., 2013).

Examples of guidelines or recommendations for practice can be accessed from the following sites:

Emergency Nurses Association (ENA): https://www.ena.org/practice-research/research/CPG/Pages/Default.aspx

Guideline Central: https://www.guidelinecentral.com/summaries/specialties/nursing/

National Guideline Clearinghouse: http://www.guideline.gov/syntheses/index.aspx

Adoption of DNP project practice guidelines is strongest when stakeholders and majority users within the intended context support the recommended action or actions emerging from your project. The intent is for the recommendations to be contextually relevant and clearly written. Customizing the practice recommendation for a particular organization can contribute to acceptance (Straus & Leung, 2013).

The next section highlights avenues for dissemination of your evidence findings, synthesis, and recommendation. Keep in mind that dissemination can, and should, occur at many points throughout your DNP project.

DISSEMINATION OF SYNTHESIS FINDINGS

Dissemination of information from the EBP synthesis report and recommendations is crucially important in growth and development of nursing practice. Practice recommendations and decisions based on best evidence must stay current for nursing practice to be effective and efficient.

Target populations for dissemination of your evidence and recommendations include (1) stakeholders, peers, and your DNP project committee and (2) other professionals in similar settings (Zaccagnini & White, 2014). Stakeholders play important roles during your project development and implementation. Stakeholders may be representatives of the local healthcare institutions and provide assistance for accessing relevant information such as documents, policies, and electronic health records data. Stakeholders are considered experts to assist your understanding of the context. Stakeholders are people who have an interest in your DNP project and open doors for implementation of your recommendations for practice. Developing a working relationship with appropriate stakeholders therefore is essential (Polit & Beck, 2012).

Venues for dissemination such as presentations and manuscripts for the broader professional population also exist for sharing your evidence search, findings, and recommendations for practice. Manuscripts can be written at any time during the process of your DNP project, from idea and background, evidence search, and implementation and evaluation of project (Oermann, Tanner, & Carman, 2014). See Chapter 15 for more information related to writing for professional journals and conference presentations.

Basic elements that make a presentation appealing, no matter the venue, include the following (Melnyk & Fineout-Overholt, 2014):

- Know your audience

- Make your presentation interesting. Grab your audience's attention.

- Show how your topic is relevant. Ideas rarely occur in isolation, and your audience may be looking for similar ideas.

- Organize your presentation to increase clarity of your ideas.

- Demonstrate the quality and rigor that went into your efforts.

- Visual appeal is important! Follow guidelines for effective construction of posters or PowerPoint presentations.

- Write and speak clearly.

Venues to consider for public dissemination include the following:

- Professional conference presentations
  - Podium or oral presentation
  - Panel presentation
  - Roundtable presentation
  - Poster presentation
- Small group presentations
  - Hospital or institutional meetings
  - Professional committee meetings
  - Community meetings

- Journal clubs
  - On-site
  - Online
- Publications
  - Peer-reviewed professional journals
  - Public media (e.g., newspaper or journal editorials)
  - Web page (personal or college)

CHAPTER SUMMARY AND AFTERTHOUGHTS

The importance of a well-written synthesis report and executive summary cannot be overstated. The quality and effectiveness of your evidence search are demonstrated with meaningful connections of best evidence that lead to development of a persuasive academic argument that addresses your EBP question or statement and concludes with a well-developed practice recommendation. Dissemination of your EBP findings and recommendations for practice are the next steps toward building your career as a DNP scholar. Dissemination is exceedingly important because you become part of the continuing cycle and legacy of scientific and practice knowledge.

Chapter 9 segues the EBP synthesis and practice recommendations into planning for implementation. When plans are finalized and written into a proposal (see Chapter 13) for your DNP project committee, real-time implementation begins.

WRITING REMINDERS...

Writer's Block

Confronting "writer's block" can be accomplished by writing every day. Setting aside even 15 minutes to focus on writing a manuscript can lead to a finished product. Hints for quality writing include the following: (1) write an entire first draft, then go back to edit and polish; (2) have a colleague review your written product; (3) use a thesaurus to find good words; and (4) refer to a writing guide to help with sentence and paragraph structure (Polit & Beck, 2013; Purdue Owl, 2014). Examples of good writing guides include the Purdue Owl Writing Guide or Joshua Schimel's (2012) *Writing Science*.

REFERENCES

Akl, E.A., Maroun, N., Guyatt, G., & Schunemann, H.J. (2007). Symbols were superior to numbers for presenting strength of recommendations to health care consumers: A randomized trial. *Journal of Clinical Epidemiology, 60,* 1298–1305.

American College of Physicians (ACP). (2014). *ACP clinical recommendations.* Retrieved from http://www.acponline.org/clinical_information/guidelines/

Branson, R.C. (2004). Anatomy of a research paper. *Respiratory Care, 49*(1), 1222–1228.

Brouwers, M., Kho, M.D., Browman, G.P., Cluzeau, F., Feder, G., Fervers, B., Hanna, S., & Makarski, J., On behalf of the AGREE Next Steps Consortium. (2010, updated 2013). *AGREE II: Advancing guideline development, reporting and evaluation in healthcare. Canadian Medical Association Journal, 182*(18):E839–E842. Retrieved from http://www.agreetrust.org/wp-content/uploads/2013/10/AGREE-II-Users-Manual-and-23-item-Instrument_2009_UPDATE_2013.pdf

Davis, D., Goldman, J., & Palda, V. (2007). *Handbook on clinical practice guidelines.* Ottawa, ON: Canadian Medical Association. Retrieved from https://www.cma.ca/Assets/assets-library/document/en/clinical-resources/CPG%20handbook-e.pdf

Dictionary.com. (2014). Retrieved from http://dictionary.reference.com/browse/

Emergency Nurses Association (ENA). (2016). *Clinical practice guidelines.* Retrieved from https://www.ena.org/practice-research/research/CPG/Pages/Default.aspx

Grove, S.K., Burns, N., & Gray, J.R. (2013). *The practice of nursing research: Appraisal, synthesis, and generation of evidence* (7th ed.). St. Louis, MO: Elsevier Saunders.

Guideline Central. (2016). *Guideline summaries.* Retrieved from https://www.guideline-central.com/summaries/specialties/nursing/

Institute of Medicine (IOM). (2011). *Clinical practice guidelines we can trust.* Washington DC: National Academies Press.

Jamieson, S. (1999). *Synthesis writing.* Drew University. Retrieved from http://www.users.drew.edu/sjamieso/synthesis.html

Joanna Briggs Institute (JBI). (2014a). *Joanna Briggs Institute reviewers' manual 2014.* University of Adelaide, Australia: Joanna Briggs Institute. Retrieved from http://joannabriggs.org/assets/docs/sumari/ReviewersManual-2014.pdf

Joanna Briggs Institute (JBI) Levels of Evidence and Grades of Recommendation Working Party. (2014b). *Supporting document for the Joanna Briggs institute levels of evidence and grades of recommendation.* University of Adelaide, Australia: Joanna Briggs Institute. Retrieved from http://docplayer.net/10190053-Supporting-document-for-the-joanna-briggs-institute-levels-of-evidence-and-grades-of-recommendation.html

McMaster University. (2014). *Health evidence: Practice tools.* Retrieved from http://www.healthevidence.org/practice-tools.aspx

Melnyk, B., & Fineout-Overholt, E. (2014). *Evidence-based practice in nursing and healthcare: A guide to best practice* (3rd ed.). Philadelphia, PA: Wolters Kluwer Health.

Moher, D., Liberati, A., Tetzlaff, J., & Altman, D.G. (2009). Preferred reporting items for systematic reviews and meta-analysis: the PRISMA Statement. *PLoS Medicine, 6*(6), e1000097.

National Guideline Clearinghouse. (2014). *Guideline synthesis.* Retrieved from http://www.guideline.gov/syntheses/index.aspx

Oermann, M.H., Tanner, K., & Carman, M. (2014). Preparing quality improvement research and EBP practice manuscripts. *Nursing Economics, 21*(2), 57–63.

Patten, M.L. (2012). *Understanding research methods: An overview of the essentials* (8th ed.). Glendale, CA: Pyrczak Publishing.

Polit, D.F., & Beck, C.T. (2012). *Nursing research: Generating and assessing evidence for nursing practice* (9th ed.). Philadelphia, PA: Wolters Kluwer/Lippincott Williams & Wilkins.

Purdue Owl. (2014). *The report abstract and executive summary.* Retrieved from https://owl.english.purdue.edu/owl/resource/726/07.

Schimel, J. (2012). *Writing science: How to write papers that get cited and proposals that get funded.* New York, NY: Oxford University Press.

Schünemann, H.J., Best, D., Vist, G., & Oxman, A.D. (2003). Letters, numbers, symbols, and words: How to communicate grades of evidence and recommendations. *CMAJ, 169,* 677–680.

Straus, S.E., & Leung, E. (2013). Section 3.1: The action cycle. *KT Clearinghouse.* Retrieved from http://ktclearinghouse.ca/files/knowledgebase/kt_in_health_care_chapter_3.1_e.pdf

Timmermans, S., & Berg, M. (2003). *The gold standard: The challenge of evidence-based medicine and standardization in health care.* Philadelphia, PA: Temple University Press.

Titler, M.G., Steelman, C., Rakel, V.J., Burdreau, B.A., Everett, L.Q., Buckwalter, K.C., Walden University Writing Center. (2014). *Synthesis.* Retrieved from http://writing-center.waldenu.edu/synthesis.htm#sthash.8GiYgt7u.dpuf.

Woolf, S., Schünemann, H.J., Eccles, M.P., Grimshaw, J.M., & Shekelle, P. (2012). Developing clinical practice guidelines: Types of evidence and outcomes; values and economics, synthesis, grading and presentation and deriving recommendations. *Implementation Science,* 7(61). Retrieved from http://www.implementationscience.com/content/7/1/61

World Health Organization (WHO). (2012). *WHO handbook for guideline development.* Retrieved from http://apps.who.int/iris/bitstream/10665/75146/1/9789241548441_eng.pdf

Zaccagnini, M.E., & White, K.W. (2014). *The doctor of nursing practice essentials: A new model for advanced practice nursing.* Minneapolis, MN: Jones & Bartlett.

IF YOU WANT TO READ MORE...

Davis, D., Goldman, J., & Palda, V. (2007). A guide to the *Canadian Medication Association Handbook on Clinical Practice Guidelines. CMAJ,* 177(10), 1221–1226. Retrieved from https://www.cma.ca/Assets/assets-library/document/en/clinical-resources/CPG%20handbook-e.pdf

Joanna Briggs Institute (JBI). (2014). *Reviewers' manual 2014*. University of Adelaide, Australia: Joanna Briggs Institute. Retrieved from http://joannabriggs.org/assets/docs/sumari/ReviewersManual-2014.pdf

World Health Organization. (2012). *WHO handbook for guideline development*. Retrieved from http://apps.who.int/iris/bitstream/10665/75146/1/9789241548441_eng.pdf

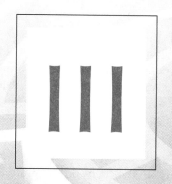

Leadership

PURPOSES

The aims of Section III are as follows: to provide information, rationale, and tools for successful planning, evaluation, and implementation of evidence-based practice recommendations for practice, and to review leadership and management skills for successful implementation of your DNP project

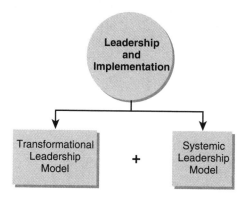

Section III focuses on planning for implementation, evaluation, budgets, and sustainability.

Planning and evaluating are complex processes and actions that require quality leadership and management skills (Rycroft-Malone et al., 2012).

Chapter 9 provides conceptual models and frameworks for consideration in thinking about the complexity of implementation. Chapter 10 begins the explanation about planning for implementation. Specifically,

Chapter 10 focuses on the importance of planning and organizing for implementation by building a detailed logic model showing relationships of actions, resources, and outcomes. A logic model is an integral part of implementation and evaluation because it precisely articulates practice activities and anticipated outcomes (Work Group, 2013). Chapter 11 continues the focus on planning with information related to evaluation. A review of quantitative and qualitative evaluation methods is provided in Appendices A and B at the end of the book. Chapters 12 and 13 continue the focus on planning by examining the details of economic considerations (e.g., budgets). Chapter 14 targets creation of the written proposal based on planning as described in Chapters 9 to 13. Chapter 15, the last chapter in Section III, focuses on review of project management and leadership skills for actualization of the implementation plan. Planning for all segments of your DNP project is complex and time consuming, yet the value of time spent planning contributes to quality and greater chance for success of your DNP project.

REFERENCES

Rycroft-Malone, J., Harvey, G., Seers, K., Kitson, A., McCormack, B., & Titchen, A. (2004). An exploration of the factors that influence the implementation of evidence into practice. *Journal of Clinical Nursing, 13*(8), 913–924.

Work Group for Community Health and Development. (2013). Developing a logic model or theory of change. *The Community Tool Box.* University of Kansas. Retrieved from http://ctb.ku.edu/en/table-of-contents/overview/models-for-community-health-and-development/logic-model-development/main

9

Implementation Frameworks

It is not always what we know or analyzed before we make a decision that makes it a great decision. It is what we do after we make the decision to implement and execute it that makes it a good decision.

WILLIAM POLLARD

OUTCOME OBJECTIVES

- Discuss implementation of evidence-based practice (EBP) recommendations within the broader structure of translational science.
- Compare and contrast implementation frameworks associated with EBP practice recommendations.

TERMS

Context	Framework	Implementation
Evidence	Function	science
Facilitation	Implementation	Translational science

Implementation is action based on recommendations from the evidence-based practice (EBP) process. Review of the EBP process conveys that it is linear and begins with an idea that leads to rigorously searching for, finding, and synthesizing best evidence. Recommendations for practice based on the written synthesis are then shared with your DNP committee and identified stakeholders. However, "guidelines alone do not lead to change in practice" (Kirchhoff, 2004, p S7). Action and leadership are required. Implementation is a complex, iterative, overlapping, and interactive process that encompasses integration, evaluation, and sustainability. Planning for implementation is an essential segment in your DNP project because of its importance in clinical decision making.

This chapter provides frameworks for thinking and strategizing about implementation of your project. Chapters 11 and 12 subsequently provide narrative and tools for process and action related to planning the integration into practice of your EBP recommendation followed by planning for evaluation and sustainability.

IMPLEMENTATION FRAMEWORKS

Recall that a framework is a place to think and strategize. That means a framework is a conceptual or theoretical model that provides structure to your thinking as you strategically plan the implementation process. Three frameworks are presented in this chapter. The selected frameworks are frequently cited for strategic thinking about implementation projects and are created by nursing experts and leaders in the areas of EBP and implementation science. Other frameworks exist, but the three presented in this chapter are the most widely cited.

Planning for implementation into the practice setting encompasses three elements: integration of evidence-based recommendations into the practice setting; evaluation of process, actions, and outcomes; and adoption of recommendation or sustainability evaluated through continuous and timely evaluation. The research element of implementation is termed *implementation science* and is described as:

> ... *the study of methods to promote the integration of research findings and evidence into healthcare policy and practice. It seeks to understand the behavior of healthcare professionals and other stakeholders as a key variable in the sustainable uptake, adoption, and implementation of evidence-based interventions. ... Implementation science is a new field of research. Its focus is to address barriers or bottlenecks that impede effective implementation, test new approaches to improve health programming, as well as determine a causal relationship between the intervention and its impact (Fogarty International Center [FIC], 2013; Health Sciences Research and Information Center [HSRIC], 2015).*

Examples of implementation science include the following:

- Comparisons of multiple evidence-based interventions

- Identification of strategies to promote the integration of evidence into policy and program decisions

- Appropriate adaptation of interventions according to context (population and setting)

- Development of innovative approaches to improve healthcare delivery

- Setting up an impact evaluation for a population-based intervention (FIC, 2013; HSRIC, 2015)

Implementation into practice and science fits within the construct of translational science by focusing on integration processes and actions for the DNP and for the nurse scientist. See Table 1.2 in Chapter 1 for a review of the translational science model. Translational science is described as "the multidirectional and multidisciplinary integration of basic research, patient-oriented research, and population-based research, with the long-term aim of improving the health of the public" (Rubio, Schoenbaum, & Esposito, 2010, p 470). The importance of quality and safety in health care is actualized with increased attention to strength of evidence and time considerations in dissemination and integration of evidence into practice. The result is a narrowed emphasis on goals, models, and terminology leading to the desired outcomes of quality and safety. Indeed, the fields of practice and implementation science are embracing the future.

The three implementation frameworks presented in this chapter include the implementation model (Titler, 2008; Titler, 2010; Titler & Everett, 2001; Titler, Everett, & Adams, 2007), the PARiHS model (Kitson et al., 1998; Rycroft-Malone et al., 2013), and the Knowledge-to-Action cycle (Graham et al., 2006; Straus & Leung, 2014; WHO, 2012). Each framework brings a different approach to implementation, thereby increasing comprehension of the topic. Table 9.1 provides an overview of similarities and differences among the implementation frameworks.

Implementation Model

Dr. Marita Titler is a prolific author and contributor to publications, clinical research, and conceptual models related to EBP, translating research into practice, and implementation science. Refer to Figure 3.2 in Chapter 3 for a review of the Iowa model of evidence-based practice (Titler et al., 2001). Note that the Iowa model flowchart concludes with *implementation* by focusing

Text continued on page 162

TABLE 9.1 Comparison of Implementation Frameworks

Implementation Model	Promoting Action on Research Implementation in Health Services: PARiHS Conceptual Framework	Knowledge-to-Action Cycle: KTA
Focus The implementation model: • Addresses lag time between dissemination of research evidence and implementation into practice by identifying potential barriers of process and actions of integration • Is interactive and iterative within a context of participative change • Is validated by numerous clinical research studies (Titler, 2010; Titler et al, 2007)	PARiHS implies an interpretivist approach for planning successful implementation of evidenced recommendations as a function of the interplay of (1) level and nature of the evidence, (2) context, and (3) facilitation of process. Each element is of equal importance for successful implementation (Kitson et al., 1998; Rycroft-Malone et al., 2013).	• KTA means knowledge creation followed by an iterative, bidirectional cycle of actions specific to implementation. • KTA focuses on the real-life complexities that create barriers for implementation. • "For the process to run efficiently, it is imperative to remain vigilant to problems at each stage of the knowledge generation, synthesis, exchange process, and to document the problems in reports, discussion forums, clinical logs, or research papers [collaboration with science and practice] so they can be identified by researchers and or the experts who can develop a solution" (WHO, 2012). • KTA is a clearly written process that identifies strategies for identifying real-life barriers to implementation and evaluation, thereby enhancing action(Straus & Leung, 2014).

Continued

| Concepts | *Characteristics of the clinical practice guideline (CPG)*: type and strength of evidence and recommendation for change or improvement
• Type and strength of evidence
• Relevance of the recommendation(s) for practice

Contextual fit: organizational factors, social systems, environment
• Perceived tension around a specific clinical or work issue that can be addressed with best evidence guidelines or recommendations is more likely to assimilate the evidence, thereby reducing the tension.

Communication and the manner in which information is presented
• "Education is necessary but not sufficient to change practice" (Titler, 2008, p 1–118). | $SI = f(E,C,F)$
SI = *successful implementation* suggests a relationship among the evidence, context, and mechanisms of facilitated change.
f = *function* implies the mechanisms (process and actions) of facilitated change. A high-functioning implementation plan is the desired outcome of the PARiHS Model.
E = *Evidence characteristics*:
1. *Evidence* implies verification or strength of practice recommendations.
2. *Characteristics* are features of strength and quality.
3. Examples include research strength established with critique and hierarchal level of evidence; strength of professional opinion established with high expert consensus; strength of patient opinions established through EHRs and patient input into decision making. | *Knowledge creation*
• *Knowledge inquiry*
• *Synthesis*
• *Product or tools*

Action cycle
• *Identify problem; review and select knowledge.*
• *Adapt knowledge to local context.*
• *Assess barriers to knowledge use.*
• *Select, tailor, and implement interventions.*
• *Monitor knowledge use.*
• *Evaluate outcomes.*
• *Sustain knowledge use.* |

TABLE 9.1 Comparison of Implementation Frameworks—cont'd

Implementation Model	Promoting Action on Research Implementation in Health Services: PARiHS Conceptual Framework	Knowledge-to-Action Cycle: KTA
• Opinion leaders from local peer group—respected source of influence, considered competent, trusted, and educated—are influential across microsystems, with influence to alter group norms. A key characteristic of an identified opinion leader is that he or she is trusted to evaluate new information in the context of group norms (e.g., "hallway chats," one-on-one discussions, answering and addressing questions). • Change champions are practitioners within the local context and social group who are expert clinicians, passionate about the innovation, on the committee to improving quality of care, and have a positive working relationship with other healthcare professionals. They circulate information, encourage peers to adopt the innovation, arrange demonstrations, and orient staff to the innovation. They believe in the idea and are persistent.	C = *Contextual readiness for EBP implementation* means the context is receptive to change or improvement. Context includes a culture of valuing learning, patients, continuing education. Context also includes leadership that is clearly defined and an organization that is effectively structured. Measurement falls under the concept of *context* because ongoing measurements are a function of a well-run organization focused on patient-centered care. F = *Facilitation* suggests that "one person makes things easier for another" (Kitson, 1998, p 152) through demonstrations of respect, empathy, authenticity, and credibility. Being a leader who is accessible, supportive, and consistent is an important role for change (Kitson et al., 1998; Rycroft-Malone et al., 2013; Stetler et al., 2011).	

- An identified core group working varied shifts assists the change champion and opinion leader with disseminating information and reinforces the practice change on a daily basis—this group provides positive feedback. Critical mass is a core-group approach in conjunction with a change champion.
- The group functions within a context of participative change.

Users of the evidence: practitioners, staff nurses, end users
- Implementation topic, process, and actions are compatible with users' values, norms, work, and perceived needs.
- Complexity of EBP recommendation: simple is more easily adopted than complex,

Role and extent of EBP adoption: evaluation and sustainability
- Evaluation data and feedback must be timely, nonpunitive, and perceived as valid to establish credibility.
- Sustainability of data feedback must persist and be integrated within the organization context to improve and change performance (Titler, 2010).

Continued

TABLE 9.1 Comparison of Implementation Frameworks—cont'd

	Implementation Model	Promoting Action on Research Implementation in Health Services: PARiHS Conceptual Framework	Knowledge-to-Action Cycle: KTA

Usefulness	The implementation model:
	• Assists in planning for implementation, such as the needs assessment, by identifying potential barriers to implementation
	• Provides methods for implementing practice change or improvement through identification of staff roles and communication models
	• Emphasizes the importance of including end users in all parts of implementation
	• Identifies *useful feedback* of evaluation data as a core concept
		The PARiHS framework
		• Is an interpretive model for understanding and comparing varying degrees of success for EBP implementation (Kitson et al., 1998; Rycroft-Malone et al., 2013)
		• Evaluates intensity of facilitation
		• Assists in keeping focus for implementation planning and action on context, evidence, and facilitation (Phipps, n.d.)
		• Informs research but has little dissemination history of use as a framework in research or evaluation of practice (Stetler et al., 2011)
			The seven phases of the action cycle:
			1. Identification of KTA gaps
			  • Needs assessment
			    Purpose
			    Resources
			    Measurement data are subjective or objective
			  • Needs perspective
			    Population
			    Organization
			    Healthcare provider
			2. Adapting knowledge to context for relevance and feasibility

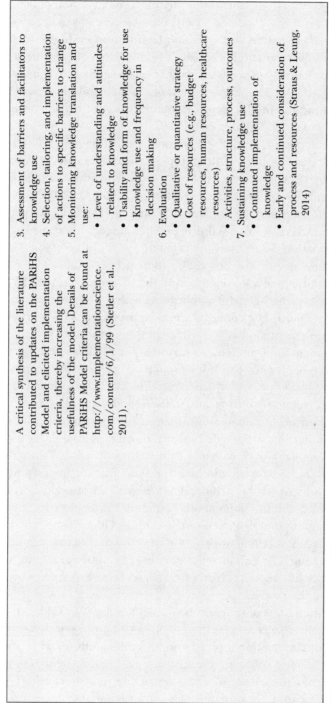

A critical synthesis of the literature contributed to updates on the PARiHS Model and elicited implementation criteria, thereby increasing the usefulness of the model. Details of PARiHS Model criteria can be found at http://www.implementationscience.com/content/6/1/99 (Stetler et al., 2011).

3. Assessment of barriers and facilitators to knowledge use
4. Selection, tailoring, and implementation of actions to specific barriers to change
5. Monitoring knowledge translation and use:
   • Level of understanding and attitudes related to knowledge
   • Usability and form of knowledge for use
   • Knowledge use and frequency in decision making
6. Evaluation
   • Qualitative or quantitative strategy
   • Cost of resources (e.g., budget resources, human resources, healthcare resources)
   • Activities, structure, process, outcomes
7. Sustaining knowledge use
   • Continued implementation of knowledge
   • Early and continued consideration of process and resources (Straus & Leung, 2014)

EBP, evidence-based practice; EHRs, electronic health records.

on instituting, evaluating, and disseminating evidence. Subsequently termed *Translating Research Into Practice,* or TRIP, the objective was to decrease the time lag between dissemination and clinical integration of evidence, in addition to evaluation and dissemination of research findings that affect patient outcomes and clinical practice (Agency for Healthcare Research and Quality [AHRQ], 2013; AHRQ, 1999). The implementation model and succeeding research studies validating the model focus on identification of barriers to integration of evidence (Titler, 2008; Titler et al., 2007).

The implementation model was adapted from Rogers' (1962) *Diffusion of Innovations.* Rogers' model is built on three basic influences: (1) perceptions of the innovation, (2) characteristics of the people who adopt or fail to adopt the innovation, and (3) contextual factors (Berwick, 2003; Orr, 2003; Rogers, 2003; Titler, 2010). Concepts of the implementation model by Titler & Everett (2007) begin with characteristics of the clinical practice guideline because the guideline or recommendation determines the rate and extent of adoption. Concepts of implementation include the communication process, the social system, end users of the clinical practice guideline, and the role and extent of EBP adoption. The concepts are intended for application within a context of participative change (Titler, 2008). The concepts are to be used interactively and iteratively, as needed. Implementation is, indeed, a complex process.

The implementation model also provides for establishment of assessment criteria before beginning the implementation process. An implementation plan establishes baseline performance indicators on which change or improvement can be measured during and following the implementation process. Collected data provide valuable information for practitioners and should be actively communicated at specific intervals throughout the process. This form of active communication of data and findings, versus passive written feedback reports, establishes your credibility in the implementation process and enhances integration and sustainability. Indeed, *useful feedback* of evaluation and audit data was identified in the implementation model as a core concept for acceptance and integration of EBP recommendations (Titler, 2008). The implementation model is a useful framework for the DNP project because it conceptualizes variables that inhibit or enhance the efficiency of application and integration of best evidence into practice. Numerous clinical research studies by Titler and others validate the model.

As a DNP student, you will likely be implementing your evidence-based recommendations in one context with a small, purposefully selected group of end users. Therefore, evaluation indicates use of a pilot study for a specified period of time (Titler, 2008). "Piloting the EBP as part of implementation has a positive influence on the extent of adoption of the new practice" (Titler, 2008, p 115) and fits within the structure of T_2 (translational science, phase 2).

PARiHS Conceptual Framework

The PARiHS (Promoting Action on Research Implementation in Health Services) model represents an interpretivist approach for addressing the overlap and integration of elements involved in implementation of evidence recommendations for change or improvement in the practice setting. PARiHS as a conceptual framework is neither linear nor hierarchal, but it is considered to be simultaneous and used for situational analyses of implementation (Kitson, Rycroft-Malone, & Titchen, 2008; Rycroft-Malone, 2004). PARiHS implies that organizational context has a greater effect in using evidence because context implicates the complexity and characteristics of implementation (Melnyk & Fineout-Overholt, 2011).

The PARiHS conceptual framework proposes that *successful implementation* is a product of the functioning relationships among *evidence, context,* and *facilitation,* formulated as SI = f (E,C,F). Initially published in 1998, the PARiHS framework has undergone additional development and analysis that currently contributes to a more practical framework for implementation (Rycroft-Malone et al., 2013; Stetler, Damschroder, Helfrich, & Hagedom, 2011). See Table 9.1 for detail on concepts and potential use of the PARiHS model as a framework for implementing your DNP project.

The intent of the PARiHS conceptual framework is to make sense of the complexities of the interactive concepts that comprise successful implementation. The PARiHS Diagnostic and Evaluation Grid is a three-dimensional 2×2 box (similar to a two-dimensional risk ratio). The PARiHS diagram is intended for use in planning successful implementation (SI) of EBP recommendations. The horizontal or x axis represents context, and the vertical or y-axis represents the evidence. Strength of the x axis moves from left (weak) to right (strong). Strength of the y axis moves from bottom (weak) to top (strong). Intensity of facilitation is represented by an arrow conveying a directional method of strength between context and evidence. The closer the facilitation arrow gets to the upper right box, the stronger is the potential for facilitating a successful intervention (Dougherty, Harrison, & Graham, 2010; Kitson et al., 2008).

Challenges related to usefulness of the initial PARiHS model included lack of understanding related to the interactive complexities among the concepts (Rycroft-Malone, 2002; Rycroft-Malone et al., 2013; Stetler, et al., 2011). A revision based on a critical systematic review enhanced conceptualization, and therefore usefulness, by identifying meaningful criteria explaining the elements and subelements of the concepts (Stetler et al., 2011). The strength of the updated PARiHS framework is that it "represents the complexity of implementation by considering subelements to be dynamic and interrelated" (Rycroft-Malone et al., 2013, p 2 of 13).

The advantages of considering the updated PARiHS conceptual model as a framework for implementation of your DNP project are the recognition provided for the variability of context and leadership choices for facilitating implementation. Variability of EBP practice recommendations influences the complexity of implementation planning.

Knowledge-to-Action Cycle

The knowledge-to-action (KTA) framework was initially proposed by Graham et al. (2006) to address the confusion and misunderstandings connected with multiple terms and labels connected to moving best evidence into the practice setting. The result was a conceptual framework for thinking and strategizing about process, action, and differing roles between those who create knowledge and those who apply knowledge (Graham et al., 2006; WHO, 2012).

The KTA framework is composed of two major concepts: knowledge creation and action cycle. The process has no boundaries between the two parts or phases. Indeed, action may occur sequentially or simultaneously with knowledge creation, and the phases may influence each other. The knowledge creation step reflects different developmental stages of knowledge: knowledge inquiry, knowledge synthesis, and knowledge tools or products. The action cycle represents activities necessary for knowledge application. Action phases include problem identification, identifying appropriate knowledge, applying knowledge to the local context, assessment of barriers to knowledge use, developing and implementing interventions, monitoring, evaluating, and sustaining the use of knowledge (Graham et al., 2006; WHO, 2012).

The KTA framework is a decision-making process that builds on theories of planned action and promotes the importance of local context as the focus for adapting knowledge. However, the framework does not portray the complexities of making change (WHO, 2012). See Table 9.1 for an analysis of KTA. Considerations for selecting the KTA framework are ease in use and well-documented action steps presented as a bidirectional cycle.

The next step in your DNP scholarly journey is selection of a framework to guide implementation. As noted in the quotation at the beginning of Chapter 10, time spent planning and making decisions about process and actions will result in better decisions and successful implementation of your EBP practice recommendations.

CHAPTER SUMMARY AND AFTERTHOUGHTS

Before reading Chapters 11 and 12, consider the implementation frameworks presented in this chapter as well as other frameworks that may influence your thinking and strategizing about your DNP project. Consider one or a combination of two or more frameworks that meet your needs to begin building your implementation plan. The cornerstone of Chapters 11 and 12 is to provide tools and explanations to assist development of an implementation plan for your EBP project. An implementation plan is a management or business tool for the purpose of providing a plan for process and action related to implementation of your EBP recommendation. A well-developed implementation plan for integration, evaluation, and sustainability of your EBP recommendations is a readiness process for success. Remember that "the learning that occurs during the process of translating research into practice is valuable information to capture and feed back into the process, so that others can adapt the evidence-based guideline and/or the implementation strategies" (Titler, 2008, pp 1–113).

CASE STUDY

Brad is the unit manager in the emergency department (ED) of a busy urban medical center. He is currently working on a post-master's DNP degree in leadership. Brad requested that a unit policy be developed for the purpose of providing guidelines for family members to be present during resuscitation and/or invasive procedure(s) performed on a family member. Brad asked for and received permission from the unit manager to write an evidence-based policy and evaluate its effectiveness. A unit-based evidence-based practice (EBP) team was formed to draft the policy. The team consisted of Brad, two nurses, an emergency physician, a nurse researcher, and a chaplaincy services representative. The following question was created to guide the search process: In a large medical center emergency department (P), will creation and implementation of a unit policy (I) versus practicing without a policy (C) enhance family presence experiences and increase healthcare workers' support of resuscitation and/or invasive procedures with family members present (O)?

The literature search for best evidence yielded 34 publications, but the evidence was weak or did not fit the context. Themes in the literature included both benefits and barriers to family presence. However, there was a gap in the literature about the patient's perspective regarding family presence, and no studies about family presence had been conducted in an ED.

A policy was subsequently written by the EBP committee, followed by education for the healthcare team, including nurses, emergency and trauma physicians, respiratory therapists, radiology technicians, social workers, and chaplaincy. Before implementation of the policy, a pilot study was endorsed by the ED staff, nurse manager, and medical director to evaluate end-user acceptance of the policy. A research measurement tool was adapted with permission from the authors of a 2007 publication.

Analysis of collected data showed that nurses and chaplaincy were strong supporters of the policy. Radiology technicians and respiratory therapists were mixed between support and nonsupport of the policy as written. Physicians were adamantly against the policy as written. A Cronbach's alpha found that questions containing the phrase "resuscitation and/or invasive procedures" were controversial and accepted by nurses and chaplaincy but rejected by physicians. The result was that the policy was not ratified at that time and returned to the committee for additional work (Adapted from Dougal, Anderson, Reavy, & Shirazi, 2011).

- *Select an implementation framework that reflects your thinking for building an implementation strategy for Brad.*

- *Discuss how an implementation framework could assist Brad in successful implementation of a new policy.*

WRITING REMINDERS...

The Outline: Why Is It So Important?

- An outline is a writing tool. The intent is to assist the order of your information.

- An outline keeps your writing organized. Organization of content assists comprehension and makes reading easier.

- An outline provides structure for development of concepts. Orderly organization of content increases the strength of the message.

- An outline increases thoroughness of your message and decreases the chance of omitting important information.

- An outline keeps you, the writer, focused on the topic.

- An outline motivates and measures progress.

- An outline contributes to development of a regular writing schedule (Serafinn, 2012).

REFERENCES

Agency for Healthcare Research and Quality (AHRQ). (1999). *Translating research into practice II.* Agency for Healthcare Research and Quality. Retrieved from http://grants.nih.gov/grants/guide/rfa-files/RFA-HS-00-008.html

Agency for Healthcare Research and Quality (AHRQ). (2013). *Translating research into practice.* Rockville, MD: AHRQ. Retrieved from http://www.ahrq.gov/research/findings/factsheets/translating/

Berwick, D.M. (2003). Disseminating Innovations in health care. *JAMA, 289*(15), 1969–1975.

Dougal, R.L., Anderson, J.H., Reavy, K., & Shirazi. C.C. (2011). Family presence during resuscitation and/or invasive procedures in the emergency department: one size does not fit all. *Journal of Emergency Nursing, 37*(2), 152–157.

Dougherty, E., Harrison, M.B., & Graham, I.A. (2010). Facilitation as a rule and process in achieving evidence-based practice in nursing: Review of concept and meaning. *World Views on Evidence-Based Practice, 7*(2), 76–89.

Fogarty International Center. (2013). *Frequently asked questions about implementation science.* Bethesda, MD: National Institutes of Health (NIH). Retrieved from http://www.fic.nih.gov/News/Events/implementation-science/Pages/faqs.aspx\

Graham, I.D., Logan, J., Harrison, M., Straus, S., Totroe, J., Caswell, W., & Robinson, N. (2006). Lost in knowledge translation: Time for a map? *Journal of Continuing Education in the Health Professions, 26*(1), 13–24.

Health Sciences Research and Information Center (HSRIC). (2015). *Dissemination and implementation science.* Bethesda, MD: U.S. National Library of Medicine. Retrieved from http://www.nlm.nih.gov/hsrinfo/implementation_science.html

Kirchhoff, K.T. (2004). State of the science of translational research: From demonstration projects to intervention testing. *Worldviews on Evidence-Based Practice, 1*(Supplement 1), S6–S12.

Kitson, A., Harvey, G., & McCormack, B. (1998). Enabling the implementation of evidence-based practice: A conceptual framework. *Quality in Health Care, 7,* 149–158.

Kitson, A.L., Rycroft-Malone, J., & Titchen, A. (2008). Evaluating the successful implementation of evidence into practice using the PARiHS framework: Theoretical and practical challenges. *Implementation Science, 3*(1). Retrieved from http://www.implementationscience.com/content/3/1/1

Melnyk, B.M., & Fineout-Overholt, E. (2011). *Evidence-based practice in nursing and healthcare* (2nd ed.). Philadelphia, PA: Wolters Kluwer/Lippincott Williams & Wilkins.

Orr, G. (2003). *Review of Dissemination of Innovations, by Everett Rogers (1995).* Retrieved from http://www.stanford.edu/class/symbsys205/Diffusion%20of%20Innovations.htm

Rogers, E. (1962, 2003). *Diffusion of innovations* (5th ed.). New York, NY: Free Press.

Rubio, E.M., Schoenbaum, E.E., & Esposito, K. (2010). Defining translational research: Implications for training. *Academic Medicine: Journal of the Association of American Medical Colleges, 85*(3), 470–475.

Rycroft-Malone, J. (2004). The PARiHS framework: A framework for guiding the implementation of evidence-based practice...promoting action on research implementation in health services. *Journal of Nursing Care Quality, 29*(4), 297–304.

Rycroft-Malone, J., Kitson, A., Harvey, G., et al. (2002). Ingredients for change: Revisiting a conceptual framework. *Quality Safe Health Care, 11,* 174–180.

Rycroft-Malone, J., Seers, K., Chandler, J., Hawkes, C.A., Crichton, N., Allen, C., & Strunin, L. (2013). The role of evidence, context, and facilitation in an implementation trial: Implications for development of the PARiHS framework. *Implementation Science, 8*(28), 13 pages. Retrieved from http://www.implementationscience.com/content/8/1/28

Serafinn, L. (2012). *Top 10 reasons (plus 1) why an outline is important when writing a book.* Retrieved from http://spiritauthors.com/news/top-10-reasons-plus-1-why-an-outline-is-important-when-writing-a-book/

Stetler, C.B., Damschroder, L.J., Helfrich, C.D., & Hagedom, H.J. (2011). A guide for applying a revised version of the PARiHS framework for implementation. *Implementation Science, 6*(99). Retrieved from http://www.implementationscience.com/content/6/1/99

Straus, S.E., & Leung, E. (2014). Section 3.1: The action cycle. *Knowledge base.* Canadian Institute of Health Research: KT Clearinghouse. Retrieved from http://ktclearinghouse.ca/knowledgebase/ktinhealthcare/3/1

Straus, S.E., Tetroe, M.A., & Graham, I. (2009). Defining knowledge translation. *CMAJ, 181*(3–4), 165–168.

Titler, M.G. (2008). The evidence for evidence-based practice implementation. In R.G. Hughes (Ed.). *Patient safety and quality: An evidence-based handbook for nurses.* Rockville, MD: Agency for Healthcare Research and Quality (AHRQ). Retrieved from www.ncbi.nlm.nih.gov/books/NBK2659

Titler, M.G. (2010). Translation science and context. *Research and Theory for Nursing Practice: An International Journal, (24)*1, 35–55.

Titler, M.G., & Everett, L.Q. (2001). Translating research into practice: Considerations for critical care investigators. *Critical Care Nursing Clinics of North America, 13*(4), 587–604.

Titler, M.G., Everett, L.Q., & Adams, S. (2007). Implications for implementation science. *Nursing Research, 56,*(4 Supplement), S53–S59.

Titler, M.G., Steelman, C., Rakel, V.J., & Good, C. (2001). The Iowa model of evidence-based practice to promote quality care. *Critical Care Nursing Clinics of North America, 13*(4), 497–509.

World Health Organization (WHO). (2012). *Knowledge translation framework for ageing and health.* Retrieved from http://www.who.int/ageing/publications/knowledge_translation.pdf

IF YOU WANT TO READ MORE ...

Kitson, A., Harvey, G., & McCormack, B. (1998). Enabling the implementation of evidence-based practice: A conceptual framework. *Quality in Health Care, 7,* 149–158.

Rubio, E.M., Schoenbaum, E.E., & Esposito, K. (2010). Defining translational research: Implications for training. *Academic Medicine: Journal of the Association of American Medical Colleges, 85*(3), 470–475.

Rycroft-Malone, J. (2004). The PARiHS framework: A framework for guiding the implementation of evidence-based practice. *Journal of Nursing Care Quality, 19*(4), 297–304.

Straus, S.E., & Leung, E. (2014). Section 3.1: The action cycle. *Knowledge Base.* Canadian Institute of Health Research: KT Clearinghouse. Retrieved from http://ktclearinghouse.ca/knowledgebase/ktinhealthcare/3/1

Titler, M.G. (2008). The evidence for evidence-based practice implementation. In R. G. Hughes (Ed.). *Patient safety and quality: An evidence-based handbook for nurses.* Rockville, MD: Agency for Healthcare Research and Quality (AHRQ). Retrieved from www.ncbi.nlm.nih.gov/books/NBK2659

10

Planning for Implementation: Integration, Management, and Leadership

There are not two sciences. There is science and the application of science, and the two are linked as the fruit is to the tree.

LOUIS PASTEUR

OUTCOME OBJECTIVES

- Describe the steps of implementation.
- Discuss the importance of planning before real-time implementation.
- Evaluate the functional use of a logic model for implementation.
- Assess the significance of project management.
- Analyze leadership skills and behaviors that contribute to successful implementation.

Evidence-based practice (EBP) guidelines or recommendations are professional coordination tools to guide actions related to patient-centered care (Timmermans & Berg, 2003). However, the process of implementing guidelines or recommendations for practice is more complex compared with the linear construct of EBP. Implementation occurs and is influenced by contextual levels of "providers, social networks, work units, delivery systems, and the broader sociopolitical environment" (Leeman & Sandelowski, 2012, p 76). Recall that implementation of guidelines or recommendations at the practice level fits within phase T_2 of the translational science model (see Chapter 1). Translational science phase 2 (T_2) is the initial step for implementation, adjustment, refinement, and establishment of value gleaned from best evidence (Sampselle, 2010; Titler, 2008; Woods & Magyary, 2010; Woolf, 2008). This chapter focuses on planning, organizing, and leadership responsibilities in preparation for real-time integration of recommendations into the practice setting. Subsequent chapters focus on planning for implementation of evaluation and sustainability.

THE IMPORTANCE OF PLANNING

Planning is a responsibility of project management and therefore an important step in implementation of practice recommendations. A plan furnishes strategy and direction for process, actions, efficiency, evaluation, and outcomes. Risks and barriers for implementation are often identified during the planning process, thereby allowing for adjustments before real-time integration. Project planning is a proactive endeavor that contributes to decision making and prioritization of tasks. Box 10.1 is a list reviewing the underlying rationale for why planning is important.

PLANNING FOR IMPLEMENTATION

Implementation implies action, beginning with a plan. An implementation plan is a proactive management strategy describing the steps and pace of the

---

BOX 10.1 The Importance of Planning

- Planning increases overall efficiency and avoids duplication.

- Planning identifies risks and barriers and helps in decision making to avoid risk.

- Planning facilitates coordination locally and systemically.

- Planning assists organization of resources.

- Planning provides direction and useful guidance.

- Planning helps achieve expected outcomes.

- Planning identifies leadership roles and tasks to motivate healthcare personnel during the intervention phase.

- Planning inspires creativity and innovation to achieve outcomes.

- Planning helps with strategizing and decision making to achieve best outcomes.

- Planning is important for effective and efficient implementation.

Source: Akrani, 2015; Hill, 2015; Pujari, 2015.

---

following: applying and integrating recommendations; evaluating process, actions, effect, and/or outcomes; assessing economic costs and creating a budget; and strategizing for sustainability. Implementation also includes consideration of your leadership roles for entry and exit strategizes in addition to communication processes for participants and end users during and at the conclusion of the project. This section provides considerations and tools for efficiency and organization of implementing EBP recommendations.

Framing the Project

Why does nursing emphasize the importance of identifying or implying a framework for DNP projects? The answer relates to the purpose of a framework. For example, the justification for a conceptual framework is to (1) explore key relationships among EBP recommendations or to (2) explain the implementation process with an implementation framework (see Chapter 9). A framework is a place for the author to think and strategize about his or her project during the planning stage. A framework also assists the reader to better understand the author's approach to operationalizing of EBP recommendations and/ or the action plan that describes the underlying assumptions about implementation and evaluation regarding the project that introduces change or revision to a practice setting (Kellogg, 2004; Wholey, Hatry, & Newcomer, 2010).

Framework examples from nursing and other disciplines include theory of human caring, adult learning theory, health education theories, behavioral science theories, marketing or business theories, and organizational and leadership theories (Farquhar, Stryer, & Slutsky, 2002; Watson, 1979). Examples of implementation frameworks include Rogers' (2003) diffusion of innovation model, Titler & Everett's (2001) implementation model, the PARiHS (Promoting Action on Research Implementation in Health Services) MODEL (Kitson, Rycroft-Malone, & Titchen, 2008), and Knowledge-to-Action (KTA) cycle (Graham, Logan, & Robinson, 2006; WHO, 2012). The Plan, Do, Study, Act (PDSA) is an organizational framework for quality improvement (QI) and focuses on continual improvement of product, process, policy, or program (Speroff, James, Nelson, Headrick, & Brommels, 2004). Sometimes a physiological framework is implied. For example, a DNP-prepared nurse practitioner may be trialing a new device for splinting tibial fractures. The framework is the scientific basis for external fixation and is considered common knowledge for healthcare providers. The framework for the practice project is therefore implied. To summarize: (1) a framework is a real, conceptual, or implied mental structure that serves as a place to think and strategize; and (2) the search and synthesis of evidence, recommendations for practice, and framework are interrelated (Grove et al., 2013).

Building a Logic Model

A basic tool of an implementation plan is the logic model because it visually describes decisions and strategies for thinking, planning, and communicating about the project's goals and deliverables. The logic model creates a picture of your assumptions about implementing the EBP recommendations (Kellogg, 2004).

A *logic model* has been compared to a road map that will guide you to an expected destination in an efficient amount of time. It is a visual tool that is rooted in systems theory and connects the parts to demonstrate the complexity of the whole (Kellogg, 2004; Oxford Dictionaries, 2014). Figure 10.1 is an example of a logic model that can be adapted for use in your DNP project.

The purpose of a logic model is to show relationships of resources, processes, and actions that meet desired outcomes and affect decision making. Another way to describe a logic model is to call it a *flowchart* that summarizes key

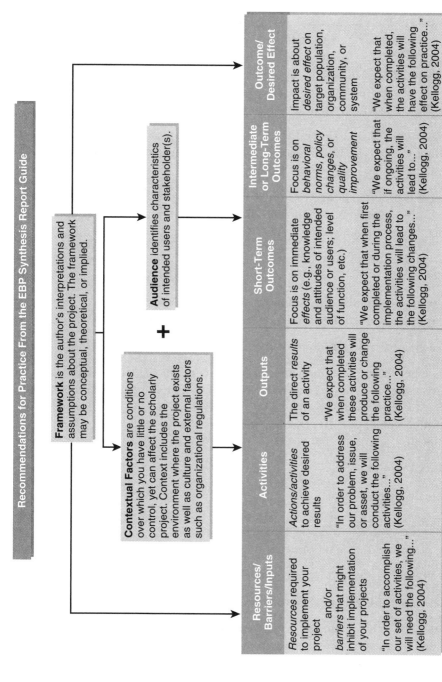

FIGURE 10.1 Example of a logic model for implementation.

elements of the project and the cause-and-effect relationships within identified contexts. The logic model is an important communication tool for discussions with stakeholders because it demonstrates the plan for accountability and management of results. Logic models are a process, not a one-time event, and they should involve stakeholders and your project committee in the building process (Kellogg, 2004; McLaughlin & Jordan, 2010; Wholey et al., 2010).

The value of using a logic model when planning the implementation is described as follows (Wholey et al., 2010):

- The model focuses on evaluation of issues and performance measurement points, thereby improving data collection that is useful for management and staff.

- It assists program design or improvement through identification of activities that are essential to attain identified goals or that may be redundant or inconsistent with identified goals.

- It describes the place and fit of a program within an organization or problem hierarchy.

- The model builds understanding of the proposed intervention, resource expectations, identified audience, and projected outcomes.

- It increases understanding for the intended audience.

Remember that logic models are working documents similar to a blueprint for construction of a house. The logic model is an organizational tool that should be flexible and updated as needed. Components of a logic model include the following elements (CDC Division for Heart Disease and Stroke Prevention, 2013 p 1):

- Displayed on one page

- Visually engaging

- Audience specific

- Appropriate in its level of detail

- Useful in clarifying program and activities and expected outcomes

- Reflective of the context in which the program operates

Strategizing and thinking about implementation of assumptions and ideas are visually represented in the logic model. Real-time action of implementation needs management and leadership. The next section focuses on planning the actions of management, leadership, and the significance of communication.

PROJECT MANAGEMENT

Principles of project management parallel implementation of healthcare projects in organizations. *Project management* is a term frequently used with civil engineers and construction management and is an increasingly common term applied in healthcare organizations.

A closer look at the term, *project management*, is helpful to understand its significance to your DNP project. A *project* is defined as a "temporary endeavor undertaken to create a unique product, service, or result" (PMI, 2013, p 5). *Management* is associated with production consisting of organizing, planning, controlling, and directing within the framework of an organization. Project requirements typically under the control of business management are scope, quality, schedule, budget, resources, and risk. The definition of *manager* indicates a power structure with responsibility for decision making to achieve identified objectives (Association for Project Management [APM], 2015; Business Dictionary.com, 2015; Project Management Institute [PMI], 2013).

The PMI, a leader in education related to project management, described five phases of managing a project from initiation to closure (PMI, 2013). The phases interact and overlap, thereby allowing for adjustments as needed. The five phases are described in Box 10.2.

Closely correlated with successful project management are leadership roles and communication skills.

PLANNING A LEADERSHIP STRATEGY

Leadership that is both individual *and* systematic is an essential partner with management for implementation of your DNP project (Tate, 2013). Chapter 2 identified two leadership models that serve as the framework for leadership needs in evidence-based practice (EBP) and project management: the systematic leadership model and the transformational leadership theory. Together, the models provide understanding and structure to empower best leadership practices for implementation of practice recommendations. *Systematic leadership* focuses on organizational development to meet the desired outcomes of stakeholders, clients or customers, and markets. Systematic leadership is practiced with humanistic and democratic values to ensure balance within the organization. Systematic leadership includes guidance for leadership correlated with management. Specific elements include the following (Tate, 2013, pp 35–36):

- A leader's application of change requires courage to lead as well as obtain management consent and support.

BOX 10.2 Five Phases of Project Management

1. Initiating

- After careful examination, the project is officially recognized and determined whether it will benefit the organization and can be completed in a realistic time frame. The project comes to life!

2. Planning

- This is a critical function in the project. Planning puts detail into the scope of the project and the work to be performed. An in-depth logic model is a useful tool that demonstrates the project plan.

- Deliverables:

  - Project scope and performance. *Scope* is conceptualized product acceptance criteria, project deliverables, project exclusions, project constraints, and project assumptions (PMI, 2013).

  - Budget

  - Process and activities

  - Schedule and timeline

  - Determination of resource needs, skills, and talents

- Articulate communication plans.

- Underline potential risks.

- Identify evaluation criteria.

3. Executing

- The work of the project happens here!

- Managing the process ensures the project is in alignment with identified goals, approved changes are implemented, and adjustments to the plan and schedule are made as needed.

- Deliverables:

  - Form, direct, and lead project teams. Project functions and responsibilities are distributed among project teams.

  - Obtain identified resources.

BOX 10.2 Five Phases of Project Management—cont'd

- Communicate information to identified stakeholders and the academic committee.

- Conduct regular status meetings.

4. Monitoring and Controlling

- Identified criteria and performance measurements are evaluated, measured, and verified. Results are accepted, or corrective actions taken to return the project to alignment with plans.

- Deliverables:

  - Performance measurements are made against baseline measurements.

  - Based on monitoring of the project's progression, corrective action may be taken to keep the project on track.

5. Closing

- A formal and orderly conclusion to the project transpires. A formal closure is the most overlooked process of the project, but it is significant to increase knowledge and understanding.

- Deliverables

  - Final project report of findings is completed and submitted to identified stakeholders and committee members.

  - Final acceptance of the project occurs.

  - Contracts and agreements are finalized.

Source: Cleland & Ireland, 2007; PMI, 2013; PMI, 2015; Project Insight, 2015.

- Leadership is a relational activity.

- Issues can be best analyzed and explained with a multidisciplined understanding of the complexity and dynamics of the system.

- Leadership should be particularly aware of the culture because it sends powerful messages about leadership values, ethics, and how managers are expected to perform.

Transformational leaders build cultures that are conducive to implementation of EBP recommendations. Transformational leaders move themselves and others to exceed their practice expectations and achieve better outcomes, including emotional and intellectual satisfaction. Transformational leaders are authentic and communicate often and honestly (Bass, 1995; Bass & Riggio, 2006; Doody & Doody, 2012; Ryeroft-Malone, 2012).

Leadership Skills and Behaviors for Managing a Project or Program

What are the right leadership behaviors for project and program management success? This question was asked of 650 program and project management practitioners. The project management structure of the survey was based on PMI's (2013) publications. Findings from the survey were consistent regardless of role, experience, organizational size, or geography. One identified difference found that program managers focused more on understanding organizational dynamics. Key leadership behaviors adapted from the survey are presented in Box 10.3.

Three major themes resonate for successful leadership. First is *communication*. The significance of communication cannot be overstated when leadership skills and behaviors are needed. *Trust* is another essential skill; trust inspires credibility. Demonstrations of trust include maintaining confidences and keeping commitments. Finally, a successful leader of projects has *integrity*. Be ethical, honest, and straightforward (Carter et al., 2013).

CHAPTER SUMMARY AND AFTERTHOUGHTS

The importance of planning for implementation helps you focus on prioritizing process, action, and intervention. Details of your plan are essential components of the written proposal for your academic committee, for the stakeholders, and for the application to the Institutional Review Board. (See Chapter 14 for information regarding writing the project proposal.) Creation of a well-designed logic model enhances understanding and decision making for your project committee. The logic model should be an appendix to your project proposal. In summary, the importance of a well-designed plan for implementation cannot be overstated. Abraham Lincoln is reported to have stated, "If I had 60 minutes to cut down a tree, I would spend 40 minutes sharpening the ax and 20 minutes cutting it down" (Stack, 2000).

BOX 10.3 Leadership Skills and Behaviors for Program and Project Managers

Strong Communication Skills

- Promote two-way communication: Be a respectful listener and speaker.

- Keep stakeholders, academic committee members, and your working teams informed on a regular basis. Remember that *useful feedback* is a core concept of the implementation model and increases acceptance (Titler, 2008).

Independent Actions

- Results: Meet personal commitments.

- Proactive: Take appropriate actions without being told.

- Flexibility: Adjust and adapt to change.

Team or Group Leadership

- Empower others to take action.

- Set challenging, achievable short- and long-term goals.

- Monitor activities and track progress.

- Build trust and credibility: Maintain confidences and keep commitments.

- Motivate others to higher levels of performance.

- Demonstrate integrity: Be straightforward and honest; demonstrate ethical standards.

Organizational Awareness

- Think strategically: Understand the long-term effects of your decisions.

- Be cognizant of the context including interpersonal and group dynamics.

- Help construct improvement by motivating others to work through change.

Continued

BOX 10.3 Leadership Skills and Behaviors for Program and Project
Managers—cont'd

Commitments to the Organization

* Keep stakeholders updated of relevant information (PMI, 2013).

* Use wise judgment for effective decision making.

* Be goal driven and meet deadlines.

* Communicate successes, evaluation results, and progress directly with
  those implementing the actions. Organize or be a presenter in planned,
  regular meetings.

* Achieve objectives by holding others accountable.

Source: Carter, Tull, & VanRooy, 2013.

CASE STUDY

*Melissa is a baccalaureate-prepared school nurse currently enrolled in a DNP
program. She works with elementary school children in kindergarten through fifth
grade. During the summer, Melissa works as the camp nurse in a beautiful moun-
tain setting. The camp is designed for healthy elementary school children, and
Melissa is the only healthcare worker at the camp. Every week during the 11 weeks
of summer, approximately 170 different children attend the camp. Thirty staff
members, mostly younger than 20 years of age, work with the children and perform
duties such as cooking and maintenance. Melissa often feels as though her load is
200 children per week.*

*Before arriving at the camp, parents of the children complete hard copies of the
general health history form, medical records form, and contact information. When
parents drop off their children at camp, they are required to check in with Melissa
to validate that the forms are completed. Melissa also validates the information
with parents and asks questions as needed. Nearly 40% of the children take a
medication. Many are prn medications such as common antiallergy medications.
Other medications include epinephrine pens and medications for attention-deficit
disorder and autism. It is common to see big buckets of medications and health
forms at the close of registration on the first day of camp. Melissa then files the
health forms and organizes the medications according to the times due. Times for*

medication administration generally include breakfast, lunch, and bedtime. In the afternoon of the first day at camp, Melissa checks for head lice. During the remainder of the week, Melissa administers medication and applies first aid. At the end of the fun week at camp, Melissa returns the unused medications to the parents. All of Melissa's nursing actions are charted.

Melissa has several concerns about the check-in process: security, data inscription, data integrity, and Health Insurance Portability and Accountability Act (HIPAA) violation. She envisions an interactive Website for parents to complete the health forms online and allow parents to check that their child received the appropriate medication and dose. If first aid is provided, parents can go online and follow the treatment and the child's response.

Melissa makes the decision that her DNP project will address the practice issues of the camp nurse. She follows the evidence-based practice process of creating a PICO(T) question based on the camp issues, completes a thorough evidence search, and concludes with a written synthesis and the following recommendations or guidelines for practice:

Summer camps for elementary aged school children should implement a computer program for parents to submit the health history form, medical records form, and contact information before dropping their child off at camp. Research indicates that a child's health information is more accurate and more easily accessible to the camp nurse, thus resulting in fewer medical errors and better care.

- *Select a framework for Melissa's plans for implementation. Consider whether Melissa's project will include direct or indirect care.*

- *Assess Melissa's needs for project management.*

- *Create a logic model for Melissa's implementation actions.*

- *Analyze leadership skills that Melissa should adapt.*

(Case study provided by Kelley Connor.)

WRITING REMINDERS...

Grammar

Grammar is paramount to keeping a captive audience. Good grammar disguises the fact that there is even an author and instead focuses the reader on the content. Good grammar is the ultimate manipulation for the writer to hide in well-constructed sentences and steer the reader toward the writer's academic argument. However, good writing and avoiding the pitfalls of bad grammar take practice. Helpful references for application of good grammar for reports and publications include the following:

American Psychological Association (APA). (2010). *Publication manual of the American Psychological Association.* Washington, DC: APA.

Schimel, J. (2012). *Writing science: How to write papers that get cited and proposals that get funded.* New York, NY: Oxford University Press.

Wilson, K., & Wauson, J. (2010). *The AMA handbook of business writing: The ultimate guide to style, grammar, usage, punctuation, construction, and formatting.* New York, NY: American Management Association.

REFERENCES

Akrani, G. (2015). *Importance of planning.* Retrieved from http://kalyan-city.blogspot.com/2012/02/importance-of-planning-why-planning-is.html

Association for Project Management (APM). (2015). *What is project management?* Retrieved from https://www.apm.org.uk/WhatIsPM

Bass, B.M. (1995). Theory of transformational leadership. *Leadership Quarterly, 6*(4), 463–478.

Bass, B.M., & Riggio, R.E. (2006). *Transformational leadership* (2nd ed.). Mahwah, NJ: Lawrence Erlbaum Associates.

BusinessDictionary.com. (2015). *Management.* Retrieved from http://www.businessdictionary.com/definition/management.html

Carter, L., Tull, K., & VanRooy, D. (2013). *Key leadership behaviors necessary to advance in project management.* Berea, OH: Baldwin Wallace University. Retrieved from https://www.bw.edu/academics/cpd/Key%20Leadership%20Behaviors%202013%20BW%20PRADCO.pdf

Centers for Disease Control and Prevention (CDC) Division for Heart Disease and Stroke Prevention. (2013). *Evaluation guide: Developing and using a logic model.* Washington, DC: Department of Health and Human Services. Retrieved from http://www.cdc.gov/dhdsp/programs/spha/evaluation_guides/logic_model.htm

Cleland, D.I., & Ireland, L.R. (2007). *Project management: Strategic design and implementation* (5th ed.). New York, NY: McGraw-Hill.

Doody, O., & Doody, C.M. (2012). Transformational leadership in nursing practice. *British Journal of Nursing, 21*(2), 1212–1218.

Farquhar, C.M., Stryer, D., & Slutsky, J. (2002). Translating research into practice: The future ahead. *International Journal of Quality Health Care, 14*(3), 233–249.

Graham, I.D., Logan, J., & Robinson, N. (2006). Lost in knowledge translation: Time for a map? *Journal of Continuing Education in the Health Professions, 26*(1), 13–24.

Grove, S.K., Burns, N., & Gray, J.R. (2013). *The practice of nursing research: Appraisal, synthesis, and generation of evidence* (7th ed.). St. Louis, MO: Elsevier Saunders

Hill, B. (2015). The importance of planning in an organization. *Houston Chronicle.* Retrieved from http://smallbusiness.chron.com/importance-planning-organization-1137.html

Kellogg Foundation. (2004). *Logic model development guide.* Battle Creek, MI: W.K. Kellogg Foundation. Retrieved from http://www.smartgivers.org/uploads/logicmodelguide pdf.pdf

Kitson, A.L., Rycroft-Malone, J., & Titchen, A. (2008). Evaluating the successful implementation of evidence into practice using the PARIHS framework: Theoretical and practical challenges. *Implementation Science, 3*(1). Retrieved from http://www.implementationscience.com/content/3/1/1

Leeman, J., & Sandelowski, M. (2012). Practice-based evidence and qualitative inquiry. *Journal of Nursing Scholarship, 44*(2), 171–179.

McLaughlin, J.A., & Jordan, G.B. (2010). Using logic models. In: S.H. Wholey, H.P. Hatry, & K.E. Newcomer, (Eds.). *Handbook of practical program evaluation* (3rd ed.). San Francisco, CA: Jossey-Bass.

Oxford Dictionaries. (2014). Retrieved from http://www.oxforddictionaries.com/definition/english/

Project Insight. (2015). *5 basic phases of project management.* Retrieved from http://www.projectinsight.net/project-management-basics/basic-project-management-phases

Project Management Institute (PMI). (2013). *A guide to the project management body of knowledge* (5th ed.). Newtown Square, PA: PMI.

Project Management Institute (PMI). (2015). *What is project management?* Retrieved from http://www.pmi.org/About-Us/About-Us-What-is-Project-Management.aspx

Pujari, S. (2015). *What is the importance of planning in management?* Retrieved from http://www.yourarticlelibrary.com/planning/what-is-the-importance-of-planning-in-management/903/

Rogers, E. (2003). *Diffusion of innovations* (5th ed.). New York, NY: Free Press.

Rycroft-Malone, J. (2012). Leadership matters. *Worldviews on Evidence-Based Practice, 9*(3), 127–128.

Sampselle, C.M. (2010). The Michigan Center for Health Intervention (MICHIN): facilitating translational science. *Research and Theory for Nursing Practice: An International Journal, 24*(1), 6–8.

Speroff, T., James, B.C., Nelson, E.C., Headrick, L.A., & Brommels, M. (2004). Guidelines for appraisal and publication of PDSA quality improvement. *Quality Management Health Care, 13*(1), 33–39.

Stack, L. (2000). *The importance of planning and prioritizing.* Retrieved from http://www.theproductivitypro.com/FeaturedArticles/article00017.htm

Tate, W. (2013). *Managing leadership from a systemic perspective.* London: Centre for Progressive Leadership. Retrieved from http://www.londonmet.ac.uk/media/london-metropolitan-university/london-met-documents/faculties/guildhall-faculty-of-business-and-law/london-metropolitan-business-school/research-centres/cpl/publications/CPL-WP---Managing-leadership-from-a-systemic-perspective—(William-Tate).pdf

Timmermans, S., & Berg, M. (2003). *The gold standard: The challenge of evidence-based medicine and standardization in health care.* Philadelphia, PA: Temple University Press.

Titler, M.G. (2008). The evidence for evidence-based practice implementation. In R. G. Hughes (Ed.). *Patient safety and quality: An evidence-based handbook for nurses.* Rockville, MD: Agency for Healthcare Research and Quality (AHRQ).

Titler, M.G., & Everett, L.Q. (2001). Translating research into practice: Considerations for critical care investigators. *Critical Care Nursing Clinics of North America, 13*(4), 587–604.

Watson, J. (1979). *Theory of human caring.* Retrieved from http://watsoncaringscience. org/images/features/library/THEORY%20OF%20HUMAN%20CARING_Website. pdf

Wholey, J.S., Hatry, H.P., & Newcomer, K.E. (Eds.) (2010). *Handbook of practical program evaluation* (3rd ed.). San Francisco, CA: Jossey-Bass.

Woods, N.F., & Magyary, D.L. (2010). Translational research: Why nursing's interdisciplinary collaboration is essential. *Research and Theory for Nursing Practice: An International Journal, 24*(1), 9–24.

Woolf, S.H. (2008). The meaning of translational research and why it matters. *JAMA, 292*(2), 211–213.

World Health Organization (WHO). (2012). *Turning research into practice: Suggested actions from case studies from sexual and reproductive health research.* Geneva: WHO. Retrieved from http://whqlibdoc.who.int/publications/2006/9241594837_eng.pdf

IF YOU WANT TO READ MORE...

Centers for Disease Control (CDC). (n.d.). *Logic models: Step 2b.* Retrieved from http:// www.cdc.gov/oralhealth/state_programs/pdf/logic_models.pdf

Kellogg Foundation. (2004). *Logic model development guide.* Battle Creek, MI: W.K. Kellogg Foundation. Retrieved from http://www.smartgivers.org/uploads/logicmodel-guidepdf.pdf

Project Management Institute (PMI). (2013). *A guide to the project management body of knowledge* (3rd ed.). Newtown Square, PA: PMI.

Wholey, J.S., Hatry, H.P., & Newcomer, K.E. (Eds.) (2010). *Handbook of practical program evaluation* (3rd ed.). San Francisco, CA: Jossey-Bass.

Planning for Implementation: Evaluation

If we want more evidence-based practice, we need more practice-based evidence.

GREEN & OTTOSON, 2004

OUTCOME OBJECTIVES

- Discuss the importance of evaluation.
- Compare and contrast the meaning and purpose for project evaluation and research analysis.
- Describe types of evaluation.
- Examine evaluation tools and determine appropriate application.
- Recommend practices for disseminating evaluation findings.

TERMS

Analysis	Formative evaluation	Outcome evaluation
Data	Interpretation	Pilot study

Continued

TERMS—cont'd

Process evaluation   Quality improvement   Research analysis
Project evaluation   Quantitative analysis Summative evaluation
Qualitative analysis

Chapter 10 focuses on planning for project integration, management, and leadership of evidence-based practice (EBP) recommendations within a specific context. This chapter continues presentation of information related to the broad topic of planning for implementation with the focus on project evaluation. Project evaluation is about developing information to explain activities and processes as well as answer questions about feasibility and effectiveness. Evaluation identifies problems as they arise, thereby allowing adjustments to be made. The outcome goal of project evaluation is to demonstrate improvement or change in a specified context. Evaluation is, indeed, an integral component of the practice project (Grove, Burns, & Gray, 2013; Harvey & Wensing, 2003; Polit & Beck, 2012; Stern, 2005).

Content in this chapter establishes the importance of evaluation and then proceeds to offer information about types of evaluation. Review of methods for data collection, analysis, and interpretation is also included. Finally, hints for using evaluation results are provided.

THE IMPORTANCE OF PROJECT EVALUATION

This section begins with a review of terms because definitions enhance understanding. Differentiating the terms *project evaluation* from *research analysis* contributes to understanding the focus of building an evaluation plan for a practice project. Recall that a *project* relates to an identified set of activities set in a specific context and performed within a specified time (Victoria Local Sustainability Accord, 2010). *Project evaluation* is described as a structured process for systematically collecting information about activities, processes, attributes, and outcomes for the purpose of learning, decision making, and improvement related to a specific context (Kellogg Foundation, 2004; Victoria Local Sustainability Accord, 2010). *Research* is described as a "diligent, systematic investigation to validate and refine existing knowledge and generate new knowledge" (Grove et al., 2013, p 1). *Analysis* is the scrutiny or detailed examination of parts or variables about a specific topic or hypothesis for the purpose

---

BOX 11.1 Importance of Project Evaluation

- Evaluation *during* the project

  - Allows for tracking progress and identifying problems; adjustments or corrective action can be addressed, thereby allowing for continual improvement or change

  - Provides useful information about process and activities

  - Demonstrates transparency and accountability for stakeholders

  - Enhances understanding of the context where the project occurs

  - Enhances understanding of the target population

- Evaluation of project *outcomes*

  - Increases understanding of *how* outcomes were achieved

  - Identifies efficiency of resources and activities

  - Increases understanding of meaningfulness of process and activities and change or improvement for project participants

  - Informs sustainability plans

  - Informs practice

Sources: CDC, 2011; Victoria Local Sustainability Accord, 2010; Zarinpoush, 2006.

of interpretation and making predictions. Box 11.1 contributes to understanding the importance of a well-planned project evaluation.

DEVELOPING THE PLAN FOR PROJECT EVALUATION

The purpose of an evaluation plan is to assess the process, actions, context, outcomes, and impact of integrating identified EBP recommendations into the practice setting. However, there is a great deal of complexity in this task. The best approach to untangling the complexity of evaluation is to create a written plan to understand how the program works and assumptions underlying the process. The written evaluation plan is an important section of your project proposal (see Chapter 14). The written evaluation plan informs your academic committee and stakeholders by providing clarification about priorities, resources, time, and skills (Centers for Disease Control and Prevention [CDC], 2011).

Types of Evaluation

Selection of an evaluation method provides direction and development for your evaluation. An evaluation method keeps you focused on the primary purpose for the evaluation and guides the evaluation questions to be answered and the data to be collected. The best-known model for planning evaluation of projects consists of formative and summative evaluations because it considers evaluation from multiple perspectives (Kellogg Foundation, 2004; Titler, Everett, & Adams, 2007; Victoria Local Sustainability Accord, 2010; Zarinpoush, 2006).

Formative evaluation begins early and is an ongoing evaluation throughout the implementation of the project. The purpose of formative evaluation is to assess or monitor actions and process before and during the project. Formative evaluation strengthens decision-making abilities by increasing the understanding of the project's parts, processes, objectives, and costs. A needs assessment of context is often completed before implementation as part of the formative evaluation. Monitoring of the context, process, and actions to assess operational aspects of the project and suggest ways to improve or change occurs during implementation. *Process evaluation* is a term complementary to formative evaluation, and you may see it used in other publications. Process evaluation focuses on input, activities, and output when evaluating whether the project is operating as planned or not (LoBiondo-Wood & Haber, 2010; Polit & Beck, 2012; Victoria Local Sustainability Accord, 2010; Wholey, Hatry, & Newcomer, 2010; Zarinpoush, 2006; Zint, 2010).

Summative evaluation occurs at the end of the project or after the project is completed. Summative evaluation assesses the overall effectiveness or impact of the project's achievements or outputs and whether the defined goals or outcomes were accomplished or not. Summative evaluation is outcome focused rather than process focused and assesses the goals of the project, determines what was learned, and makes suggestions for improvement (Victoria Local Sustainability Accord, 2010; Polit & Beck, 2012; Zarinpoush, 2006; Zint, 2010).

Two terms often used with types of healthcare project evaluations are *pilot study* and *quality improvement (QI)*. Both terms are similar in meaning to formative and summative evaluation, yet with subtle differences. The terms are described here for the purpose of increased understanding of meaning and use.

Box 11.2 is a description of a *pilot study*. A pilot study is a small-scale, preliminary research study to assess feasibility, time, cost, risks, benefits, and predict effect size for a larger research study.

BOX 11.2 Description of a Pilot Study

- The sample size is small because recruitment is based on accessibility of participants and budgetary constraints.

- Pilot studies generally occur in one setting or context that is specific to your practice.

- One context limits generalizability.

- Pilot studies are short in duration.

- Pilot studies are sometimes referred to as *feasibility studies*. Feasibility information assists in making program or project modifications to plan and design larger efficacy trials and generate evidence for wider use.

- Pilot studies can identify potential problems about implementation, process, data collection, and evaluation methods.

- Pilot studies are useful to assess specific parts of a project or program that are new or unclear.

- Pilot studies describe or explore.

- Pilot study results are useful in decision making because results increase understanding of underlying assumptions, project activities, process, and results.

- Pilot study findings affect decisions about the usefulness of the project, ways to improve the project, and assess the significance of change and implementation.

Sources: Grove, Burns, & Gray, 2013; Leon, Davis, & Kraemer, 2011; Lewis-Beck, Bryman, & Liao, 2004; Polit & Beck, 2012; Timmermans & Berg, 2003; Wholey, Hatry, & Newcomer, 2010.

QI projects focus on "How are we doing?" and "How can we do it better?" (Edwards, 2008). QI evaluates process and desired outcome because *quality* is linked to service delivery and performance. *Continuous QI (CQI)* is a continuous monitoring system that evaluates progress. CQI is a method for evaluation of project sustainability (see Chapter 13). Successful QI and CQI:

- Work as systems and processes

- Focus on patient safety and care

- Focus on teamwork

- Focus on using collected data for improvement (Health Resources and Services Administration [HRSA], 2011)

Establishing Questions for Evaluation

The first step in creating an evaluation plan is to identify questions specific to your project. Evaluation questions are based on anticipated outcomes of the EBP recommendations for practice. Questions assist identification of specific criteria for project evaluation. Box 11.3 provides example questions for evaluation planning.

Answers to evaluation questions must be reliable and believable. Therefore, collection and evaluation of information must be consistent, thorough, and thoughtful (Kellogg Foundation, 2004). The next section provides suggestions for collection of information.

Figure 11.1 is an example of building an evaluation plan. This example is useful as a reference while reading the text narrative.

Collection of Data for Evaluation

Methods for making decisions about what data to collect for evaluation are based on your evaluation questions. Decide what information is needed to answer the questions, how the information will be collected and from whom, and how the information will be analyzed. A good plan decreases the risk of collecting irrelevant information and keeps your data collection and analysis plan focused on the question. Make the plan "simple, flexible, and responsive to changing needs of the project" (Kellogg Foundation, 2004, p 70).

Quantitative, qualitative, and mixed methods are the categories for collecting and analyzing data for project evaluation. A mixed methods approach for project evaluation is encouraged for the purpose of fully informing decision making with depth and breadth of information. However, both quantitative and qualitative data sources have strengths and weaknesses. Combining the two designs provides a method to understand process and context related to change and improvement more fully (Zarinpoush, 2006). For example, a quantitative survey can provide aggregate information about how many pregnant refugee patients attend a group prenatal clinic. However, a quantitative survey does not provide individual information about why the patients attend a group clinic instead of an individual office visit with a healthcare provider.

Qualitative methods of evaluation use words, conversations, interviews, and stories to collect information. However, personal interactions for collection of

---

BOX 11.3 Examples of Questions for Evaluation Planning

Formative Evaluation Questions

- Are the recommended actions of project participants performed as planned?

- Is implementation of the recommendations reaching the intended patient population?

- Are project participants satisfied with their involvement?

- Are planned activities working for the project participants or should modifications be implemented?

- What lessons can be learned during implementation?

Summative Evaluation Questions

- Are the intended numbers of patients participating?

- Are project participants' actions leading to the anticipated EBP recommendations?

- Are unexpected outputs occurring for patients or project participants?

- Do project participants note any changes in their skills, knowledge, attitudes, or behaviors?

- Do patients note any changes or improvements in their care?

- What changes or improvements were noted?

- Did the project meet the needs of the stakeholders?

- Did the EBP recommendations meet the needs that led to the project?

- What other needs were identified that the EBP recommendations did not address?

EBP, evidence-based practice.
Adapted from Zarinpoush, 2006.

evaluation data take more time. On the other hand, the quantity and depth of information provide a wider scope of understanding. Information is analyzed by looking for repetitive themes in the stories, conversations, and interviews. Qualitative designs are built from different philosophical paradigms and

EBP Recommendation(s) for Practice: Summer camps for elementary aged school children should implement a computer program for parents to submit the health history form, medical records form, and contact information before dropping their child off at camp. Research indicates that a child's health information is more accurate and more easily accessible to the camp nurse, thus resulting in fewer medical errors and better care. **Strong** recommendation rating

Type of Evaluation	Questions for Evaluation	Method(s) for Information Collection	Methods for Data Analysis	Interpretation and Presentation
Formative Evaluation	Are the recommended actions of parents performed as planned?	Observation notes	Theme analysis (qualitative)	Story telling
		Focus group; Semi-structured interviews	Theme analysis (qualitative)	Verbal presentation with PowerPoint
	Are the camp nurses satisfied with the online registration or are adjustments needed?	Focus group; Semi-structured interviews; Post-project written questionnaire using open-ended questions	Theme analysis (qualitative)	Written report
	What lessons can be learned from camp nurses and parents regarding the process of submitting health histories online?			
Summative Evaluation	Are the parents participating in the online health history submissions?	Demographics; Survey	Mean, SD (quantitative)	Graphs (e.g., pie graph, bar graph)
	Did the project meet the needs of the camp administrators (stakeholders)?	Electronic health records	Mean, SD, t-test or Chi-square (quantitative)	Verbal presentation with PowerPoint
		Likert-style questionnaire	Theme analysis (qualitative)	Written report
	Were other needs identified from camp nurses, camp administrators, and parents regarding online submission of health histories?	Written questionnaire with open-ended questions; Semi-structured interview		

Distribution of Evaluation Report: Stakeholder(s); Academic committee; End-users; Project participants

FIGURE 11.1 An Example of a Project Evaluation Plan. The intent of this template is to assist development, organization, and meaningfulness for project evaluation. Suggestions for use include adding the completed form to the program logic model and as an appendix to the academic project proposal and stakeholder executive summary. EBP, evidence-based practice.

attempt to construct meaning from experiences or phenomena. Qualitative evidence is useful for understanding details of an implementation process in the contextual reality of the lived experience. Qualitative information is especially useful for understanding an intended user's lived experiences regarding a new project or delivery method. Qualitative methods are considered complex and interpretive (Leeman & Sandelowski, 2012; LoBiondo-Wood & Haber, 2010; Polit & Beck, 2012; Victoria Local Sustainability Accord, 2010). See Appendix A in this textbook for a review of qualitative collection and evaluation methods.

Quantitative evaluation methods collect information with numbers. Quantitative research enrolls large numbers of participants, but there is little personal interaction. Quantitative research is divided into three major design categories, with numerous subcategories within each:

1. Experimental evaluation *must* have randomization, control, and manipulation.

2. Quasiexperimental evaluation does not contain all three elements. Subjects are not randomly assigned and may not have a control group, instead serving as its own control.

3. Quantitative nonexperimental designs have no randomization, control, or manipulation. Nonexperimental designs provide descriptive information that is useful from data collected through observation of participants, process, and actions.

Quantitative evaluation methods usually involve short interactions with participants compared with qualitative methods, which are time intensive (LoBiondo-Wood & Haber, 2010; Polit & Beck, 2014). Descriptive analyses of quantitative data are useful for end users and stakeholders when reporting findings. For example, bar graphs and frequencies are more understandable and meaningful for demonstrating improvement or change. See Appendix B in this textbook for a review of quantitative collection and analysis methods.

Suggested *evaluation tools for collection of project information* are presented in Box 11.4.

With so many options for collection of data, how do you prioritize which tools to use? Your focus should be on the priorities of the key stakeholders. Next, consider feasibility and cost of collecting the information. For example, if the information is easy to obtain, is inexpensive, and has a high priority for the stakeholder, then the data must be collected. If the information source is unclear or inaccessible and the stakeholder gives it a low priority, then reconsider collection of that data (Grove, Kibel, & Hoss, 2005; Zarinpoush, 2006).

BOX 11.4 Suggested Evaluation Tools for Collection of Data

Qualitative Evaluation Tools

- Anecdotal records: stories and narratives about the project from participants
- Electronic health records: documentation of patient safety and care
- Field notes or observation notes: notes taken by evaluator following observation of participants or context
- Focus group: a group guided discussion to explore perceptions of project topics or process
- Interviews: questions between a participant and the evaluator
  - Interviews: informal and conversational
  - Semistructured interviews: open-ended questions and follow-up questions
  - Structured interviews: narrow questions in a specific order and no follow-up questions
- Journal recordings: participants' written self-report of contextual and process activities
- Observation notes
- Questionnaire: printed self-report form to obtain information about a specific topic; short answers
- Site visits: combination of observation and unstructured interviews with participants

Quantitative Evaluation Tools

- Demographics: numeric description of project participants (e.g., age, sex, cultural identity, number of hospitalized days)
- Electronic health records: documentation of patient safety and care
- Preproject survey and postproject survey: quasiexperimental design for evaluation of an intervention

> **BOX 11.4** Suggested Evaluation Tools for Collection of Data—cont'd
>
> - Postproject survey: assessment of achievement of project goals
> - Questionnaire: printed self-report form to obtain information about a specific topic; use of Likert scale for measurement
> - Survey: predetermined questions about a specific topic

Sources: Grove, Burns, & Gray, 2013; Kellogg Foundation, 2004; Zarinpoush, 2006.

Data Analysis and Interpretation

Analysis of collected data follows standard quantitative and qualitative procedures and is beyond the scope of this textbook. Appendixes A and B provide a short review of qualitative and quantitative analyses that are useful and meaningful for the practice setting. You are encouraged, however, to review your textbooks related to quantitative statistical analysis and qualitative theme analysis. Suggestions for useful textbooks or other resources are included with Appendixes A and B.

Time and resources committed to analysis and interpretation are essential because interpretation of the data analysis influences decision making and subsequent actions. *Interpretation* means looking beyond data analysis and making judgments about the meaning of the data related to implementation of the EBP recommendations. Interpretation focuses on how the pieces of the project fit together with contextual considerations. Analysis without interpretation leads to premature conclusions. Interpretation questions to ask about analyzed data might include the following: What do the results mean? What led to the findings? Are the findings significant? Reviewing interpretation of findings with stakeholders will enhance your insight (Kellogg Foundation, 2004).

INTERPRETATION AND COMMUNICATION OF EVALUATION RESULTS

Use and application of results from practice evaluation involve interpretation and communication. Communicating your interpretation of evaluation results to stakeholders within the healthcare organization contributes to decision making about the current project and facilitating strategic planning. The nursing adage, "If it wasn't charted, it wasn't done" applies to project evaluation results. If evaluation results are not interpreted and communicated, evaluation is a waste of time and money for you and the healthcare organization (Zarinpoush, 2006).

Box 11.5 is a list of suggestions for planning how to use evaluation findings during and at the end of project evaluation. This list is helpful in planning for communication with stakeholders, your project committee, end users, and project participants. Use of data results and interpretation are integral parts of your project because transparency contributes to acceptance.

Finally, consider *reporting styles* for communication of the final evaluation and interpretation of results. The intended audiences will be groups or individuals of organizational stakeholders, academic groups, or end users. Your reporting

---

BOX 11.5 Suggestions for Communication of Evaluation Findings and Interpretation

- Identification of strengths and weaknesses of process and actions

- Clarification of options for decision making

- Identification of key contextual features that affect the project

- Identification of ways to improve the work process, setting, or context

- Facilitation of change

- Preparation of process reports and final reports

- Planning for sustainability of project

- Increased knowledge about contextual influence on process and actions

- Increased knowledge about the target population

- Planning for additional projects

- Making evidence-based practice decisions for the organization

- Demonstration of the healthcare organization's ability to perform project evaluations

- Demonstration of organizational accountability of successful project implementation and evaluation

Sources: Kellogg Foundation, 2004; Victoria Local Sustainability Accord, 2010; Zarinpoush, 2006.

and presentation style will depend on the audience's preference, the information to be presented, and the allotted time. Examples of reporting styles include a full written evaluation report, an executive summary, or a PowerPoint presentation (Kellogg Foundation, 2004; Zarinpoush, 2006). See Chapter 15 for detailed information about dissemination of your project results.

CASE STUDY QUESTIONS

Review the Chapter 10 case study. Recall that Melissa, the camp registered nurse and current DNP student, is planning a DNP project using interactive computer technology for parents to complete the health information form for their child. Discuss the following questions about project evaluation for Melissa's DNP project.

- *Select the type of evaluation that will best meet Melissa's needs to implement change and improvement.*

- *Identify evaluation questions or criteria for Melissa's project evaluation.*

- *What evaluation tools will provide the most useful results? Provide rationale.*

- *Describe how Melissa can use and share the evaluation results.*

WRITING REMINDERS...

Plagiarism

"As a member of an intellectual community you are expected to respect the ideas of others in the same way that you would respect any other property that didn't belong to you, and this is true whether you plagiarize on purpose or by accident" (Harvard College Writing Program).

Plagiarism can be avoided by following these easy steps:

- Paraphrase in your own words.

- Cite the source of the paraphrase in the body of the manuscript. Follow APA rules.

- If quoting a source, state it exactly as written. "No one wants to be misquoted" or accused of plagiarism. Avoid long *block quotes*. Strive to keep quotes less than 40 words.

- Cite the source of the quotation, including the page number. Follow APA rules.

- Cite yourself if you are using a paper you previously wrote for a current or previous class.

- References: Be sure all of your in-text citations lead the reader to the reference page of your paper.

- Edit your paper! Carefully review your writing to be sure you have given credit where credit is due (WriteCheck, 2014).

What is considered common knowledge? *Common knowledge* is information considered widely known and therefore does not need a reference or in-text citation. An example is the molecular symbol for water (H_2O). However, recognizing whether or not something is common knowledge can be difficult. If you are uncertain, always err on the side of caution and give credit to the most reliable source or the source you relied on most (Harvard College Writing Program, 2015).

References

Harvard College Writing Program. (2015). What constitutes plagiarism? *Harvard guide to using sources.* Retrieved from http://isites.harvard.edu/icb/icb.do?keyword=k70847&pageid=icb.page342054

WriteCheck (2014). *6 ways to avoid plagiarism in research papers.* Retrieved from http://en.writecheck.com/ways-to-avoid-plagiarism/

APA, American Psychological Association.

CHAPTER SUMMARY AND AFTERTHOUGHTS

Creation of an evaluation plan before implementing your practice project increases the clarity of your project's purpose and direction, thus contributing to a quality project that will be meaningful and useful to your organization and to the practice of nursing. Chapter 12 continues the topic of evaluation by focusing on economic issues important to the value and strength of the project.

REFERENCES

Centers for Disease Control and Prevention (CDC). (2011). *Developing an effective evaluation plan: Setting the course for effective program evaluation.* Atlanta, GA: CDC. Retrieved from http://www.cdc.gov/obesity/downloads/cdc-evaluation-workbook-508.pdf

Edwards, P.J., Huang, D.T., Metcalfe, L.N., & Sainfort, F. (2008). Maximizing your investment in EHR: Utilizing EHRs to inform continuous quality improvement. *Journal of Healthcare Management, 22*(1), 32-37. Retrieved from http://www.ncbi.nlm.nih.gov/pubmed/19267005

Grove, S.K., Burns, N., & Gray, J.R. (2013). *The practice of nursing research: Appraisal, synthesis, and generation of evidence* (7th ed.). St. Louis, MO: Elsevier Saunders.

Grove, J.T., Kibel, B.M., & Hass, T. (2005). *EvaluLead: A guide for shaping and evaluating leadership development programs.* Oakland, CA: The Public Health Institute.

Harvard College Writing Program. (2015). What constitutes plagiarism? *Harvard guide to using sources.* Retrieved from http://isites.harvard.edu/icb/icb.do?keyword=k70847&pageid=icb.page342054

Harvey, G., & Wensing, M. (2003). Methods for evaluation of small scale quality improvement projects. *Quality and Safety in Health Care, 12*(3), 210-214. Retrieved from http://www.ncbi.nlm.nih.gov/pmc/articles/PMC1743722/

Kellogg Foundation. (2004). *Evaluation handbook: Philosophy and expectations.* Battle Creek, MI: Kellogg Foundation. Retrieved from https://www.wkkf.org/resource-directory/resource/2010/w-k-kellogg-foundation-evaluation-handbook

Health Resources and Services Administration (HRSA). (2011). *Quality improvement.* Washington, DC: US Department of Health and Human Services. Retrieved from http://www.hrsa.gov/quality/toolbox/508pdfs/qualityimprovement.pdf

Leeman, J., & Sandelowski, M. (2012). Practice-based evidence and qualitative inquiry. *Journal of Nursing Scholarship, 44*(2), 171-179.

Leon, A.C., Davis, L.L., & Kraemer, H.C. (2011). The role and interpretation of pilot studies in clinical research. *Journal of Psychiatric Research, 45,* 626e-629e.

Lewis-Beck, M.S., Bryman, A., & Liao, T.F. (2004). *The SAGE encyclopedia of social science research methods.* Thousand Oaks, CA: SAGE Publications.

LoBiondo-Wood, G., & Haber, J. (2010). *Nursing research: Methods and critical appraisal for evidence-based practice* (7th ed.). St. Louis, MO: Mosby Elsevier.

Polit, D.F., & Beck, C.T. (2012). *Nursing research: Ggenerating and assessing evidence for nursing practice.* (9th ed.). Philadelphia, PA: Lippincott Williams & Wilkins.

Stern, E. (2005). *Evaluation research methods.* Thousand Oaks, CA: SAGE Publications.

Timmermans, S., & Berg, M. (2003). *The gold standard: The challenge of evidence-based medicine and standardization in health care.* Philadelphia, PA: Temple University Press.

Titler, M.G., Everett, L., & Adams, S. (2007). Implications for implementation science. *Nursing Research, 56*(4), S53-S59.

Victoria Local Sustainability Accord. (2010). *Community sustainability engagement evaluation toolbox.* Victoria, AU: Art9th. Retrieved from http://evaluationtoolbox.net.au

Wholey, J.S., Hatry, H.P., & Newcomer, K.E. (Eds.). (2010). *Handbook of practical program evaluation* (3rd ed.). San Francisco, CA: Jossey-Bass.

WriteCheck (2014). *6 ways to avoid plagiarism in research papers.* Retrieved from http://en.writecheck.com/ways-to-avoid-plagiarism/

Zarinpoush, F. (2006). *Project evaluation guide for nonprofit organizations: Fundamental methods and steps for conducting project evaluation.* Imagine Canada. Retrieved from http://sectorsource.ca/sites/default/files/resources/files/projectguide_final.pdf

Zint, M. (May 2010). *My environmental education evaluation resource assistant (MEERA).* *Science Direct, (33)*2, 178-179.

IF YOU WANT TO READ MORE...

Kellogg Foundation. (2004). *Evaluation handbook: Philosophy and expectations.* Battle Creek, MI: Kellogg Foundation. Retrieved from http://www.wkkf.org/resource-directory/resource/2010/w-k-kellogg-foundation-evaluation-handbook

Victoria Local Sustainability Accord. (2010). *Community sustainability engagement evaluation toolbox.* Victoria, Australia: Art9th. Retrieved from http://evaluationtoolbox.net .au

Wholey, J.S., Hatry, H.P., & Newcomer, K.E. (Eds.). (2010). *Handbook of practical program evaluation* (3rd ed.). San Francisco, CA: Jossey-Bass.

Zarinpoush, F. (2006). *Project evaluation guide for nonprofit organizations: Fundamental methods and steps for conducting project evaluation.* Imagine Canada. Retrieved from http://sectorsource.ca/sites/default/files/resources/files/projectguide_final.pdf

12

Planning for Implementation: Cost Management, Economic Analysis, and Risk Management

If your actions inspire others to dream more, learn more, do more and become more, you are a leader.

JOHN QUINCY ADAMS

OUTCOME OBJECTIVES

- Discuss the similarities and differences between cost management and economic analysis.

Continued

- Describe the importance of risk management.
- Create plans for ensuring patient safety and efficient management of resources during implementation of your DNP project.

TERMS

Budget	Cost management	Economic analysis
Cost-benefit analysis	Cost-minimization	Efficiency
Cost-effectiveness	analysis	Risk management
analysis	Cost-utility analysis	Risk indexes

Cost management of a DNP project involves estimating, budgeting, and controlling costs (American National Standards Institute [ANSI], 2004). *Economic analysis* (also called *cost analysis*) focuses on whether benefits outweigh costs (Polit & Beck, 2012). This implies that cost management includes actions that occur before and during the process of DNP project implementation, whereas economic analysis occurs with or after evaluation of DNP project outcomes. Economic analysis is a practical tool for some, but not all, DNP projects. Economic analysis for a DNP project depends on topic, process, context, and need. An economic analysis may be more useful for a translational science phase III large-scale comparative-effectiveness study as an intraprofessional, collaborative study. See Chapter 16 for information about postgraduate collaborations. Cost management, however, centers on resources and costs of supporting and sustaining implementation of the DNP project. Therefore, every DNP project should have a cost management plan. The first part of this chapter provides details about cost management and cost analysis, leading to an understanding of purpose, importance, and differences. The second half of the chapter focuses on *risk management*. Objectives of risk management are to "increase the probability and impact of positive events and decrease the probability and impact of events adverse to the project" (ANSI, 2004, p 237), including the impact of cost (ANSI, 2004).

COST MANAGEMENT

A proposal for a DNP project budget is important for business decisions of healthcare organizations because the budget proposal estimates costs or expenses, revenues, and resources over a specified period of time. A budget proposal assists in decision making for implementation of your DNP project as well as the baseline for cost control. Budgets establish parameters for the cost of performance by how funds are allocated (Lister, 2015).

The first step in cost management is estimating costs, beginning with an estimation of inputs or revenues. Estimated revenues are based on actual costs from similar projects. For example, Medicare reimbursements for appointment visits and laboratory tests can be revenue producers for a nursing-led healthcare clinic. Cost outputs in a healthcare clinic include both direct and indirect costs. Direct and indirect budget outputs have meanings similar to direct and indirect patient-centered care (see Chapter 2). Budget costs categorized as *direct costs* relate to salaries and charges of nursing care, physician time, medications, and treatments. Budget costs categorized as *indirect costs* include administrative tasks (e.g., operations, management, accountants), information technology, utilities, system structures, and processes. Depending on the topic of the DNP project, direct and indirect costs also apply to patients. Direct costs to patients include debits not covered by healthcare insurance. Indirect costs to patients focus on time off from work for self and/or family members and expenses related to travel for receipt of health care (World Health Organization [WHO], 2003). An example of a budget is presented in Table 12.1. The example uses fictitious input as an example of a budget for a clinic model that serves low-income refugee patients.

Management of budget outcomes or outputs, also called *cost control*, begins with a baseline of costs against which budget outcomes or outputs can be measured. Management of outputs also includes a time frame for measuring, monitoring, and controlling cost performance. Tasks for managing projected outcomes during implementation of the DNP project are listed here (ANSI, 2004):

- Monitor, or intervene as needed, the project activities and processes that create change or flexibility to the baseline budget.

- Decisions related to activity or process change, if requested, are made in consultation with stakeholders.

- Inform appropriate healthcare personnel of approved changes.

- Monitor for cost overruns; be sure an overrun does not exceed funding authorization or affect the total project cost.

- Monitor for variance in the baseline.

- Keep a record of all appropriate changes and costs against the cost baseline.

TABLE 12.1 Nurse-Run Clinic for Refugees—Budget Model*

Number of patients	Year 0 Startup	Year 1 20	Year 2 40	Year 3 60
Revenues (in Dollars)				
Grant	75,000	—	—	—
Midwife care; Medicaid reimbursement	—	30,000	60,000	90,000
Social worker, Medicaid reimbursement, 12 h/mth	—	7,200	7,400	7,600
Language interpreters; Medicaid reimbursement for 3 interpreters, 8 h/mth	—	7,200	7,200	7,200
Taxi service for pts; Medicaid reimbursement	—	2,000	4,000	6,000
Other revenue	—	—		
Total revenues	75,000	46,400	78,600	110,800
Operating Expenses (in Dollars)				
DIRECT CARE				
Midwife care, part time	3,000	15,000	20,000	30,000
Peer health advocates, part time	2,500	15,000	15,000	20,000
Social worker, part time	—	6,500	6,600	6,700
Language interpreters, part time	—	6,500	6,500	6,500
Registed nurses (2): 12 h/mth	—	8,600	8,800	9,000
Other direct care expenses	—			
Total Direct Expenses	5,500	51,600	56,900	72,200
INDIRECT CARE				
Office staff (1)	2,000	3,800	3,800	5,000
Clinic Manager, 18 h/mth	10,500	10,000	10,000	10,000
Other indirect care expenses	—	—	—	—
Total Indirect Expenses	12,500	13,800	13,800	15,000
Total Expenses	18,000	65,400	70,700	87,200

	Year 0 Startup	Year 1 20	Year 2 40	Year 3 60
TABLE 12.1 Nurse-Run Clinic for Refugees—Budget Model—cont'd				
Number of patients				
Expendables				
Medical supplies and equipment	40,000	3,000	3,000	3,000
Office supplies	5,000	1,000	1,000	1,000
Patient teaching material	12,000	1,000	1,000	1,000
Nonreimbursed taxi service for patient	—	3,000	3,000	3,000
Other Expenses	—	—	—	—
Total Expendable Expenses	57,000	8,000	8,000	8,000
TOTAL OPERATING EXPENSES	75,000	73,400	78,700	95,200
TOTAL NET INCOME/LOSS	0	(27,000)	(200)	15,600

Data and monetary entries are fictional.

ECONOMIC ANALYSIS

Economic analysis (also called cost analysis) is an evaluation of cost and outcome for the purpose of controlling costs associated with change of healthcare practices. Economic analysis assesses whether benefits outweigh costs, thereby affecting decisions about economic viability of a DNP project (Polit & Beck, 2012).

Note that healthcare costs vary according to context, thereby affecting the economic analysis. For example, perspectives differ regarding location of healthcare practices, monetary currencies, and available resources. Context also influences economic perspectives among patients, healthcare providers, hospitals, insurance companies, and politicians related to outcome expectations (Polit & Beck, 2012; WHO, 2003). As you read the next section, keep in mind the importance of context in the four categories of economic analysis that are useful in cost analysis of a DNP project.

Types of Economic Analyses

Types of economic analyses fall into four general categories: (1) cost-effectiveness, (2) cost-utility, (3) cost-benefit, and (4) cost-minimization. These types of analyses provide different information to assess if the benefits of the DNP project outweigh the monetary costs. Indeed, change may be expensive, but existing practices may also be expensive.

Cost-effectiveness analysis compares the relationship between resource costs of alternative interventions or courses of action and a health outcome. For example, analysis of two medications that lower blood pressure are compared in terms of cost and outcome. The findings contribute to decision making. The outcome is more difficult, however, when the outcome is assigning a dollar amount to the value of human life (Grove, Burns, & Gray, 2013; Joanna Briggs Institute [JBI], 2014; Polit & Beck, 2012; WHO, 2003).

Cost-utility analysis is similar to cost-effectiveness analysis except the outcome is focused on morbidity, mortality, and quality of life indicators. Use of cost-utility analysis allows for comparison of different outcomes over time correlated with the cost of the action or intervention (Grove, Burns, & Gray, 2013; JBI, 2014; Polit & Beck, 2012; WHO, 2003).

Cost-benefit analysis is distinguished from cost-effectiveness analysis and cost-utility analysis in that both costs and benefits are measured in monetary units. In health care, there remains a difficult challenge to assign a monetary value to a patient service (JBI, 2014; Polit & Beck, 2012).

Cost-minimization analysis has been called a practical economic analysis. Cost-minimization comparisons are assumed to be equivalent, and only the costs of intervention are compared. For example, comparison of a generic and brand name medication is made in which both dose and therapeutic outcomes are equivalent (JBI, 2014; WHO, 2003).

Economic analyses can be evaluated using *risk indexes*. A risk index assists interpretation of an economic analysis based on the comparative aspect of two dichotomous variables measured on a nominal level. A risk index employs a 2×2 contingency table to compare change. Risk indexes can be used for clinical decision making by assessing absolute change or the actual difference between two variables, as well as relative change or the comparison among groups (Polit, 2010). Detailed information and examples for calculating risk indexes to assist in economic analysis are found in Appendix B of this textbook.

RISK MANAGEMENT

Risk management is another important part of planning for your DNP project. *Risk* is defined as an "uncertain event or condition that, if it occurs, has a positive or negative impact on a project's objectives such as time, cost, scope, quality, etc." (Department of Health and Human Services [DHHS], n.d., p 1 of 6). Risk originates within an element of uncertainty. Risk management focuses on directly or indirectly reducing harm or injury to patients, staff, and visitors, thereby increasing patient safety during implementation of the DNP project while maintaining control of costs within the identified project budget. As the manager for your DNP project, a plan to prevent or minimize risk is essential. Note that risk has contextual influences, meaning that risks are assessed within the context of the environment and relationships that exist within the organization (Chartered Accountants, 2013).

To summarize, risk management planning can prevent compromises to patient care and reduce liability risks that contribute to financial losses (Elearning, 2015). In today's business and litigious environment, your personal involvement with risk management of your DNP project is increasingly important. Planning for risk increases your awareness and enhances your observation skills.

Planning for Risk Management

Risk management is a proven structure that follows a process of identification, assessment, response, communication, and monitoring of risks. A risk management plan provides information for decision making. The risk management plan for your DNP project is an iterative process that begins before implementation and continues until closure. Systematically thinking about all possible outcomes before an event and defining procedures to accept, avoid, or minimize the impact of risk on the DNP project summarizes the purpose and strength of a risk management plan. Types of risk to consider during the DNP process include the following (ANSI, 2004):

- Financial risk

- Legal risk

- Government or political risk

- Intangible risk (e.g., human resources, skill sets, relationships)

- Technical risk (e.g., infrastructure, software, information technology security)

- Security risk (e.g., documentation)

Identification of risk is the first step in a risk management plan. Identification of potential risk begins before implementation of the DNP project, but it may also occur at any time throughout the DNP project. Common methods of risk identification include brainstorming, interviewing, diagramming, and SWOT analysis. The goal of *brainstorming* is to identify and create a list of risks that may arise with implementation of the DNP project. Brainstorming with your DNP project team or a multiprofessional group whose members work within the contextual setting of the DNP project is a good source of ideas about risk. *Interviewing* staff and healthcare personnel with years of work experience and within the contextual setting of the DNP project is a main source for risk identification. A conceptual *diagram* or concept map is another method to identify contextual factors contributing to risk. Conceptual diagrams are useful for identifying cause and effect of risk. Finally, a *SWOT analysis* is an easy-to-use tool for analyzing risk. SWOT is an acronym for strengths, weaknesses, opportunities, and threats. A SWOT analysis examines the project from each SWOT perspective, thereby increasing the range of risk identification (ANSI, 2004). Figure 12.1 is an example of a SWOT analysis.

Assessment and prioritization according to level of importance occur next in the risk management process. Prioritization of risk is best illustrated with a *probability and impact* matrix that arranges each identified risk by level of probability and impact. *Probability* is the chance that a risk will occur. *Impact* is the potential effect, either positive (opportunity) or negative (threat), on a project outcome

Strengths	Weaknesses
• Support from medical staff • Support from nursing staff • Support from hospital administration • Scheduling through the computer program • Provision of charity care by hospital • Provision of wellness care and maintenance therapy for patients with an inability to pay for health care	• Target clinic population underinsured or uninsurable and frequents the emergency department for health care • Unidentified support from ancillary staff • Costs: utilities, staff, supplies
Opportunities	**Threats**
• Improved health in the community • "Give back" to the community; volunteer services • Cost savings through decreased cost of emergency department care for subacute and wellness care of underinsured and uninsured patients	• Cost of liability insurance for healthcare staff who work at the clinic • Lack of monetary resources • Hospital policies • Language barriers • Potential lack of volunteers • Perceived costs • Lack of reimbursement for patient care

FIGURE 12.1 Example of a SWOT Risk Analysis for Development of a Free Clinic. (Adapted with permission from Angela McGregor's DNP Project, 2011).

such as cost, quality (e.g., intervention, action), relevance, and time (ANSI, 2004).

Assessment of identified risks begins with qualitative assessment of impact for each identified risk, which is then quantified based on a scale of the project manager's decision. Next, a quantitative probability ranking is subjectively assigned by the project manager. Probability assesses the chance that an identified risk will occur. This means that risk data are subjective by nature but objectively recorded by you, the project evaluator. Begin by qualitatively categorizing or grouping sources or common root causes of risk. Next assess the level of urgency or time to respond, acuity of symptoms, or warning signs. These characteristics increase understanding about the impact of a risk (ANSI, 2004). Table 12.2 is an example of an objective numerical scale of subjective definitions for *impact*.

To summarize, an *impact* scale can be created to objectively assess each subjectively identified risk, and a *probability* scale is subjectively quantified. A probability and impact matrix serves as a tool by which identified risks within your practice context can be quickly visualized according to degree of risk (ANSI, 2004). The next topic presents the probability and impact matrix.

Organizing identified risks by probability and impact displayed on a cross-tabulation matrix or structure is an efficient method to assess and react to an identified risk. The American National Standards Institute (ANSI, 2004) displays both threats (negative) and opportunities (positive) on the same table. Figure 12.2 is an example of a probability and impact matrix that assesses only negative risk. A positive risk matrix can be added to the right, as desired. The upper right hand corner indicates the highest level of risk. Lowest risk is in the lower left corner. High risks require priority action and response, whereas medium risk should be monitored. Low-risk threats can be placed on a watch list (ANSI, 2004).

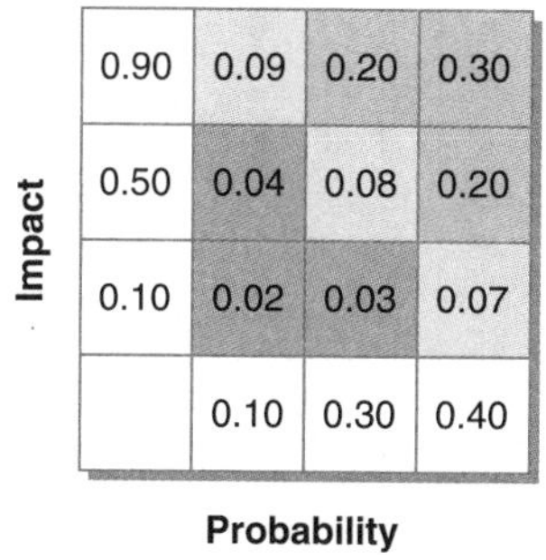

Impact			
0.90	0.09	0.20	0.30
0.50	0.04	0.08	0.20
0.10	0.02	0.03	0.07
	0.10	0.30	0.40

Probability

FIGURE 12.2 Risk Matrix. Impact (severity) is based on a quantitative numerical scale; probability (chance) is generated by the project manager. The purpose of the risk matrix is a visual representation of risk for quick reference (ANSI, 2004; Youssef & Hyman, 2010).

TABLE 12.2 Quantitative Numeric Scale for Subjective Definitions of Impact

Outcome Objective	Very Low/.05	Low/.10	Moderate/.20	High/.40	Very High/.80
Cost	Insignificant increase	<10% cost increase	10–20% increase	40–80% increase	>80% increase
Quality	Very high improvement in quality	High improvement in quality	Moderate improvement in quality	Low improvement in quality	No improvement in quality
Relevance	Very high ability to effect change	High ability to effect change	Moderate ability to effect change	Low ability to effect change	Inability to effect change
Time	No observed wasted time	Minor observation of wasted time	Moderate increase of wasted time	High increase of wasted time	Significant increase of wasted time

Adapted from American National Standards Institute (ANSI), 2004, p. 245.

The final step of risk planning is development of response options and actions. Responses must be appropriate, realistic, and significant. Communication with the stakeholders regarding the response plan is expected. Throughout the implementation of your DNP project, monitoring and control of risk are ongoing. Keep a log of identified risks, reassess existing risks for safety, and evaluate the response and outcome of any risk interventions. Above all, stay vigilant to risk throughout implementation of your DNP project (ANSI, 2004).

The following is an example of a risk analysis narrative from a DNP executive summary. The narrative is specific to building a business model for a free clinic. Thank you to Dr. Angela McGregor (2011) for giving permission to publish these portions of her DNP written report:

Risk Analysis

By Dr. Angela McGregor (2011)

The leading risk identified in operationalizing a free clinic was liability. All providers at the free clinic will be volunteers. Several healthcare personnel may need malpractice insurance in order to practice. Malpractice insurance is expensive and volunteers may not have their own coverage. Application for liability insurance under the Free Clinic Federal Torts Claim Act (FTCA) Medical Malpractice Program will be applied for. The FTCA policy, enacted by Congress, provides medical malpractice insurance for volunteer health professionals. Requirements for coverage include (1) no third-party reimbursement, (2) no fees can be imposed, only charges according to a patient's ability to pay, (3) donations may be accepted, and (4) the healthcare professional must be licensed or certified to provide health services. The FTCA status provides volunteers with immunity from medical malpractice lawsuits; claimants must file malpractice claims against the United States (Department of Health and Human Services: Health Resources and Services Administration, 2009). The FTCA does not allow underinsured patients to be seen in the free clinic; however the hospital will continue to provide charity care to help these individuals.

The second risk identified with the greatest impact potential was liquidity. The free clinic may not receive adequate donations to keep the clinic open. This risk can be avoided by using some of the Emergency Department (ED) funds allocated for charity. In 2010 the hospital ED had a loss of $337,776 (personal communication, February 1, 2011). The amount of debt incurred by uninsured patients who did not qualify for assistance through the hospital was $24,400 (personal communication, February 1, 2011). The amount of debt incurred by uninsured patients who qualified for patient financial assistance through the hospital was $56,616. The free clinic will provide a place for these uninsured patients to receive care and decrease the ED debt. The hospital apportioned 1% of annual gross revenues for charity care and allocated $24,400 for the first year of the free clinic.

The next risk identified is a potential language barrier. The county population was 4.4% Hispanic or Latino in 2010 (US Census Bureau, 2010). Many do not speak English or speak and understand little English. The hospital utilizes a language line for patient and provider communication. This 24-hour-a day telephone service will be free to the clinic because of the hospital contract.

The fourth risk identified is an issue of sustainability. The expense of supplies may exceed the contributions or donations to the free clinic and could affect the budget and overall functioning of the clinic. A cost-benefit analysis was performed to evaluate the potential savings from the ED compared to the cost of the free clinic. Vendors for hospital supplies will be contacted and negotiations for a fixed price contract and supply donations will be negotiated thereby avoiding a cost increase and supply shortages.

The fifth identified risk is an operational risk. Eight of the hospital providers have stated they will volunteer at the free clinic. The free clinic also needs nursing staff and receptionists. If the number of volunteers from the hospital is not adequate to run the free clinic, the risk can be avoided by contacting local agencies such as the public health center to assist with recruitment of volunteer nurses and receptionists. Hospital administrative personnel will also attend a city meeting to gain the support of the community and to assist in possible recruitment of volunteers. Monitoring the volunteer services of healthcare providers will be a continuing task.

The final identified risk is the potential that patients seen in the hospital ED may not utilize the free clinic. Education will be provided to the ED healthcare personnel and staff regarding referrals to the free clinic for follow-up appointments. Cost evaluations will be conducted on a monthly basis to determine cost savings to the ED, the number of patients who utilized the ED but would have gone to the free clinic if they knew about it, costs of charity care and remaining monetary amount.

CHAPTER SUMMARY AND AFTERTHOUGHTS

Planning and evaluating a budget and risk management plan for your DNP project incorporate your knowledge and leadership within the business of the healthcare organization. Working with the stakeholder during this economic and budget planning stage is important. Details of leadership and management practiced during this stage of implementation furnish important lessons that provide opportunity for enhancing your career. Time spent on the details of your DNP project are challenging but essential to demonstrate effectiveness, efficiency, and leadership.

WRITING REMINDERS...

Paraphrasing

Paraphrasing means writing something that is different from the original source yet retains the meaning of the original source. Paraphrasing is an important skill in order to avoid plagiarism.

Suggestions for paraphrasing include the following:

- First try to understand the meaning of the entire passage you are reading, then carefully choose phrases or information that make a point for your manuscript;

- Use your own words (not the author's words) to explain the selected information from the original source;

- Always give the author of the original source credit with an intext citation following a paraphrase or quotation that leads the reader to the reference list if he or she desires more information.

Data from The Writing Center at the University of Wisconsin. (2014). *Successful vs. unsuccessful paraphrases.* Retrieved from https://writing.wisc.edu/Handbook/QPA_paraphrase.html

REFERENCES

American National Standards Institute (ANSI). (2004). *A guide to the project management body of knowledge* (3rd ed.). Newtown Square, PA: Project Management Institute.

Bates College. (2012). *Almost everything you wanted to know about making tables and figures.* Lewiston, ME: Bates College, Department of Biology. Retrieved from http://abacus.bates.edu/~ganderso/biology/resources/writing/HTWtablefigs.html

Centers for Disease Control and Prevention (CDC). (2006). Risk management. *CDC Unified Process Practices Guide.* Retrieved from http://www2a.cdc.gov/cdcup/library/practices_guides/CDC_UP_Risk_Management_Practices_Guide.pdf

Chartered Accountants. (2013). *Establish the context.* Retrieved from https://survey.charteredaccountants.com.au/risk_management/small-firms/context.aspx

Elearning. (2015). *The purpose of risk management in health care.* University of Scranton Online Resource Center. Retrieved from http://elearning.scranton.edu/resource/business-leadership/purpose-of-risk-management-in-healthcare

Grove, S.K., Burns, N., & Gray, J.R. (2013). *The practice of nursing research: Appraisal, synthesis, and generation of evidence* (7th ed.). St. Louis, MO: Elsevier Saunders.

Joanna Briggs Institute (JBI). (2014). *The Joanna Briggs Institute reviewers' manual 2014: The systematic review of economic evaluation evidence.* Retrieved from http://www.joannabriggs.org/assets/docs/sumari/ReviewersManual-The-Systematic-Review-of-Economic-Evaluation-Evidence-2014_v2.pdf

Lister, J. (2015). *What is a budget proposal?* eHow. Retrieved from http://www.ehow.com/info_8162458_budget-proposal.html

McGregor, A. (2011). *Increasing access to healthcare: Development of a free clinic business proposal.* University of Iowa, unpublished DNP project.

Polit, D.F. (2010). *Statistics and data analysis for nursing research* (2nd ed.). Boston, MA: Pearson.

Polit, D.F., & Beck, C.T. (2012). *Nursing research: Generating and assessing evidence for nursing practice* (9th ed.). Philadelphia, PA: Wolters Kluwer Health/Lippincott Williams & Wilkins.

Vanderbilt Institutional Research Group. (2010). *Reporting quantitative results.* Retrieved from http://virg.vanderbilt.edu/AssessmentPlans/Results/Reporting_Results_Quantitative.aspx

World Health Organization (WHO). (2003). Economic aspects of drug use. In *Introduction to drug utilization research.* Retrieved from http://apps.who.int/medicinedocs/en/d/Js4876e/5.html

Youssef, N., & Hyman, W.A. (2010). Risk analysis: Beyond probability and severity. *MD+DI, 32*(8). Retrieved from http://www.mddionline.com/article/risk-analysis -beyond-probability-and-severity

IF YOU WANT TO READ MORE...

American National Standards Institute (ANSI). (2004). *A guide to the project management body of knowledge* (3rd ed.). Newtown Square, PA: Project Management Institute.

Centers for Disease Control and Prevention (CDC). (2006). Risk management. *CDC Unified Process Practices Guide.* Retrieved from http://www2a.cdc.gov/cdcup/library/practices_guides/CDC_UP_Risk_Management_Practices_Guide.pdf

Polit, D.F. (2010). *Statistics and data analysis for nursing research* (2nd ed.). Boston, MA: Pearson.

13

Writing the DNP Project Proposal

Ideas are cheap—making something of them is difficult.

ANNE SIGISMUND HUFF (1998)

OUTCOME OBJECTIVES

- Discuss the purpose of a DNP project proposal.
- Describe the content and process for writing a successful DNP project proposal.
- Compare and contrast content and utilization of a DNP project proposal, an IRB proposal, and a grant proposal.

TERMS

Collaborative Institutional Training Initiative (CITI)	Funding grant Health Insurance Portability and Accountability Act (HIPAA)	Institutional Review Board (IRB) Proposal
Ethics		

Consider your progress this far in creation of your DNP project. Beginning with evidence-based practice (EBP) recommendations based on synthesis of evidence (see Section II) and strategizing a master plan for implementation (see Section III, Chapters 9 through 12), you are now ready to complete the DNP project proposal.

Recall that Chapter 8 provided details and tools to assist in writing an analysis and synthesis of the evidence. The synthesis report answered your PICO(T) question and led to recommendations for the practice setting. You are now ready to build onto your synthesis report and complete your DNP project proposal by providing the details of your implementation and evaluation plan. This chapter provides information and resources to increase your understanding and assist in writing and presenting a successful DNP project proposal.

THE DNP PROJECT PROPOSAL: OVERVIEW

A proposal is written along with verbal communication identifying the major elements of your EBP recommendations for practice and implementation plan. A good proposal is a fair and balanced argument about the significance of your DNP project. The intended audiences for your DNP project proposal are your DNP project committee, peers, and the institutional stakeholders where the project will be implemented. Be prepared therefore for suggestions and requests for clarification or modification before final approval for implementation of your DNP project. On approval, the proposal will serve as a contract regarding how the DNP project will be carried out (Denzin & Lincoln, 1994; Polit & Beck, 2012).

Types of Proposals

This chapter focuses on the proposal for implementation of your DNP project. The general concept of a proposal is communication. However, the written proposal also serves as a template for other uses such as completing an application for the ethics committee or Institutional Review Board (IRB), as well as writing a grant for funding your project. A DNP project proposal requires depth and detail to meet the rigorous standards of your university and generally requires more detail than a proposal written for a grant or an IRB application. Therefore, time spent writing, completing, and reviewing a successful DNP project proposal is a valuable use of your time (Grove, Burns, & Gray, 2013; Tappen, 2011).

THE DNP PROJECT PROPOSAL

DNP project proposals accomplish important functions. A proposal describes and justifies the importance of implementing a practice change or improvement, then proposes a suitable recommendation for practice. Finally, the DNP project proposal generates support for the project (Grove et al., 2013).

The proposal is a purposeful, reasonable, and knowledgeable process. Presentation of the proposal may be in the form of a written document, a verbal presentation, or both. A verbal presentation provides additional opportunity for your peers and DNP project committee to evaluate your understanding and knowledge of the proposed change or improvement. Therefore, use logical explanations in the written and verbal presentations. Presentations are professional interactions, so dress accordingly and demonstrate competence by appearing calm, confident, and in control. Presentations may be timed. Practice and be prepared with audiovisuals (Grove et al., 2013; Johnson-Sheehan, 2015).

Content criteria for your DNP project proposals are established by your university, college, school, or department. This means that proposal guidelines for layout, depth, and detail may vary, but content remains basically the same. Table 13.1 provides a comparison between proposal focus and content for a DNP project and a PhD dissertation.

Writing hints for the DNP project proposal are similar or generic to most forms of proposals. The following list supplies information to assist you in writing a proposal.

- Develop ideas logically. Remember that each section builds on the previous section.

- Identify critical points in the proposal.

- Use transitional sentences for smooth reading.

- Show the qualifications of the practitioner, and generate support for the project.

- Demonstrate attention to detail and rigor.

TABLE 13.1 Comparison of a DNP Project Proposal and a PhD Dissertation Proposal

DNP Project Proposal	PhD Dissertation Proposal
Focus • Practice • Direct and indirect patient-centered care, quality, and safety • Implementation and evaluation of EBP based on best evidence	*Focus* • Research • Contribute to nursing's body of knowledge • Rigorous scientific studies appropriate for generalizability or transferability of findings
Title *Table of contents* *Executive summary* *Introduction* • Background and identification of a practice issue or problem • Significance of problem for nursing practice • PICO(T) question or statement	*Title* *Table of contents* *Abstract* *Introduction* • Background of a research issue • Significance and magnitude of problem for nursing • Purpose statement
Evidence search and synthesis • Search statement • Analysis and synthesis of relevant evidence • EBP recommendations for practice • Conceptual, physiological, or theoretical	*Literature review* • Search statement • Analysis and summary of relevant research evidence • Identification of gaps in the literature • Conceptual, philosophical, or theoretical framework
Implementation planning • Plan for integration, management, and leadership • Plan for evaluation • Plan for economic analysis • Plan for sustainability *Timeline*	*Researh methodology* • Description of research design • Description of sampling • Plan for measurement tool(s) • Plan for data analysis *Timeline*

EBP, evidence-based practice; HIPAA, Health Insurance Portability and Accountability Act; RCT, randomized controlled trial.

Sources: Grove, Burns, & Gray, 2013; Johnson-Sheehan, 2015; Knafl & Deatrick, 2005; McLaughlin, 2014; Pan, 2013; Polit & Beck, 2012.

• A concise, clear, complete, and well-written executive summary should precede the proposal. This may be the first introduction of your proposal to stakeholders and other decision makers. Make it count.

• Proposals are written using future tense verbs (e.g., "the context for implementation *will be* the medical-surgical unit ..."). The final report builds on the proposal and uses past tense verbs.

- Development of your proposal should be logical, with adequate depth and detail of content.

- Support your idea with best evidence.

- Justify use of the identified participants and context.

- Identify how rigor is built into evaluation and sustainability of your project.

- Use correct spelling, grammar, punctuation, headings, and subheadings. Follow American Psychological Association (APA) format. Proofread! Do not depend on *spell check* and *grammar check.*

- Include appropriate tables and figures to clarify essential information.

- "Begin and end with a flourish" (Polit & Beck, 2012, p 714). The executive summary, background information, and concluding section of the proposal should trigger excitement and confidence in you and your project.

- Provide a realistic timetable of your intended implementation and evaluation processes.

- Finish early. Let your proposal sit for a day or two and then reread and enhance it as needed. Others should read and critique your proposal before final submission to your committee (Grove et al., 2013; Knafl & Deatrick, 2005; Levinson & McLaughlin, 2011; Offredy & Vickers, 2010: Polit & Beck, 2012).

THE INSTITUTIONAL REVIEW BOARD APPLICATION

Your academic proposal is a useful template for writing the application for the IRB. An IRB is a formal group of qualified people designated to formally review and monitor research involving human subjects. According to federal policies and regulations, an IRB has the authority to approve applications, require modifications to secure approval, or disapprove an application to implement your DNP project. The purpose of IRBs is to ensure, before implementation of the project begins and as needed during the implementation process, that appropriate patient safety and protection procedures are in place and are followed for the rights and welfare of human subjects participating in the practice project. The IRB committee is charged with approving and reviewing project protocols, materials, and implementation plan (Department of Health and Human Services [DHHS], 2014). The next section presents information related to ethical considerations, Collaborative Institutional Training Initiative (CITI) training, submission of the IRB application, and adherence to IRB requirements.

Ethics is a branch of philosophy associated with moral values and conduct (Offredy & Vickers, 2013; Porter, 2000). Ethics is commonly described as "norms for conduct that distinguish between acceptable and unacceptable behavior" (Resnick, 2011). Although people generally recognize common norms, interpretation and actions vary based on lived experiences. Ethics is considered to comprise broad and informal values, as opposed to laws that are enforceable. Ethical norms guide or govern different disciplines specific to the goals of the identified professions. Normal ethical behaviors include the following (Resnick, 2011):

- Ethical behaviors promote the aims of projects and research (e.g., knowledge, truth, avoidance of error).

- Ethical behaviors promote the values that are essential to collaborative work (e.g., trust, accountability, mutual respect, fairness).

- Ethical behaviors promote accountability to the public (e.g., obedience to federal policies on projects and research misconduct, conflicts of interest, and human subjects protection).

- Ethical behaviors build public support for DNP projects (e.g., trust in quality and integrity).

- Ethical behaviors promote moral and social values.

In the United States, the Belmont Report (initially published in 1979 and last revised in 2008) remains an essential reference for IRBs. The report identified three fundamental ethical principles for projects and research that involve human subjects: respect for persons, beneficence, and justice (DHHS, 2008). The principle of *respect for persons* means that research participants have the right to self-determination and therefore the right to decide whether or not to participate in your project. The decision should be based on the right to full disclosure before signing, or not signing, an informed consent to participate. *Beneficence* is the principle that requires a practitioner or researcher to maximize benefits, which implies decrease of risk. Nonmaleficence is the opposite of beneficence and requires that the research or project do no harm. The third principle is *justice*. Justice is the right to fair treatment and the right to privacy (Grove et al., 2013; DHHS, 1979; DHHS, 2008; Polit & Beck, 2012).

The Health Insurance Portability and Accountability Act (HIPAA), published in 1996, expanded a patient's right to privacy of his or her health information (Grove et al., 2013; DHHS, 1979; DHHS, 2008; Polit & Beck, 2012). Healthcare institutions are required to enforce control over how personal health information is used and disclosed. The federal rules specify administrative, technical, and physical security safeguards to ensure confidentiality of electronic protected health information. Authority to enforce the Security Rule was given to the Office for Civil Rights (OCR) in July of 2009 (DHHS, 2015). Therefore, as you prepare the application for IRB review, check with the healthcare institution's IRB office regarding organizational policies and procedures that demonstrate compliance with HIPAA privacy rules. Document your actions on the IRB application as well as in your project proposal.

Formal training or education is required of all practitioners, clinicians, managers, or assistants who will lead or be involved with leading a DNP project. Training is required because of incidents of regulation noncompliance. The CITI is a provider of the required education. Compliance of a CITI course is required *before* you are eligible to submit an application to an IRB (CITI, 2014). The CITI course is available online (https://www.citiprogram.org). Universities and hospitals are subscribing CITI institutions. Check with your IRB office for assistance in subscribing to the CITI Internet site.

Institutional Review Board Application Content

Your DNP proposal is a valuable asset for the IRB application because most of the proposal content addresses the same criteria as the IRB proposal. Table 13.2 provides a general overview of criteria requested for the form. Be clear and detailed when writing.

Institutional Review Board Review Process

After the IRB application is completed, the process for approval begins. There are three levels of IRB review. *Exempt* review implies no risk to human subjects. The following quotation from DHHS regulations (2010) provides a more detailed explanation of the term *exempt*.

> ... *research involving the use of educational tests (cognitive, diagnostic, aptitude, achievement), survey procedures, interview procedures or observation of public behavior unless (i) information obtained is recorded in such a manner that human subjects can be identified, directly or through identifiers linked to the subjects; and (ii) any disclosure of the human subjects' responses outside of the research could reasonably place the subjects at risk of criminal or civil liability or be damaging to the subjects' financial standing, employability or reputation (DHHS, 2010, 46.101[b][2]).*

Expedited means minimal risk to human subjects. An expedited review is reviewed by only one member of the IRB committee. Examples of categories identified as minimal risk include evaluation of hair, saliva, or dental plaque samples, evaluation of blood samples from healthy volunteers, and analyses of voice recordings (University of California, Irvine, 2014). This category includes

TABLE 13.2	Important Components of an Institutional Review Board Application
Purpose of evaluation	• What are the evidence-based practice recommendations for practice implementation? • What do you plan to evaluate? • Who is the target population for evaluation? • Who are the end users?
Selection of sample or participants	• Will recruitment of the sample or participants be equitable and unbiased? • How and where will sample or participants be recruited? • What is the setting for the evaluation? • Is the target population protected or vulnerable? • Are there potential risks to the sample or participants? • How will confidentiality be maintained?
Procedures and processes	• Provide a detailed description and rationale of the implementation plan. • Will identity of sample/participants be protected?
Evaluation data	• Describe what data you plan to collect and how you plan to collect it. • What is the source of data? • Where will the data be stored? • How long will the data be stored? • How will data be destroyed after the required length of storage time?

Consent document	• Attach a copy of the informed consent.
	• An informed consent includes the following criteria:
	  • Participant should understand differences between intended practice change or improvement and current practices.
	  • Process, actions, and outcome goals are written clearly and at a level of understanding for participant.
	  • Describe type of data to be collected.
	  • Describe data collection procedures.
	  • Description of implementation is clearly described.
	  • Participant should understand expected time commitment.
	  • Any sponsor or funding agency should be named.
	  • Explain how sample or participants are selected.
	  • Discuss potential risks. Note that all change or improvement has risks, but they are generally minimal.
	  • Discuss potential benefits specific to the participant as well as others.
	  • If compensation will be paid, discuss payment arrangements with each participant.
	  • Participant must know that participation is strictly voluntary and no coercion is implied. Participant must be given adequate time for consideration whether or not to participate. Refusal to participate will not result in any penalty. Participant must be informed that he or she has the right to withdraw from participation or to withhold information without penalty.

TABLE 13.2	Important Components of an Institutional Review Board Application—cont'd
	• Provide your name, credentials, and contact information for each participant, and encourage participants to contact you if there are additional questions, comments, concerns, or complaints.
Risks and benefits	• What are the potential risks to participants (e.g., exposure to physical harm; exposure to emotional or mental trauma through questions or observations)? • How will risks be minimized? • What are potential benefits of the implementation project? Will participants be benefited?
Conflicts of interest	• Identify any financial grants received and the source of the grant. • Identify whether you will make money on the evaluation findings or implementation project. • Identify whether you work for a company that will make money on your DNP project.

"employment of survey, interview, focus group program evaluation, human factors evaluation or quality assurance methodologies" (Polit & Beck, 2012, p 166).

Full board review means that there is more than minimal risk to human subjects. In other words, all members of the ethics board will review your IRB application when it is submitted and falls under neither expedited nor exempt review criteria.

GRANT PROPOSAL FOR FUNDING

Seeking funding early in your doctoral career is a strategy to launch your scholarly trajectory. As a DNP student, your focus on implementation projects and evaluation of process, actions, and/or effect in one context lends the DNP project evaluation to pilot studies. Therefore, as a student and in the early stages of your career, begin writing for small grants and building collaborative teams to write for large-scale grants following graduation with your DNP degree. See Chapter 15 for information related to professional collaboration.

Experiential knowledge gained from *doing* a DNP project advances your capacity of internal resources and enhances successful dissemination of knowledge gained and lessons learned (Grove et al., 2013). Dissemination of outcomes fosters communication and collaboration with other practice experts and researchers, thereby contributing to efficient use of the translational science model: collaboration of practice and research. Small grants can launch your scholarly pathway and potentially lead to winning grants that provide funding for clinical practice projects and research. Writing for grants, no matter the size, is a demonstration of commitment to the profession of nursing. Chapter 16 discusses the methods and resources for dissemination and collaboration within the framework of translational science.

Sources for Funding

Categories of funding sources are listed in this section, followed by examples. You are encouraged to do a *Google* search using the headers listed here. In addition, access grants.gov to gain information about federally funded grant opportunities.

- Local funding
  - College
  - University
  - Local chapters of nursing organizations
- Professional nursing organizations
  - American Association of Colleges of Nursing (AACN)
  - American Organization of Nurse Executives (AONE)
  - American Nurses Association (ANA)
  - Emergency Nurses Association (EMA)
  - National Association of Clinical Nurse Specialists (NACNS)
  - Sigma Theta Tau International (STTI)
- Organizations focused on a specific disease
  - Arthritis Foundation
  - American Heart Association
  - National Kidney Foundation
- Foundations
  - The Aetna Foundations
  - The Bill and Melinda Gates Foundation

- The Kresge Foundation

- Robert Wood Johnson Foundation

- Corporations

  - Genzyme.com

  - Pfizer

- U.S. federal agencies

  - Agency for Healthcare Research and Quality (AHRQ)

  - Health Resources and Services Administration (HRSA)

  - National Institute of Nursing Research (NINR)

  - Patient-Centered Outcomes Research Institute (PCORI)

Writing Hints

Hints for writing grants are similar to those presented for writing the DNP project proposal. A few additional hints, specific to grant writing, are as follows:

- Assume that the reviewer knows nothing about your project and may be from another discipline. This means to write clearly with adequate description and detail using terms that can be understood by professionals outside of nursing.

- Read the directions. Follow the directions. Grant proposals differ from the proposal for your DNP project committee and IRB. Therefore, focus on your audience.

- Size matters. Create a clear, concise proposal that meets the needs of the recipient. Think quality, not quantity (i.e., number of pages).

- Update your biographical sketch and curriculum vitae that will be submitted with a grant proposal. Highlight the skills and talents that demonstrate your qualifications.

- "Don't let your claims outdistance your true capabilities" (Levinson & McLaughlin, 2011).

- "A *skilled* grant writer will have one proposal funded for every five submitted" (Grove et al., 2013, p 671). Most have far fewer. Be committed to addressing reviewer comments and resubmit your grant (Grove et al., 2013; Knafl & Deatrick, 2005; Levinson & McLaughlin, 2011; Polit & Beck, 2012).

CHAPTER SUMMARY AND AFTERTHOUGHTS

Writing the proposal for your DNP project is hard work, but the importance of a well-constructed proposal cannot be overlooked. Indeed, time spent developing practice recommendations and an implementation plan is foundational for a successful proposal. A successful proposal informs your DNP project committee and leads to acceptance of your implementation plan. Writing a DNP project proposal is also experiential learning for future scholarly activities. Once the proposal is accepted by your DNP project committee and stakeholders and IRB approval is received, you are ready to begin the real-time implementation.

CASE STUDY

There is no case study with discussion questions because the intent of this chapter is to encourage you to write.

WRITING REMINDERS...

Intext Citations

The purpose for intext citations is to guide the reader to your reference list at the end of your manuscript. This allows the reader to search for additional information about your topic. The reference list also demonstrates the quality and rigor of your evidence search, thereby enhancing trust in your written manuscript.

Reference

Medaille College Libraries. (2015). *APA intext citations.* Retrieved from http://libraryguides. medaille.edu/apaintext

---

REFERENCES

Collaborative Institutional Training Initiative (CITI). (2014). *CITI program.* Retrieved from https://www.citiprogram.org

Denzin, N.K., & Lincoln, Y.S. (Eds.). (1994). *Handbook of qualitative research.* Thousand Oaks, CA: SAGE Publications.

Department of Health and Human Services (DHHS). (1979). *The Belmont Report.* Retrieved from http://www.hhs.gov/ohrp/humansubjects/guidance/belmont.html

Department of Health and Human Services (DHHS). (2008). *The Belmont Report.* Retrieved from http://www.hhs.gov/ohrp/humansubjects/guidance/belmont.html

Department of Health and Human Services (DHHS). (2010). *Code of federal regulations.* Retrieved from http://www.hhs.gov/ohrp/humansubjects/guidance/45cfr46 .html

Department of Health and Human Services (DHHS). (2014). *Health information privacy.* Retrieved from http://www.hhs.gov/ocr/privacy/

Department of Health and Human Services (DHHS). (2015). Enforcement highlights. *Health Information Privacy.* Retrieved from http://www.hhs.gov/ocr/privacy/hipaa/ enforcement/highlights

Grove, S.K., Burns, N., & Gray, J.R. (2013). *The practice of nursing research: appraisal, synthesis, and generation of evidence* (7th ed.). St. Louis, MO: Elsevier Saunders.

Johnson-Sheehan, R. (2015). *Planning and organizing proposals and technical reports.* Indiana University: Purdue Owl. Retrieved from https://owl.english.purdue.edu/ media/pdf/20080628094326_727.pdf

Knafl, K., & Deatrick, J. (2005). Top 10 tips for successful qualitative grantsmanship. *Research in Nursing and Health, 28*(6), 441-443.

Levinson, J.D., & McLaughlin, M.S. (2011). *Guerilla marketing for consultants: Breakthrough tactics for winning profitable clients.* Hoboken, NJ: John Wiley & Sons, Inc.

Offredy, M., & Vickers, P. (2013). *Developing a healthcare research proposal: An interactive student guide.* West Sussex, United Kingdom: Wiley-Blackwell.

Pan, M.L. (2013). *Preparing literature reviews* (4th ed.). Glendale, CA: Pyrczak.

Polit, D.F., & Beck, C.T. (2012). *Nursing research: Generating and assessing evidence for nursing practice* (9th ed.). Philadelphia, PA: Wolters Kluwer/Lippincott Williams & Wilkins.

Porter, J. (2000). Responsibility, passion, and sin. *Journal of Religious Ethics, 28*(3), 367-395.

Resnick, D.B. (2011). *What is ethics in research and why is it important?* National Institute of Environmental Health Sciences. Retrieved from http://www.niehs.nih.gov/ research/resources/bioethics/whatis/

Tappen, R.M. (2011). *Advanced nursing research: From theory to practice.* Sudbury, MA: Jones & Bartlett.

University of California, Irvine, Office of Research. (2014). *Levels of review.* Retrieved from http://www.research.uci.edu/compliance/human-research-protections/ researchers/levels-of-review.html

IF YOU WANT TO READ MORE...

Funk, S.G., & Tornquist, E.M. (2015). *Writing winning proposals for nurses and health care professionals.* New York, NY: Springer Publishing Company.

Skloot, T. (2010). *The immortal life of Henrietta Lacks.* New York, NY: Random House.

14

Managing Actualization of the Project

A goal without a plan is just a wish.

LARRY ELDER

OUTCOME OBJECTIVES

- Review your strategic plan for implementation of evidence-based practice (EBP) recommendations.
- Describe the DNP roles and responsibilities for successful actualization of your EBP practice recommendations.
- Prepare a final written report.
- Discuss plans for reporting intermittent and final DNP project findings.

TERMS

Project management   Project manager

Detailed strategic planning for implementation of your evidence-based practice (EBP) recommendation is now complete and ready for actualization. Managing actualization of a DNP project involves your role and responsibilities as the project manager. On completion of your project's implementation and evaluation, a final written report will be submitted to your DNP project team, project participants, stakeholders, and other identified personnel or community partners associated with the project. This chapter concludes with a review of the importance of written reports. Section IV provides information related to dissemination of findings. Although dissemination occurs throughout your academic journey to achieve a DNP degree, professional dissemination and collaborations of your scholarship continue after graduation as work and time commitments change.

PROJECT MANAGEMENT

The aim of project management is to manage change for the purpose of achieving "greater efficiency with less risk and uncertainty" (Cleland & Ireland, 2007, p 17). Projects within a healthcare organization possess unique characteristics, yet health care can learn from engineering and business disciplines regarding management of projects. Indeed, implementation of EBP recommendations for practice follows the process of project management within a healthcare organization. For example, project management meets one or more of four basic purposes:

1. Create change

2. Implement strategic plans

3. Fulfill contractual agreements

4. Solve specified problems (Cable & Adams, 1997)

Key responsibilities of a project manager include application of "organizational methodologies to plan, coordinate, and integrate activities and resources across functional lanes of responsibility necessary for successfully delivering project outcomes" (Centers for Disease Control and Prevention [CDC], 2010, p 1 of 2). This means that you are essential to the project and are responsible to deliver the project outcomes. During the implementation stage, the project manager delivers on the actions and processes identified in the strategic plan. You, the project manager, are also responsible for delivering instructions, identifying and communicating about problems and risks, and monitoring participant actions in implementation of EBP recommendations. Throughout implementation, project management is also responsible to the organization for patient safety and satisfaction in the delivery of quality care. Project management is a challenging role (CDC, 2010).

Key roles associated with being the *project manager* include the following:

- Set the implementation plans in motion to achieve outcomes within the identified timeline.

- Organize all the parts: resources, participants, activities, processes. Project managers identify and classify activities and assignment of human resources (i.e., project participants, registered nurses). Project managers create responsibility and assign authority for specified activities (Norman, 2015).

- Transformative leaders motivate and empower the project participants to achieve the identified project goals (see Chapter 2). "Effective leaders are students of human personalities, motivations, and communication" (Norman, 2015).

- Control involves measuring and reporting actions and achievements against identified outcome goals. Corrective action by managers is required when actions toward goals are not followed. Managers must also control for continued focus on patient safety, satisfaction, and quality of healthcare services (Norman, 2015; Snyder, 2013).

Reminders about *leadership skills* that can be applied during the DNP project's implementation to enhance motivation and empowerment include the following:

- Clearly communicate the goals and direction for the DNP project.

- Celebrate achievement of goals during and at the conclusion of the DNP project.

- Use open communication to assess issues, risks, and solutions.

- Support leadership by recognizing change champions.

- Communicate on a regular basis the progress, or lack of, regarding the DNP project (White, n.d.).

FINAL WRITTEN REPORT AND PRESENTATION

Final written reports of DNP projects focus on collection of project data and interpretation of findings. Remember that your project goals and plans were grounded in implementation of EBP recommendations for practice. The final report therefore must stay focused on bringing closure to implementation and evaluation of the EBP recommendations for practice. Depending on the type of project and identification of evaluation criteria, focus of the findings section will vary. Suggested subheadings for interpretation of practice project findings that should be included in the final report include the following:

- Project successes

- Unexpected events

- Lessons learned

- Project process, actions, and outcomes

  - Effectiveness of practice change or improvement with emphasis on patient safety and quality

  - Efficiency of time and resources

  - Quality of product (e.g., the degree to which the project met the expected outcomes)

- Summary: achievement of expectations (Carleton University, 2015)

DISSEMINATION OF FINDINGS

Following conclusion of your DNP project and final written report, dissemination of findings begins with presentations and discussions of project outcomes. Initial identified audiences for presentation are those with direct involvement, interest, or oversight of your project: your DNP project team, stakeholders, peers, project participants, and funding agency if applicable. Recall that dissemination was encouraged for findings from your evidence search, synthesis, and EBP recommendations for practice (see Chapter 8). Colleges of nursing generally require poster or podium presentations at professional conferences. Publications in peer-reviewed professional journals before graduation may also be encouraged by your DNP project chair. Dissemination during your academic years therefore remains within the construct of learning. Dissemination of your DNP project findings after graduation provides opportunity for interprofessional communicatation. You are directed to Chapter 16 for details on the preparation of written and verbal presentations. Dissemination of information leads to communication and fosters collaboration for future scholarly activities.

CHAPTER SUMMARY AND AFTERTHOUGHTS

Your journey from idea to recommendations for practice to strategic planning and actualization of the DNP project is concluding. Take this time to reflect on your growth in knowledge, leadership, and practice. Congratulate yourself on the accomplishment of completing a rigorous DNP project that contributes to accomplishment of the DNP degree.

WRITING REMINDERS...

Field Notes

Question: What are field notes?
- Field notes are your written notes about observations, conversations, and reflections during the actualization of implementing your DNP project.

- Field notes help you remember and make meaning because field notes are written as soon as possible after leaving the field site.

- Field notes capture descriptive and reflective information about actions, dialogue, and context.

Question: What is the process for collecting field notes?
- Use a spiral bound or hardcover notebook, not single pages, for organization and sequential entries. Page numbers help keep observed events in order of occurrence.

- At the conclusion of each day, review your notes. Look for repetition of themes and actions. Organize daily findings by creating a code.

Question: What information should be included in written field notes?
- Date, time, and place for each observation

- Objective, coherent detailed descriptions (e.g., who, what, when, where, how)

- Contextual observations and sensory impressions (e.g., smells, room temperature, noise, other activities)

- Details of pertinent phrases or questions from conversations

- Your questions and thoughts about people, actions, and/or behaviors for future observation

- Contact information in case you need additional information

- Reflections on the personal nature and meaning of the event (e.g., Did your leadership style connect with the people? Did you feel uncomfortable in the setting? Were your management suggestions well received?)

- Analysis of what you learned

Data from Chiseri-Strater & Sunstein, 1997; Foster, A., 2011; Grieve, n.d.; Polit & Beck, 2012; Sanjek, 1990.

REFERENCES

Cable, D.P., & Adams, J.R. (1997). Organizing for project management. In *Principles of project management*. Newtown Square, PA: Project Management Institute.

Carleton University. (2015). *Doing the right things … doing things right*. Project Management Office. Retrieved from http://carleton.ca/ccs/project-office/

Centers for Disease Control and Prevention (CDC). (2010). Project roles and functions. *Project Management Newsletter: Supporting a Common Project Delivery Framework 4*(11). Retrieved from http://www2.cdc.gov/cdcup/library/newsletter/CDC_UP_Newsletter_v4_i11.pdf

Chiseri-Strater, E., & Sunstein, B.S. (1997). *Fieldworking: Reading and writing research*. Upper Saddle River, NJ: Blair Press.

Cleland, D.I., & Ireland, L.R. (2007). *Project management: Strategic design and implementation* (5th ed.). New York, NY: McGraw-Hill.

Foster, A. (2011). The art and science of good field notes. *National Geographic*. Retrieved from http://voices.nationalgeographic.com/2011/08/22/the-art-and-science-of-good-field-notes

Grieve, G.P. (n.d.). *How to write field notes*. Retrieved from http://www.gpgrieve.org/PDF/How_to_write_Field_Notes.pdf

Norman, L. (2015). What are the four basic functions that make up the management process? *Chron*. Hearst Newspapers LLC. Retrieved from http://smallbusiness.chron.com/four-basic-functions-make-up-management-process-23852.html

Polit, D.F., & Beck, C.T. (2012). *Nursing research: Generating and assessing evidence-for nursing practice* (9th ed.). Philadelphia, PA: Wolters Kluwer/Lippincott Williams & Wilkins.

Sanjek, R. (Ed.). (1990). *Fieldnotes: The making of anthropology*. Ithaca, NJ: Cornell University Press.

Snyder, C.S. (2013). *A user's manual to the PMBOK guide* (5th ed.). Hoboken, NJ: John Wiley & Sons, Inc.

White, L. (n.d.). *What leaders do: Five actions that make a difference.* The Education Group. Retrieved from http://educationgroup.com/pdf/leadersdo.pdf

IF YOU WANT TO READ MORE...

Snyder, C.S. (2013). *A user's manual to the PMBOK guide* (5th ed.). Hoboken, NJ: John Wiley & Sons, Inc.

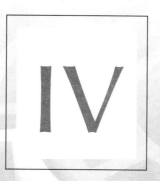

IV

Looking Forward

PURPOSE

The aim of Section IV is to increase understanding and motivation of postgraduate scholarly activities involving intradisciplinary and interdisciplinary collaboration within the structure of translational science.

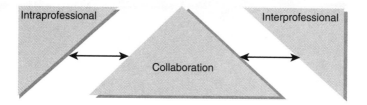

Completion of academic requirements related to the DNP project does not terminate your professional responsibility for postgraduate scholarly activities in practice. It is only the beginning. Section IV presents information about the professional phase of scholarship beginning in Chapter 15 with the topics of dissemination and collaboration. Dissemination is grounded in communication and leads to collaboration within a structure of translational science. Dissemination is a final action for the academic DNP project as well as a beginning of new collaborations within your healthcare organization. Chapter 16 focuses on the structure of translational science. Translational science effectively models the cyclic nature of creating, finding, and using evidence in practice. The statement attributed to Green and Ottoson (2004), "If we want more evidence-based practice, we need more practice-based evidence" (Leeman & Sandelowski, 2012), emphasizes the need for translational science.

REFERENCES

Green, L.W., & Ottoson, J.M. (2004). From efficacy to effectiveness to community and back: evidence-based practice vs. practice-based evidence. Paper presented at *From Clinical Trials to Community: The Science of Translating Diabetes and Obesity Research,* January 12-13, 2004, Bethesda, MD.

Leeman, J., & Sandelowski, M. (2012). Practice-based evidence and quality inquiry. *Journal of Nursing Scholarship, 44*(2), 171-179.

15

Dissemination and Collaboration

The strength of the team is each individual member.
The strength of each member is the team.

PHIL JACKSON

OUTCOME OBJECTIVES

- Formulate a plan for dissemination and collaboration of your DNP project findings.
- Review the steps of getting a manuscript ready for publication in a peer-reviewed professional journal.
- Discuss the importance of communicating your DNP project findings.
- Appraise the relevance of teaching and learning the concept of collaboration.

TERMS

Collaboration	Interdisciplinary	Intradisciplinary
Dissemination	Interprofessional	Intraprofessional

Reflecting on completion of your DNP project should generate understanding and wisdom about your scholarship for the future. You put a lot of time into planning, applying, and evaluating for the purpose of making change or improvement in direct or indirect patient-centered care and safety. As a DNP leader in the practice setting, you are now expected to continue scholarly activities as part of your advanced practice role.

This chapter is about your professional and scholarly future following successful completion of a DNP degree. Your responsibility in implementing and evaluating practice knowledge is a valued partnership role that enhances ideas and leads to collaborative opportunities for large-scale randomized controlled trials and generalization of findings. Responsibility rests with you, the DNP, to contribute your knowledge and effort for scholarly activity and knowledge in practice. Achievement of these goals is grounded in continued dissemination of your DNP project findings. Formal and informal communication in multiple settings leads to collaboration. This chapter reflects on opportunities for continued actions for new programs and projects that can arise from collaborative efforts.

DISSEMINATION

Dissemination implies circulation of information to your intended audience through written, verbal, and visual avenues. Dissemination leads to communication, a central component of nursing's discipline (Woods & Magyary, 2010). Communication leads to interdisciplinary and interprofessional partnerships and collaborations, and collaboration is a motivator because of the cooperative nature of recognizing and sharing interests. Herein is the basis of respect and trust. Dissemination is like marketing to promote and influence practice. In marketing, remember the importance of your peers and local audience. Individual conversations and comments or presentations at staff meetings are good avenues for beginning the dissemination process (Leeman & Sandelowski, 2012; Woods & Magyary, 2010).

The purposes of dissemination are as follows: (1) to clarify the purpose of your project; (2) to identify processes, actions, and other types of useful support and information for potential use by others; (3) to generate positive publicity for the practice change or improvement; and (4) to generate interest for collaboration, grants, expansion, and large-scale research.

Planning for dissemination leads to useful information regarding what to disseminate. Before you create the content for your written or verbal presentation, consider the needs, time, and abilities of your intended audience or end users.

Examples of audiences and dissemination products include the following (Centers for Disease Control and Prevention [CDC], 2009):

- Stakeholders: executive summary, technical reports

- End users in your organization: Facebook, LinkedIn, Web page

- Peers: printed brochures, newsletters

- Workshops: printed materials

- Conference presentations: PowerPoint slides, handouts, posters

- Public: guest editorials, news releases in print or on public radio stations

- Global: websites

Multiple methods of dissemination are needed because no single strategy will meet the needs of all audiences. Recall that evidence-based healthcare practices use best evidence and act on best recommendations. Therefore, present your data clearly (Agency for Healthcare Research and Quality [AHRQ], 2013; CDC, 2009; Polit & Beck, 2012). Planning for effective dissemination is enhanced when you reflect on the following questions (AHRQ, 2013; CDC, 2009, p 2 of 2):

- What are your outcome goals and objectives for dissemination?

- Who are your audience and end users?

- What does your audience need to know, or what are their specific interests?

- What do you hope to gain through dissemination?

- Who will be most affected by your findings?

- Are the findings of interest to the broader community, or are findings specific to stakeholders?

- How can you communicate effectively about the project or program?

- What are the most effective ways to reach your intended audiences?

- When should dissemination occur (e.g., after completion of evidence-based practice recommendations; after planning and before implementation; after project evaluation is completed)?

- What resources and materials do you need for each presentation?

- What networks, organizations, or individuals can help you reach the end users?

Answers to the questions will vary depending on the makeup of your audience (e.g., patients, parents, staff nurses, nurse management, healthcare personnel who deliver direct patient care, healthcare personnel who deliver indirect patient care, politicians, business leaders, community events).

The *purpose of publishing* is to make your information available to the practice and scientific communities. Hints for successful publishing are intended as reminders for planning and writing a publishable manuscript. First, however, selecting an appropriate professional journal is essential. The following bulleted points provide a guideline to help you make decisions.

- *Select a professional journal* that meets the needs of your intended audience *and* meets your needs. Select a journal that your intended audience generally reads (MacDonald, Ford-Jones, Friedman, & Hall, 2006).

- *Professional journals* are published as print copies, online publications, and open access publications.

- The professional rigor and quality of *print journals* can be established by reviewing the credentials of the journal's editorial board, the reputation and name recognition of the publisher, and a statement that the journal's content is peer reviewed.

- *Online publications* are journals that have no print copies or may have both a hard copy and a print copy available for readers. The content of numerous online journals demonstrates professional rigor and quality. Examples include *Clinical Simulations in Nursing,* published in the United States, and *Journal of Rural and Remote Health,* published in Australia.

- *Predatory journals,* on the other hand, should be avoided. Predatory journals are advertised as open access journals but require a publishing fee from you, the author. Predatory journals are not legitimate professional or scholarly publications because there is minimal or no peer review of the manuscript. New authors are particularly vulnerable to predatory journals, but even well-published scholars have been lured into paying for publication or sitting on an editorial board that uses the scholar's credentials to advertise legitimacy of the journal. A list of predatory publishers was created by J. Beall, the librarian credited with coining the term *predatory publisher.* The list can be found at http://scholarlyoa.com/publishers (Fitzpatrick, 2015; Gennaro, 2014).

- Before making your final journal selection for submission of a manuscript, *read and follow the fine print,* ask questions, consult a colleague who has experience with publications, and/or write to the journal editor (Fitzpatrick, 2015).

Problems frequently noted with manuscripts submitted by new authors relate to clarity of writing, grammar, and organization. The following list offers recommendations for writing manuscripts for publication (Grove, Burns, & Gray, 2013; MacDonald et al., 2006; Oermann, Turner, & Carman, 2014):

- Avoid manuscripts that are "too wordy, too long, and . . . difficult to follow" (MacDonald et al., 2006, p 341).

- Use the active voice, not the passive voice.

- Use technical, professional skills. Refer to Purdue Owl: Professional, Technical Writing at https://owl.english.purdue.edu/owl/resource/560/01/

- Use correct grammar, spelling, and punctuation; proofread before submitting.

- Read and follow directions as published by the journal.

- Page length and formatting generally include a 20-page limit of double-spaced, 1-inch margins, 11 or 12 point size. This includes references, tables, and figures.

- The final report of your DNP project is *not* a publishable manuscript. However, the final report has information for one or more professional publications. Rewrite as needed according to journal requirements.

- Use headings and subheadings throughout your manuscript for organization and increased clarity for your reader.

- Include transition sentences at the end of every section to indicate you are moving to another idea.

- Review the correct use of in-text reference citations. Then be sure your reference list includes all in-text reference citations. Different reference formats (i.e., American Psychological Association [APA], Modern Language Association [MLA]) are used in publications. Remember to follow the directions for the selected journal.

- If your project evaluation used statistics, have them reviewed by a statistician.

- Continuously, read journal publications for formatting and style for examples of good writing.

A review of information to include for each section of your manuscript follows.

- *Introduction*
  - Succinctly and clearly, describe:
    - The problem or issue

- Why there is a need for intervention

- Characteristics of the context

- Conclude with your PICO(T) question adapted to the specific content of your manuscript and intended audience (Grove et al., 2013; MacDonald et al., 2006; Oermann, 2014).

- *Evidence review*

  - Describe the literature search strategy for the purpose of establishing trust in the evidence on which practice recommendations are made:

    - Search terms

    - Expanders and limiters

    - Databases searched

    - Screening and selection criteria for publications

      - Eligibility criteria for publications

      - Number of publications screened

      - Number and type of publications included

      - Critique of publications

        - Risk for bias

        - Quality, leveling, and grading of research publications

  - Describe the screening and selection criteria for other types of evidence.

  - Synthesize only the evidence that is specific to your manuscript topic.

    - Remember to group ideas together, thereby leading the reader in the direction of your evidence-based recommendations.

    - Limit the use of direct quotations for emphasis and for when the meaning of the original author's words might be lost.

    - Conclude with your recommendations for practice improvement or change based on your PICO(T) question or statement (Grove et al., 2013; MacDonald et al., 2003; Oermann, 2014).

- *Implementation and evaluation plan*

  - Describe how, where, when your recommendations for practice will be implemented.

- Notify your reader that Institutional Review Board or ethics committee approval has been received.

- Describe what will be evaluated from your implementation (process, action, outcome).

- Describe methods for the project evaluation (Grove et al., 2013; MacDonald et al., 2003; Oermann, 2014).

- *Discussion and recommendations*

  - Describe and discuss the important findings specific to the PICO(T) question and context.

  - Describe limitations, barriers, and facilitators to the project implementation.

  - Make recommendations for use of the findings, including but not limited to:

    - Application in other settings

    - Research collaborations with intraprofessional and/or interprofessional, scientists (Grove et al., 2013; MacDonald et al., 2003; Oermann, 2014)

Table 15.1 describes useful tools for writing a publishable manuscript followed by helpful hints for an oral presentation. These tools are helpful as you, the practitioner, collaborate with scientists and advance your scholarly activities in the practice setting.

Preparation for an oral presentation requires time. The aims of an oral presentation are to keep your audience's attention and deliver a take home message. Unlike a publication, the audience of an oral presentation is looking at you as well as listening to you. It can be intimidating. *Hints for a successful oral presentation* begin with creation of an engaging PowerPoint slide show. Consider the following hints for successful PowerPoint slides (Sieber, 2009):

- Select a background design, and use it consistently. The design should be simple and not distract from your oral presentation.

- Black print on a white background is easy to read, but it also can be boring. If you choose to use color, use contrasting colors between print and background design for your audience to see the slide's content easily.

- Keep the content of the slide simple. That means keywords or symbols only and no sentences.

- Use images to reinforce, complement, visualize, and explain.

TABLE 15.1 Manuscript Preparation Tools for Practitioners and Scientists

Evidence-based practice	PRISMA (Preferred Reporting Items for Systematic Reviews and Meta-Analyses)	Usefulness: (1) improved reporting of systematic reviews and meta-analyses; (2) framework for EBP literature review (Oermann, Turner, & Carman, 2014)
Quality improvement	SQUIRE (Standards for Quality Improvement Reporting Excellence)	Usefulness: (1) framework for reporting about improvement studies; (2) design and plan of study intended for publication (Oermann, 2009)
Research	IMRAD (Introduction, Methods, Results, and Discussion)	Usefulness: structure for research reports (Sollaci & Pereira, 2004)
Randomized controlled trial (RCT)	CONSORT (Consolidated Standards of Reporting Trials)	Usefulness: improvement of *completeness* related to RCT (Turner et al., 2012)
Qualitative research	COREQ (Consolidated Criteria for Reporting Qualitative Research)	Usefulness: guidelines for reporting interviews and focus groups (Oermann et al., 2014)
Epidemiology	STROBE (Strengthening Reporting of Observational Studies in Epidemiology)	Usefulness: reporting of cohort, case-control, and cross-sectional studies (Oermann et al., 2014)

- The last slide is your take home message. Remember the adage "*A picture is worth a thousand words.*"

- Remember copyright laws whether your speech is at a public event or a closed meeting.

- Use animations sparingly and appropriately. Humor can add relevance, but silliness distracts.

- Limit the number of slides. Make each slide relevant.

- Always keep your audience in mind.

Presentation of your speech can be enhanced by applying the following helpful hints (American Association of College if Nursing [AACN], n.d.):

- Be prepared. Rehearse!

- *Never* read your PowerPoint slides. A PowerPoint slide show is for support and does not replace what you say.

- Speak slowly, clearly, and enthusiastically.

- Begin with a purpose statement, and end with a take home message.

- Be logical. Organize your ideas.

- Similar to a written publication, use summary and transition sentences.

The importance of disseminating your DNP project is the provision of opportunities for communication, both in writing and in person. Communication, in turn, opens the door to collaboration on future projects.

COLLABORATION

Strategic dissemination of your DNP project findings leads to communication opportunities for collaboration and partnerships. Collaboration draws energy from others and initiates opportunities for postgraduation scholarly activities. Synergistic opportunities contribute significantly to practice evidence and enhance population health and patient-centered care (Montero, Lupi, & Jarris, 2015). Put another way, collaboration begins with a good conversation. Collaborative conversations illuminate processes for continuing scholarly work in intraprofessional and interprofessional programs and projects.

Collaboration means working with others to create something. Collaboration is further modified as interdisciplinary, interprofessional, intradisciplinary, and intraprofessional. *Discipline* is described as specific knowledge gained from a designated program of higher education such as nursing, biology, business, or engineering, whereas *professional* is described as a person formally qualified such as a registered nurse, social worker, business manager, or structural engineer. Although the terms have different meanings, both apply to learning or working collaboratively with nurse scientists and/or other professionals and practitioners (Oxford Dictionaries, 2015).

Interdisciplinary or *interprofessional* collaboration implies teams from two or more academic or professional areas of knowledge for the purpose of integrating information to advance specialized knowledge beyond the scope of a single practice (National Science Foundation (NSF), 2004). *Intradisciplinary* or *intraprofessional* collaboration implies individual people or teams from the same discipline or profession but at different levels of education and different roles working together for a common outcome (Columbia University, n.d.; Oxford Dictionaries, 2015).

Differentiating the meaning between *discipline* and *profession* within the academy and practice is a good reminder that scholarly collaboration is learned as a student and practiced as a professional. The current healthcare culture is adjusting to change on several levels as efforts move forward to address cost, access to health care, aging, and population health. Educating students for professional careers in nursing is also undergoing change and improvement, including laying the groundwork for collaborative actions. Collaboration begins in academia through implementation of *interdisciplinary* and *intradisciplinary* teaching and learning opportunities. Curricular construction and revision grounded in best available evidence assist students in adapting to 21st century nursing health care.

A model for experientially teaching collaboration is depicted in Figure 15.1. The figure represents the Bachelor of Science in Nursing (BSN) as foundational for collaborative practice, beginning with nursing and allied health collaborating on curricular development and teaching basic healthcare skills in the simulation laboratory. *Graduate degrees in nursing* offer multiple pathways to graduation, such as BSN to DNP nurse practitioner degree (direct patient care), BSN to PhD nurse scientist degree (indirect patient care), MSN degrees (indirect patient care) before selecting a DNP leadership degree (indirect patient care) or a PhD degree (indirect patient care). Time from entry as a BSN prepared registered nurse (RN) into a graduate degree program and graduation with a completed DNP or PhD doctoral degree should reflect equity in credit loads. Intradisciplinary core courses among all nursing graduate programs should be shared. Identified interdisciplinary graduate courses within the university should also be shared, thereby providing expert knowledge needed for healthcare practice and efficient use of education funding. Examples and suggestions include DNP direct care nurse practitioner students and medical students sharing clinical courses and clinical sites or master's degree students sharing courses with business students, public health students, information technology students, biology or engineering students. Collaboration leads to greater trust and respect among professionals because of shared knowledge and learning experiences. The result leads to increased opportunities within the academies and the healthcare organizations.

Collaboration in your *professional leadership roles* builds on your academic learning and experiences. The prefix *inter* preceding *professional* is central to collaborative teamwork and leads to integration of ideas, interventions, and outcomes. Collaborative teamwork functions best in a professional environment that incorporates the following elements (O'Daniel & Rosenstein, 2008):

- Clarity of purpose

- Strategy for success or entrance plan

- Honest and open communication

- Supportive and respectful environment

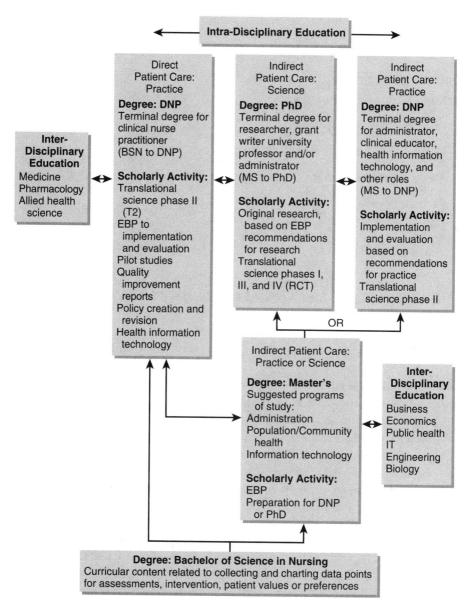

FIGURE 15.1 Suggestion for a Model for Intradisciplinary and Interdisciplinary Academic Collaboration. The model represents effectiveness, efficiency, and equity: efficiency of teaching and learning strategies and knowledge; efficiency of financial resources; equity in student time to graduation.

- Clarity in written and verbal communication
- Clarity of team role and expectations for each member
- Shared responsibility
- Rules for processing conflict
- Rules for making decisions
- Regular communication and meeting notes
- Access to identified resources
- Evaluation plan
- Exit plan

CHAPTER SUMMARY AND AFTERTHOUGHTS

Health care is consistently changing, improving, and rethinking varied approaches and opportunities affecting delivery. For example, health technology predictions include shifting more care and testing to patients' homes, made possible with computer applications and telehealth. Use of technology, especially for chronic conditions, addresses the importance of the social context and genomics. Increased creation of large volumes of patient-centered health data from individual hospital electronic health records presents opportunities and challenges for data analytics contextually specific to an organization. Finally, preparation of future nurses must include curriculum related to use of technological information tools, accurate and detailed input of patient data, analytics, and critical thinking regarding use of analytical findings. Increased collaboration and communication among all elements of health care—academic, direct patient care, indirect patient care, and translational science—provide opportunities for professional DNP leadership in continuing scholarly activities after graduation (Grumbach, Lucey, & Johnston, 2014; Skiba, 2014; Skiba, 2015). Recognition and achievement of improved population health "require building and reinforcing a continuous, iterative, and synergistic cycle of discovery, education, and care delivery in which the effect of each component is enriched by its association with and learning from the other components" (Grumbach et al., 2014, p 1110). Chapter 16 brings your scholarly project endeavors full circle by discussing the importance of translational science, a model for increasing creation and use of evidence.

WRITING REMINDERS...

Sharing Your Work With Peers

There is great value in finding someone you trust to show your written work to before sending it out into the world. A fresh set of eyes and a new perspective help find those places in our writing that might not flow or places that make sense to only you. It can be daunting to share something that is not finished. You may want to explain why one particular paragraph is not good and that you're still working on that paragraph— but don't! Just smile serenely and pass it on to a friend and give them free reign to review whatever seems out of place or confusing.

Data from Lamott, A. (1994). *Bird by bird: Some instructions on writing and life.* New York, NY: Pantheon Books.

REFERENCES

Agency for Healthcare Research and Quality (AHRQ). (2013). Section 5: Creating your dissemination plan. *Guide to evaluating health information exchange projects.* Washington, DC: AHRQ. Retrieved from http://healthit.ahrq.gov/health-it-tools-and-resources/guide-evaluating-health-information-exchange-projects

American Association of Colleges of Nursing (AACN). (n.d.). *Recommendations for effective podium presentations of abstracts.* Retrieved from http://www.aacn.nche.edu/conferences/Podium-Recommendations.pdf

Centers for Disease Control and Prevention (CDC). (2009). Disseminating program achievements and evaluation findings to garner support. *Evaluation Briefs,* no. 9. Retrieved from http://www.cdc.gov/healthyyouth/evaluation/pdf/brief9.pdf

Columbia University. (n.d.). *Presentation plan: Team health care models, focus 3, part I: The interdisciplinary healthcare team,* pp 215-218. Retrieved from http://www.columbia.edu/itc/hs/dental/cbdpp/sl2/pdf/glossary.pdf

Fitzpatrick, J.J. (2015). Predatory journals: What nurse educators need to know. *Nursing Education Perspectives,* 36(1), p 7.

Gennaro, S. (2014). Where should you share? *Journal of Nursing Scholarship,* 47(1), 1-2.

Grove, S.K., Burns, N., & Gray, J.R. (2013). *The practice of nursing research: Appraisal, synthesis, and generation of evidence* (7th ed.). St. Louis, MO: Elsevier Saunders.

Grumbach, K., Lucey, C.R., & Johnston, S.C. (2014). Transforming from centers of learning to learning health systems: The challenge for academic health centers. *JAMA, 311*(11), 1109-1110.

Leeman, J., & Sandelowski, M. (2012). Practice-based evidence and qualitative inquiry. *Journal of Nursing Scholarship, 44*(2), 171-179.

MacDonald, N., Ford-Jones, L., Friedman, J.N., & Hall, J. (2006). Preparing a manuscript for publication: A user-friendly guide. *Paediatrics and Child Health, 11*(6), 339-341.

Montero, J.T., Lupi, M.V., & Jarris, P.E. (2015). *Improved population health through more dynamic public health and health care system collaboration.* Institute of Medicine of the National Academies. Retrieved from http://www.iom.edu/Global/Perspectives/2015/Million-Hearts-Collaboration.aspx

National Science Foundation (NSF). (2004). *What is interdisciplinary research?* Retrieved from https://www.nsf.gov/od/oia/additional_resources/interdisciplinary_research/definition.jsp

O'Daniel, M., & Rosenstein, A.H. (2008). Professional communication and team collaboration. In R.G. Hughes (Ed.). *Patient safety and quality: An evidence-based handbook for nurses.* Rockville, MD: Agency for Healthcare Research and Quality (AHRQ). Retrieved from http://www.ncbi.nlm.nih.gov/books/NBK2637/

Oermann, M.H. (2009). SQUIRE guidelines for reporting improvement studies in healthcare: Implications for nursing publications. *Journal of Nursing Care Quality, 24*(2), 91-95.

Oermann, M.H., Turner, K., & Carman, M. (2014). Preparing quality improvement, research, and evidence-based practice manuscripts. *Nursing Economics, 32*(2), 57-69.

Oxford Dictionaries. (2015). Retrieved from http://www.oxforddictionaries.com/us/definition/american_english/collaboration

Polit, D.F., & Beck, C.T. (2013). *Nursing research: Generating and assessing evidence for nursing practice* (9th ed.). Philadelphia, PA: Wolters Kluwer/Lippincott Williams & Wilkins.

Sieber, T. (2009). *10 PowerPoint tips for preparing a professional presentation.* Retrieved from http://www.makeuseof.com/tag/10-tips-for-preparing-a-professional-presentation/

Skiba, D.J. (2014). The connected age: Digital tools for health. *Nursing Education Perspectives, 35*(6), 415-417.

Skiba, D.J. (2015). Health technology predictions for 2015: Ringing in the new. *Nursing Education Perspectives, 36*(1), 63-65.

Sollaci,, L.B., & Pereira, M.G. (2004). The introduction, methods, results, and discussion (IMRAD) structure: A fifty-year survey. *Journal of the Medical Library Association, 92*(3), 364-371.

Turner, K., Shamseer, L., Altman, D.G., Weeks, L., Peters, J., Kober, T., & Moher, D. (2012). Consolidated standards of reporting trials (CONSORT) and the completeness of reporting of randomized controlled trials (RCTs) published in medical journals. *Cochrane Database of Systematic Reviews, 11,* MR000030.

Woods, N.F., & Magyary, D.L. (2010). Translational research: Why nursing's interdisciplinary collaboration is essential. *Research and Theory for Nursing Practice: An International Journal, 24*(1), 9-24.

IF YOU WANT TO READ MORE...

Berkey, B., & Moore, S. (2012). Preparing research manuscripts for publication: A guide for authors. *Oncology Nursing Forum, 39*(5), 433-435.

International Committee of Medical Journal Editors. (2013). *Recommendations for the conduct, reporting, editing, and publication of scholarly work in medical journals.* Retrieved from http://www.icmje.org/icmje-recommendations.pdf

Moore, S. (2011). Can we trust your data? [Editorial]. *Oncology Nursing Forum, 38*(6), 615.

Oermann, M.H. (2009). SQUIRE guidelines for reporting improvement studies in healthcare: Implications for nursing publications. *Journal of Nursing Care Quality, 24*(2), 91-95.

16

Coming Full Circle: The Importance of Translational Science

What we call the beginning is often the end. And to make an end is to make a beginning. The end is where we start from.

T.S. ELIOT

OUTCOME OBJECTIVES

- Assess the purpose for translational science.
- Describe the phases of translational science.
- Discuss the usefulness of each translational science phase.
- Evaluate your responsibility for continuing practice scholarship within the framework of translational science.

TERMS

Applied research	Comparative-effectiveness research	Diffusion research
Basic research		Dissemination research

Continued

TERMS—cont'd

| Implementation research | Learning health system | Outcomes research Translational science |

Final chapters and conclusions contribute to bringing a message full circle, and that is the purpose of this chapter. Section 1 (Introduction) begins with laying the groundwork for your DNP project. Sections II and III (Inquiry and Leadership) focuses on evidence-based practice (EBP), implementation, and evaluation of your project framed in phase II of translational science (see Table 1.2 in Chapter 1). This final chapter in Section IV (Looking Forward) concludes by examining the interconnectedness of all four phases of the translational science structure for the purpose of looking at your role in collaboration and contribution to practice-based evidence.

WHAT IS TRANSLATIONAL SCIENCE?

Translational science is still commonly described as *translating research into practice*. However, translational science is much more than *bench-to-bedside* research. Recall that Dr. Steven H. Woolf (2008) wrote, "translational research means different things to different people, but it seems important to almost everyone" (p 211). Translational science is a 21st-century movement initiated by the medical profession for the purpose of addressing the needs of clinical research and health care practice. Dr. Elias A. Zerhouni (2005), author of the seminal article "Translational and Clinical Science—Time for a New Vision," wrote about the essential need for "transformation of translational clinical science and the novel interdisciplinary approaches that will advance science and enhance the health of the nation" (p 1352).

The evolutionary origins of translational science from EBP expanded the clinical research-based model. However, the issue of too many conceptualizations and terms related to *translational science* and *research translation* led to further confusion of who did what and when. Early in the translational science movement, scientists interpreted the model as developing new drugs and devices in the laboratory followed by implementation of human clinical trials. Hence, the development of the term *bench to bedside*. On the other hand, public health interpretations of translational science meant integrating new discoveries into practice settings at the population level. Translational science was in need of better communication. A rubric was needed to understand the phases in which investigators could create new ideas, evaluate processes and applications in designated clinical or practice settings followed by large-scale studies to validate practice changes and long-term outcomes. The 2007 publication by Khoury et al. proposed a "simple framework" of four translational phases, emphasizing collaborative research among multiple disciplines and professions. The four phases of translational science are bidirectional, iterative, and overlapping (Khoury et al., 2007). Box 16.1 provides definitions of the translation phases.

BOX 16.1 Translational Phases and Definitions Adapted for the DNP Project

T_1: Basic Research and Discovery

- "A systematic inquiry that uses disciplined methods to answer questions or solve problems. The ultimate goal of research is to develop, refine, and expand a base of knowledge" (Polit & Beck, 2006, p 4).

- T_1 expedites the movement between basic research and patient-oriented research (Robio et al., 2010).

- Observational studies and clinical trials are recommended (Khoury et al., 2007).

T_2: Application and Transformation of Best Evidence Into Practice

- "Evidence-based practice is the conscientious and judicious use of current best evidence in conjunction with clinical expertise and patient values to guide health care decisions" (Titler, 2010, p 36).

- Practice implementation involves adjusting or refining and establishing the value of EBP recommendations, quality improvement, or developmental projects that were identified through an EBP process (Sampselle, 2010; Titler, 2008; Woods & Magyary, 2010; Woolf, 2008).

- "T_2 facilitates the movement between patient centered research and population-based research" (Robio et al., 2010, p 471).

Continued

BOX 16.1 Translational Phases and Definitions Adapted for the DNP Project—cont'd

T$_3$: Dissemination

- The focus is on large-scale RCT dissemination research, implementation research, and diffusion research, similar to a phase IV clinical trial (Khoury et al., 2007; Woods & Magyary, 2010).

- The focus of dissemination research is to increase adoption and use of EBP practice implementation projects and practices to other workplace and community settings. Dissemination tests improvement and change in multiple sites, thereby contributing to health promotion research (ITHS, 2015).

T$_4$: Population Health Research

- Large-scale RCTs evaluate intervention effects, cost analysis, and practice utility and assesses how EBP recommendations can make an impact on real-world outcomes.

- Outcomes research and quality of life research are recommended (Khoury et al., 2007; Sampselle, 2010).

EBP, evidence-based practice; RCTs, randomized controlled trials.

Terminology

Definitions of the following research terms are intended to enhance your understanding and voice as a member of a collaborative team connected with a translational science project or research. A DNP is a significant member of collaborative teams because of his or her expertise in evaluation of direct and/or indirect patient-centered care. The following terms are extracted from the translational science model.

Basic research provides general knowledge without specific thought for practical ends, although it answers numerous questions important in practical problems. *Applied research* completes the answers for practical use (Robio et al., 2010).

Implementation research focuses on activities, strategies, and processes used for successful implementation of EBP recommendations (Khoury et al., 2007).

Dissemination research studies are large-scale studies that relate to distribution of evaluation findings from a single context to the wider population in multiple areas and can be successfully completed. The result is increased spread of information and knowledge of the evidence-based implementation in addition to the effect of the intervention (Khoury et al., 2007).

Diffusion research examines widespread, successful adoption of new practices or "the penetration of broad-scale recommendations" based on implementation of EBP recommendations (Khoury et al., 2007, p 668).

Outcomes research "describes, interprets, and predicts" end points related to the effect of the EBP intervention (Khoury et al., 2007, p 668).

Comparative-effectiveness research compares effectiveness, benefits, risks, costs, and strategies of interventions for the purpose of making healthcare decisions. Comparative-effectiveness research comprehensively collects large volumes of data from diverse populations for the purpose of informing patients, providers, and decision makers regarding effectiveness of interventions for varied patients under specific circumstances (Health Services Research Information Central [HSRIC], 2015).

Implementation and Growth of Translational Science

Past and current actions and publications to encourage system and organizational improvement of translating research into practice included the following. The National Institutes of Health (NIH) in 2006 published *Roadmap for Medical Research*, a collection of initiatives that proposed to "transform the Nation's medical research capabilities and improve the translation of research into practice" (Kantor, 2008, p 12). Box 16.2 lists the NIH roadmap initiatives applicable to nursing.

The four phases of translational science proposed by Khoury et al. (2007) were subsequently adapted with modifications for general use at translational science centers (Woods & Magyary, 2010).

Translational science centers were started for the purpose of supporting clinical research training for basic and clinical scientists from multiple disciplines. Translational science centers or institutes (e.g., The Institute of Translational Health Sciences [ITHS], Clinical and Translational Science Institutes [CTSI]) accommodate the learning and training needs for meeting the demands of translational science. These institutes are regionally located on multiple university campuses and are funded under the NIH. The purpose for the institutes is to improve and change how research and training are delivered, thereby influencing the next generation of researchers (ITHS, 2015) and "accelerating the translation of research into clinical use, medical practice, and health policy" (CTSI, 2015). *Clinical and Science Awards (CTSAs)* are offered to promote development and implementation throughout the translational science spectrum (National Center for Advancing Translational Sciences [NCATS], 2015).

BOX 16.2 National Institutes of Health Roadmap Initiative Themes Pertinent to Nursing

Research Teams of the Future

High-risk research

Interdisciplinary research

Public-private partnerships

Reengineering the Clinical Research Enterprise

Clinical research networks

Clinical outcomes assessment

Clinical research training

Clinical research policy analysis and coordination

Translational research

Source: Kantor (2008).

The *NCATS* was established near the end of 2011. Housed at the Institutes and Centers that compose the NIH, the NCATS is the newest enterprise among the institutes and centers. The NCATS describes itself as an *adapter* to enhance more effective collaborations among government, academia, industry, and non-profit organizations for the successful translation of research (NCATS, 2015). It was developed to address the obstacle of time between development of new processes, drugs, and devices and delivery to the intended patients and users. Time gaps can be multiple years (Institute of Medicine [IOM], 2012; NCATS, 2015). Obstacles identified as contributing to the time gap include the following (NCATS, 2015):

- Lack of understanding the science behind the translational process

- Shortage of qualified investigators

- Environments that do not support collaborations in the public and private sectors

- Inflexible, inefficient clinical trial designs and low participation in studies

- Regulatory issues

Implementation of the translational science model is being actualized through a *Learning Healthcare System* (LHS). The purpose of this recent initiative is to create a sizable and committed culture to continuously learn and improve a system or organization. The cyclic process of system improvements is grounded in evidence, including published evidence and analysis of data from electronic health records (Olsen, Aisner, & McGinnis, 2007; University of Michigan Health Informatics, 2013). The Institute of Medicine (IOM) held numerous round table workshops about LHSs. An important outcome from the workshops was a series of reports published between 2007 and concluding in 2013. The reports can be downloaded free of charge or purchased as hard copies from the National Academies Press (NAP). Titles from this series are included in the *If you want to read more …* section that follows the reference list. Identified needs and subsequent foci of the series include the following (IOM, 2015):

• Adaptation to the pace of change

• Stronger synchrony of efforts

• Culture of shared responsibility

• New clinical research paradigm

• Clinical decision support systems

• Universal electronic health records

• Tools for database linkage, mining, and use

• Notion of clinical data as a public good

• Incentives aligned for practice-based evidence

• Public engagement

• Trusted scientific broker

• Leadership

DNP involvement with leadership (see Chapter 2) and knowledge specific to practice (i.e., DNP project findings and professional practice involvement) are needed for transformation of knowledge into a functional learning healthcare system. A model for implementation of an LHS is published in the *Annals of Internal Medicine* (Greene, Reid, & Larson, 2012). The model is similar to the steps in your DNP project. The themes of the model reflect that research and practice are bidirectional and iterative, and they influence each other, similar to the structure of translational science wherein DNP- and PhD-prepared nurses collaborate for best practice outcomes. Themes identified for the LHS include the following (Greene et al., 2012):

1. Identification of a problem with innovative solutions

2. Design of the innovation based on evidence from publications, electronic health records, and other relevant sources

3. Implementation of the practice design as a pilot study with a comparison group

4. Evaluation of innovation actions and processes to show what works or does not work

5. Practice adjustments to make improvements, as needed, based on practice-based evidence

6. The model concluding with recommendations for dissemination.

Your efforts in learning and applying new knowledge that concluded with a successful DNP project now prepare you for collaboration and leadership within your healthcare organization. Continuation of lessons learned lead to your role as a lifelong leader.

WHAT ARE YOUR DNP ROLES IN TRANSLATIONAL SCIENCE?

The important roles of leadership and interdisciplinary collaboration are learned during your academic years. After graduation, DNPs are encouraged to continue scholarly, collaborative, and leadership roles within the model of translational science by identifying new practice issues and leading new projects to address the issues within the structure of your organization's LHS. Issues will be identified through contextual observations and communication. Introduction of recommendations for change or improvement in practice will follow the steps learned from successful completion of your DNP project. At this postgraduation stage of your career, your leadership abilities to address practice issues will initially focus on establishing interprofessional and/or intraprofessional teams and motivate end users for successful implementation.

In conclusion, promotion of translational science includes the following elements: (1) think and work in new ways; (2) collaborate and share strengths; and (3) train and educate legislators, organizations, and teams to better understand the importance of translational science (Grady, 2010).

CHAPTER SUMMARY AND AFTERTHOUGHTS

Lessons learned during the planning, implementation, and evaluation of your DNP project are expected to be used in your professional practice because you are uniquely qualified to fill the research-to-practice gap (Vincent, Johnson, Valasquez, & Rigney, 2010). Remember to pursue quality rigorously in all your professional scholarly activities for the purpose of gaining and retaining the trust of your peers and your intended audience. Your active participation and leadership in translational science following graduation with your terminal degree in nursing practice contribute valued knowledge to health care.

Contribute to the legacy of evidence: find best evidence → to use best evidence → leading to contributions of best evidence for the purpose of finding best evidence. Always remember, "if we want more evidence-based practice, we need more practice-based evidence" (Green & Ottoson, 2004).

WRITING REMINDERS...
Concluding Sentences

The first and last sentences of an evidence-based practice project are the most difficult to write. Think of the first and last paragraphs as a frame around the body of your written project. Whereas the beginning transitions you out of your current practice experiences, the ending transitions you back to your practice experiences. Conclusions help the reader envision why your knowledge and ideas are important before they put the paper down. The conclusion gives you, the writer, the last word to influence the reader with a new view or appreciation of the topic. The concluding paragraph should leave a positive impression with the reader.

Hints for writing a conclusion include the following (Haloewa, 2004):

- Create a full circle: tie the conclusion with the PICO question or recommendations for practice.

- Remind the reader of the most important key point from your paper.

- Reference the meaningfulness of the paper's topic on practice improvement or change.

- Challenge the reader to build on the conclusions.

- Leave a positive feeling with the reader.

REFERENCES

Clinical and Translational Sciences Institute (CTSI). (2015). *Tufts CTSI.* Retrieved from http://www.tuftsctsi.org

Department of Learning Health Services. (2016). *Learning health system (LHS) vision.* University of Michigan. Retrieved from http://lhs.medicine.umich.edu/lks/learninghealthsystem

Grady, P.A. (2010). News from NINR: Translational research and nursing science. *Nursing Outlook, 58*(3), 164-166.

Greene, L.W., & Ottoson, J.M. (2004). *From efficacy to effectiveness to community and back: Evidence-based practice vs. practice-based evidence.* Paper presented at From Clinical Trials to Community: The Science of Translating Diabetes and Obesity Research conference, Bethesda, MD.

Greene, S.M., Reid, R.J., & Larson, E.B. (2012). Implementing the learning health system: From concept to action. *Annals of Internal Medicine 157*(3), 207-210.

Haloewa, R. (2004). *Strategies for writing a conclusion.* St. Cloud State University: The Write Place.

Health Services Research Information Central (HSRIC). (2015). *Comparative effectiveness research (CER).* Retrieved from http://www.nlm.nih.gov/hsrinfo/cer.html

Institute of Medicine (IOM). (2015). *The learning healthcare system in America.* Washington, DC: National Academies Press. Retrieved from www.iom.edu/Activities/Quality/LearningHealthCare.aspx

Institute of Translational Health Sciences (ITHS). (2015). *About ITHS.* Retrieved from https://www.iths.org

Kantor, L.W. (2008). NIH roadmap for medical research. *Alcohol Research and Health, 31*(1), 12-13. Retrieved from http://pubs.niaaa.nih.gov/publications/arh311/12-13.pdf

Khoury, M.J., Gwinn, M., Yoon, P.W., Dowling, N., Moore, C.A., & Bradley, L. (2007). The continuum of translation research in genomic medicine: How can we accelerate the appropriate integration of human genome discoveries into health care and disease prevention? *Genetics in Medicine, 6*(10), 665-674.

National Center for Advancing Translational Sciences (NCATS). (2015). *Clinical and translational science.* Bethesda, MD: NCATS. Retrieved from http://www.ncats.nih.gov/ctsa

Olsen, L.A., Aisner, D., & McGinnis, M. (Eds.). (2007). *The learning healthcare system: Workshop summary.* Washington, DC: National Academies Press. Retrieved from http://www.nap.edu/catalog/11903/the-learning-healthcare-system-workshop-summary-iom-roundtable-on-evidence

Polit, D.F., & Beck, C.T. (2006). *Nursing research: Generating and assessing evidence for nursing practice* (8th ed.). Philadelphia, PA: Wolters Kluwer/Lippincott Williams & Wilkins.

Robio, D.M., Schoenbaum, E.E., Lee, L.S., Schteingart, D.E., Marantz, M.D., Anderson, M.D., & Esposito, K. (2010). Defining translational research: Implications for training. *Academic Medicine, 85*(3), 470-475. Retrieved from http://www.ncbi.nlm.nih.gov/pmc/articles/PMC2829707/

Sampselle, C.M. (2010). The Michigan center for health intervention (MICHIN): Facilitating translational science. *Research and Theory for Nursing Practice: An International Journal, 24*(1), 6-8.

Titler, M.G. (2008). The evidence for evidence-based practice implementation. In R.G.Hughes (Ed.). *Patient safety and quality: An evidence-based handbook for nurses.* Rockville, MD: Agency for Healthcare Research and Quality (AHRQ).

Titler, M.G. (2010). Translation science and context. *Research and Theory for Nursing Practice, 24*(1), 35-55.

Vincent, D., Johnson, C., Valasquez, D., & Rigney, T. (2010). DNP-prepared nurses as practitioner-researchers: Closing the gap between research and practice. *American Journal of Nursing Practitioners, 14*(11-12), 28-34.

Woods, N.F., & Magyary, D.L. (2010). Translational research: Why nursing's interdisciplinary collaboration is essential. *Research and Theory for Nursing Practice, 24*(1), 9-24.

Woolf. S.H. (2008). The meaning of translational research and why it matters. *JAMA, 292*(2), 211-213.

Writing Center, University of North Carolina at Chapel Hill. (2015). *Conclusions.* Retrieved from http://writing center.unc.edu/handouts/conclusions/

Zerhouni, E. (2005). US biomedical research: Basic, translational, and clinical sciences. *JAMA, 294*(11), 1352-1358.

IF YOU WANT TO READ MORE...

Alper, J., Rapporteur. (2013). *Population health implications of the Affordable Care Act: workshop summary.* Washington, DC: National Academies Press. Retrieved from http://www.nap.edu/catalog.php?record_id=18546

Berkman, N.D., Lohr, K.N., Ansari, M., McDonagh, M., Balk, E., Whitlock, E., & Chang, S. (2013). Grading the strength of a body of evidence when assessing health care interventions for the Effective Health Care Program of the Agency for Healthcare Research and Quality: an update. *Methods guide for comparative effectiveness reviews.* Publication no. 13(14)-EHC130. Rockville, MD: Agency for Healthcare Research and Quality (AHRQ). Retrieved from www.effectivehealthcare.ahrq.gov/reports/final.cfm

The Learning Health System Series (by publication year, not alphabetized)

Olsen, L.A., Aisner, D., & McGinnis, M. (Eds.). (2007). *The learning healthcare system: Workshop summary.* Washington, DC: National Academies Press. Retrieved from http://www.nap.edu/catalog/11903/the-learning-healthcare-system-workshop-summary-iom-roundtable-on-evidence

McClellan, M.B., McGinnis, J.M., Nabel, E.G., & Olsen, L.A. (Eds.). (2008). *Evidence-based medicine and the changing nature of health care: Meeting summary.* Washington, DC:

National Academies Press. Retrieved from http://www.nap.edu/catalog/12041/evidence-based-medicine-and-the-changing-nature-of-health-care

Olsen, L.A., Goolsby, W.A., & McGinnis, J.M. (Eds.). (2009). *Leadership commitments to improve value in health care.* Washington, DC: National Academies Press. Retrieved from http://www.nap.edu/catalog/11982/leadership-commitments-to-improve -value-in-health-care-finding-common

Young, P.L., Olsen, L.A., & McGinnis, J.M. (Eds.). (2009). *Value in health care: Accounting for cost, quality, safety, outcomes, and innovation.* Washington, DC: National Academies Press. Retrieved from http://www.nap.edu/catalog/12566/value-in-health-care -accounting-for-cost-quality-safety-outcomes

Goolsby, W.A., Olsen, L.A., & McGinnis, M. (Eds.). (2010). *Clinical data as the basic staple of health learning: Creating and protecting a public good.* Washington, DC: National Academies Press. Retrieved from http://www.nap.edu/catalog/12212/clinical-data-as-the -basic-staple-of-health-learning-creating

Olsen, L.A., & McGinnis, M. (Eds.). (2010). *Redesigning the clinical effectiveness research paradigm: Innovation and practice-based approaches.* Washington, DC: National Academies Press. Retrieved from http://www.nap.edu/catalog/12197/redesigning-the -clinical-effectiveness-research-paradigm-innovation-and-practice-based

Grossmann, C., Goolsby, A., Olsen, L.A., & McGinnis (Eds.). (2011). *Engineering a learning healthcare system: A look at the future.* Washington, DC: Institute of Medicine. Retrieved from https://www.iom.edu/Reports/2011/Engineering-a-Learning -Healthcare-System.aspx

Grossman, C., Powers, B., & McGinnis, M. (Eds.). (2011). *Digital infrastructure for the learning health system: The foundation for continuous improvement in health and health care.* Washington, DC: National Academies Press. Retrieved from http://www.nap.edu/ catalog/12912/digital-infrastructure-for-the-learning-health-system-the-foundation- for

Olsen, L.A., Grossman, C., & McGinnis, J.M. (Eds.). (2011). *Learning what works: Infrastructure required for comparative effectiveness research.* Washington, DC: National Academies Press. Retrieved from http://www.nap.edu/catalog/12214/learning-what -works-infrastructure-required-for-comparative-effectiveness-research-workshop

Young, P.L., Saunders, R.S., & Olsen, L.A. (Eds.). (2011). *The healthcare imperative: Lowering costs and improving outcomes.* Washington, DC: National Academies Press. Retrieved from http://books.nap.edu/openbook.php?record_id=12750

Smith, M., Saunders, R., Stuckhardt, L., & McGinnis, J.M. (Eds.). (2012). *Best care at lower cost: The path to continuously learning health care in America.* Washington, DC: National Academies Press. Retrieved from http://books.nap.edu/openbook. php?record_id=13444

Appendix: Review of Qualitative Methods for Practice Projects

Words, especially organized into incidents or stories, have a concrete, vivid, mean-ingful flavor that often proves far more convincing to a reader—another researcher, a policymaker, a practitioner—than pages of summarized numbers.

MILES & HUBERMAN, 1994

Appendix A is a review of qualitative designs and methods that are useful for evaluating practice projects. Qualitative methods are described as collecting and analyzing data with words, stories, and pictures, as opposed to quantitative methods, which collect and analyze data that can be quantified. Qualitative methods describe and evaluate processes and activities that are new or not well understood (Leeman & Sandelowski, 2012; Tripp-Reimer & Doebbeling, 2004).

Denzin and Lincoln's (1994) definition of qualitative research is helpful in understanding that the broad concept of qualitative research is valuable for evaluation of DNP practice projects.

Qualitative research is multi-method in focus, involving an interpretive, naturalistic approach to its subject matter. This means that qualitative research studies things in their natural settings, attempting to make sense of, or interpret, phenomena in terms of the meanings people bring to them. Qualitative research involves the studied use and collection of a variety of empirical materials—case study, personal experience, introspective, life story, interview, observational, historical, interactional, and visual texts—that describe routine and problematic moments and meanings in individuals' lives. Accordingly, qualitative researchers deploy a wide range of interconnected methods, hoping always to get a better fix on the subject matter at hand (p 2).

Recall that the purpose of this appendix is to review qualitative methods that are useful for your practice project (see Chapter 11). First, however, a historical overview of qualitative research and evaluation methods puts it into perspective.

HISTORICAL PERSPECTIVE OF THE IMPORTANCE OF QUALITATIVE METHODS

Quantitative approaches to methodology and research were increasingly recognized in the 20th century. In the 21st century, qualitative approaches to evaluation continue to contribute a depth of understanding and interpretation regarding lived experiences surrounding health care (Joanna Briggs Institute [JBI], 2014). The philosophical origins of qualitative approaches are credited to August Comte, a 19th-century philosopher. Comte is recognized as the first philosopher of science who paid attention to social dimensions of science and current points of view (Bourdeau, 2013). Science at the time of Comte was considered a positivistic paradigm (i.e., a worldview of objective reality) wherein knowledge was absolute, systematic, and logical.

Philosophers noted for building on Comte's writings included Edmund Husserl (1859–1938), Martin Heidegger (1889–1976), and Maurice Merleau-Ponty (1908–1961). These philosophers focused on the phenomenological understanding of people within their naturalistic state. Husserl and Merleau-Ponty surmised that humans and human activity cannot be studied in isolation but should be understood within the context of lived experiences that include personal, cultural, and social connections. These early philosophers contributed to a *postpositivist paradigm* in which understanding occurs within the naturalistic state (Blackburn, 1994; Denzin & Lincoln, 1994; University of Utah, 2014).

Constructivist paradigm is another common term indicating a reaction to the *positivist paradigm.* Constructivism is credited to writers such as Max Weber (1864–1920). The premise is that old ideas are taken apart or deconstructed and are reconstructed in a new way that gives meaning within an identified context. In other words, reality is not a fixed structure. Reality has multiple

---

BOX A.1 Qualitative Characteristics Common to Practice Evaluations

- Holistic approach to understanding participants' perspectives
- Relationships
- Naturalistic, personal, face-to-face, current
- Focus on describing and understanding a context, not predicting
- Inductive in nature
- Time-consuming data collection
- Ongoing analysis

From Denzin & Lincoln, 1994, p 212.

constructions and interpretations within a context. Constructivist findings are produced through interactions between inquirer and participants, especially when the distance between inquirer and project participant is minimized. This naturalist approach is useful for evaluation in the practice setting (Polit & Beck, 2012).

Box A.1 is a list of qualitative research characteristics that are useful to practice evaluations. The historical perspective of paradigms, or worldviews, is further categorized into qualitative designs. These approaches to understanding the intent of qualitative research methodologies are discussed in the next section.

PHILOSOPHICAL ASSUMPTIONS ABOUT QUALITATIVE DESIGNS

Philosophical paradigms and assumptions about qualitative designs are "basic sets of beliefs that guide action" (Guba, 1990, p 17). Philosophical assumptions about design influence the author's understanding of how a project should be evaluated (Denzin & Lincoln, 1994). Philosophical paradigms and assumptions of qualitative methods are based on *ontological* (the nature of being) *assumptions, epistemological* (the study of knowledge) *assumptions,* and *methodological* (data collection and data analysis) *assumptions.* Table A.1 is an overview of qualitative paradigms and designs.

TABLE A.1 Philosophical Paradigms and Assumptions or Orientation to Design

Philosophical Paradigms	Assumptions or Orientation of Qualitative Design
Positivist	Quantitative analysis See Appendix B
Constructivist or interpretivist	Phenomenology Ethnography Case study Grounded theory
Critical theory	Feminist Participatory action research (PAR)
Other qualitative research terms derived from contemporary applications	Qualitative descriptive

Data from Denzin & Lincoln, 1994; JBI, 2014; Polit & Beck, 2012.

The *constructivist* (also called *interpretivist*) paradigm is a qualitative paradigm that purports many interpretations of reality within a single context. The goal of qualitative evaluations is to objectively interpret or find meaning from the data. Stated another way, the evaluator seeks to understand how people construct meaning within their context. Interpretivist thinking arises from the hermeneutic tradition of German philosophers. *Interpretivist thinking* examines the subjective experiences of people while striving to objectify collection and analysis of data. *Constructivist thinking* posits that knowledge is a "pluralistic and plastic" (Denzin & Lincoln, 1994, p 125) nature of *knowing*. Knowing is the result of perspective, and perspective is specific to context (Denzin & Lincoln, 1994; JBI, 2014; Polit & Beck, 2012).

Specific designs within the constructivist or interpretivist paradigm frame the different approaches or orientations to qualitative methods. The following is a descriptive list of qualitative designs from the approaches or orientations of qualitative research:

Phenomenology arises from philosophy and psychology. The focus is construction of meaning from lived experiences. The phenomenological orientation is widespread in the practice setting (Denzin & Lincoln, 1994; Grove, Burns, & Gray, 2013). An example of phenomenology is seeking to understand a child's perceptions of postsurgical pain.

Ethnography originated with studies in culture and civilization that grew from anthropology and sociology. Ethnography has similarities to phenomenology, but the focus is culture, as in nursing units, inner city gangs, or tribal traditions (Denzin & Lincoln, 1994; Grove et al., 2013). An example of ethnography is seeking to understand newly arrived refugee families' expectations of prenatal care compared with families who have lived in the same city for more than one generation.

Case study is about choosing a specific case to be evaluated by looking at the parts or subsections of the case in its naturalistic setting (Burns & Grove, 2011; Denzin & Lincoln, 1994). An example of a case study is an epidemiological case. For example, a state epidemiologist receives increasing data about an outbreak of Salmonella infection in a specific population and region of the state. A researcher is sent to the site wherein substantial time is spent gathering information from a variety of sources such as interviews of people, observations of places and activities, and reading documents. The specific, unique, detailed information is analyzed and described, thereby increasing its usefulness of preventing Salmonella infection.

Grounded theory is considered a general methodology widely used by social scientists and includes "a way of thinking about and conceptualizing data" (Denzin & Lincoln, 1994, p 275). Put another way, grounded theory is about building a theory when no theory exists or the existing theory does not explain the concepts or circumstances (LoBiondo-Wood & Haber, 2010). The qualitative approach to grounded theory is considered "conceptually dense" with sets of concepts for the purpose of creating relationships or propositions. Analysis focuses on patterns of actions among variables. Analytical thinking and writing about the conceptual relationships contribute rigor to the methodology and therefore the usefulness of the relationships (Denzin & Lincoln, 1994). An example of a grounded theory study is development of a theory addressing recovery from schizophrenia from the viewpoints of patients, family members, and healthcare professionals (Grove et al., 2013; Noiseux and Ricard, 2008).

Critical theory is a paradigm that focuses on critique and transformation. Its origins lie in Germany with Jurgen Habermas (born in 1929) and other philosophers of Marxist thought. Habermas' philosophical writings focus on political domains, rationality, knowledge, and communication. The most current interpretation of critical theory and most useful for today's nursing environment is to focus on social, historical, and ideological structures that produce or limit criticism and social movement (Denzin & Lincoln, 1994; Bohman & Rehg, 2005).

Methodologies associated with critical theory include feminist theory and participatory action research. **Feminist theory** centers on gender, class, and race, with the focus on the experiences of oppressed people. **Participatory action research** is attributed to Kurt Lewin (1890–1947). Action research works with groups or communities vulnerable to oppression by a dominant or influential group. The term *participatory* implies that study participants are involved with identification of the problem, data collection and analysis, and decisions regarding use of findings. The purpose is to produce not only findings but also participants' social action and consciousness raising. A goal of participatory action research is to empower people who feel disempowered (Baum, MacDougall, & Smith, 2006; Denzin & Lincoln, 1994; Friere, 1970; Polit & Beck, 2012). An example of participatory action research is to engage newly arrived non–English-speaking female refugees to identify their personal and cultural needs related to prenatal health care.

Some qualitative practice researchers do not prescribe to a traditional classification. For example, a qualitative descriptive evaluation uses words to describe observations of a project participant following a new procedure for patient teaching. These studies are commonly referred to as *qualitative descriptive studies*. Care should be taken, however, not to name a study as qualitative descriptive after the fact because your project evaluation was poorly conceived and constructed. Descriptive methodology draws from variations of the philosophical orientations (Polit & Beck, 2012; Sandelowski, 2010).

QUALITATIVE METHODS FOR EVALUATION

Qualitative methods for collecting and evaluating data are truthful and meaningful ways of evaluation for applied fields, including health care. The *value* of qualitative research methods is best described by Miles and Huberman (1994).

> *Qualitative data are a source of well-grounded, rich descriptions and explanations of processes in identifiable local contexts. With qualitative data one can preserve chronological flow, see precisely which events led to which consequences, and derive fruitful explanations. Then, too, good qualitative data are more likely to lead to serendipitous findings than to new integrations.… Finally, the findings from qualitative studies have a quality of undeniability. Words, especially organized into incidents or stories, have a concrete, vivid, meaningful flavor that often prove far more convincing to a reader than pages of summarized numbers (p 1).*

Challenges with qualitative methods include the labor-intensive process of data collection, personal feelings of data overload, potential for evaluator bias, and the time-intensive nature of data analysis. Findings cannot be generalized because of the small sample sizes (Miles & Huberman, 1994). Additionally, the effect of context is increasingly important because the conditions or events being evaluated continually interact with each other. Understanding interactions within the context affects what is important (Agency for Healthcare Research and Quality [AHRQ], 2013). Qualitative evaluations are useful for understanding complex issues including risk factors, populations, change, process, and context. Qualitative methods provide findings about concepts, meaning, feasibility, sustainability, acceptability, process, and effectiveness (Kitson, 2002; Leeman & Sandelowski, 2012).

Participant selection for qualitative inquiry is driven by knowledge of the context and target population. Participants are selected because of their experience and their ability to provide information about implementing the recommendations for practice. Participant selection for qualitative inquiry is generally purposeful, meaning that the researcher selects participants based on his or her personal judgment of the participant (Grove et al., 2013; LoBiondo-Wood & Haber, 2010; Polit & Beck, 2012).

Sampling size for a qualitative study is determined when information gleaned from participants produces no new information and becomes redundant of previously collected data. This is called *data saturation.* Factors to consider in determining data saturation include scope of evaluation, topic, and quality of collected data. Scope infers breadth and depth, meaning that evaluation with a broad scope needs more participants for data collection, versus a study with a narrow focus in which clarity occurs more quickly (Burns & Grove, 2011; Denzin & Lincoln, 1994; Grove et al., 2013).

In qualitative evaluation, the researcher or project evaluator interacts with participants of the study. Viewed as bias in quantitative studies, researcher involvement is considered an important element in qualitative studies. Sometimes called *researcher-as-instrument* or *researcher-participant relationship,* the involvement by the researcher enhances relationship building with the participant, thereby increasing trust and participant's sharing of intimate knowledge (Burns & Grove, 2011; LeCompte, Millroy, & Preissis, 1992). The following quotation eloquently addresses the responsibilities of the qualitative researcher: "Qualitative researchers are guests in the private spaces of the world. Their manners should be good and their code of ethics strict" (Stake, 1994, p 244).

DATA COLLECTION

Qualitative inquiry focuses on *mountains of words* (Johnson, Dunlap, & Benoit, 2010). The nature of qualitative data revolves around observation, interviews, and documents. Qualitative data are collected by watching, asking, and examining. Data are collected in a natural environment, meaning that the evaluator is in close proximity to the local setting for extended periods of time. Qualitative data are concerned with actions because actions are rooted in intentions and meaning that lead to consequences. Collection of evaluation data is more complex than first appears and requires honest self-appraisal. Using multiple methods of data collection provides a means of demonstrating *triangulation.* Triangulation is a means of applying rigor to data collection (LoBiondo-Wood & Haber, 2010; Miles & Huberman, 1994).

Collecting data from *observation* is fundamental to nurses. Evaluating pain by observing signs and symptoms of a patient's facial grimace, decreased movement, or pale skin is an example of collecting data that should be documented in the patient's chart. Observing a non–English-speaking refugee patient smile when she receives ethnic food prepared by a friend may be important information to chart, especially if he or she has eaten little or no food prepared by the hospital. The importance of narratively charting *unstructured observations* cannot be overemphasized. It is the basis of establishing evidence-based data. Other types of observations used in qualitative evaluations include a more structured observation. *Structured observations* are challenging because the evaluator must gain entry and be accepted into the participant's group or culture where change is being implemented. The observer's role begins by establishing trust and rapport within the group and learning the context (Grove et al., 2013; Polit & Beck, 2012). Steps in the evolving role of observer are best described by Leininger and McFarland (2006):

- Observe and listen actively.

- Observe and participate on a limited basis.

- Participate with continued observation.

- Reflect and reconfirm with participants your findings from observation.

Observation is a data collection method to establish authenticity of participants' interviews. For example, a nursing instructor told the interviewer that her favorite method of teaching is small group activities during face-to-face time in the classroom, but when the interviewer became a classroom observer and noticed that the nursing instructor never used small group activities in class, the evaluator deduced that interview answers lacked credibility.

Interviews for collection of qualitative data can be structured, unstructured, focused, or semistructured, but the basic format for interviewing is the same: asking, listening, and recording. *Unstructured interviews* occur when the data collector has no preconceived idea for flow of information. Unstructured interviews are conversational and interactive. Participants tell their stories with little interruption. *Structured or semistructured interviews* are used when the evaluator has specific topics or questions to cover with each participant. Questions should encourage opportunities for participants to tell their stories about a topic in depth and detail. The evaluator's role is to encourage participants to speak freely and tell their stories in their own words. Preparation for the semistructured interview is to order the questions in a logical sequence. Interviewers need to listen closely because questions may be answered out of sequence to the evaluator's list, but in conjunction with other questions about which the participant is speaking. Attentive listening prompts the interviewer to ask follow-up questions to be sure he or she clearly understands the participant's story (Grove et al., 2013; Polit & Beck, 2012).

Focused group interviews comprise another venue for data collection because group interviews involve group dynamics such as stimulating subtopics for conversation, thereby increasing understanding of the practice project. Focus groups grew out of marketing research from opinions, product characteristics, delivery, or process. Your job as project leader is to act as moderator by asking unstructured, structured, or semistructured questions. Skills for the moderator are basically the same as for an interviewer. Focus groups are useful in gathering data for participatory action research (Denzin & Lincoln, 1994; Grove et al., 2013; Polit & Beck, 2012).

Life histories are written or verbal self-disclosures about lived experiences and are grounded in ethnographic philosophical designs. Histories provide useful data for evaluation of a patient-centered project because the chronology of events, actions, and process is important for understanding the participants' stories and needs. Comparative histories are helpful in providing information about cultural ethnicities, generations, or contexts that affect change. Life histories may also contain new information about patients' coping (Denzin & Lincoln, 1994; Grove et al., 2013; Polit & Beck, 2012). For example, collecting histories from patients recovering from disputed divorces, child custody battles, or financial stress and who are currently participating in a new educational program provides information about process, actions, and outcomes of the intervention.

The *think-aloud* method is a process to collect data about problem-solving and decision making. It is based on Ericsson and Simon's (1993) information processing theory. Thinking aloud is an action wherein people talk aloud into an audio recorder at the time they are problem-solving in a naturalistic setting. Thinking aloud can also be set in a simulated setting (Aitken & Mardegan, 2000; Polit & Beck, 2012). The think-aloud method is helpful in understanding change and process in the project participants.

Field notes are extremely valuable and can be used with triangulation. Field notes are your personal written or recorded observations and reflections about what happened during implementation of the project. They are broad and analytical and reflect your reactions to observations, interviews, or conversations. Field notes reflect your personal feelings or ethical dilemmas and contribute to interpretation of observations and other collected data. Field notes contribute to a holistic approach to evaluation because they help an evaluator remember events (Polit & Beck, 2012; Spindler & Spindler, 1992).

Patient chart reviews are repositories for nursing data about patients' values and preferences. Creating this base of evidence for evaluation of evidence-based practice (EBP) guidelines or recommendations is a direct example of creating evidence for use in evaluating change. Charting contributes to a legacy of evidence directly related to the definitions of EBP by Titler et al. (2001) and by Sackett, Straus, Richardson, Rosenberg, and Haynes (2000) that incorporate patients' values and clinical expertise.

Review of *policies, procedures, and other institutional documents* contributes to evaluation of context and process. Review of documents provides data on the history, philosophy, and operation of your institution or unit. Documents assist in identifying whether formal written expectations are implemented as intended. Document reviews also increase your understanding of the current program, personnel, and costs associated with the project (Centers for Disease Control and Prevention [CDC], 2009).

DATA ANALYSIS

Qualitative data collection, data management, and data analysis are iterative procedures rooted in question and answer cycles about implementation evaluation of your EBP project. This implies organization and structure. Qualitative inquiry strives to carefully build protocols for storage, retrieval, and management of data to use and analyze collected data effectively (Huberman & Miles, 1994; Johnson et al., 2010). Figure A.1 provides an overview for thinking about qualitative data and for analyzing the data.

Data management and analysis revolve around *grounded theory coding.* A code is a system of words, symbols, and numbers that contributes to deciphering and understanding qualitative data (Oxford Dictionaries, 2014). Coding is considered an analytical problem-solving technique in that it looks for patterns and relationships in the data extracted from interview transcriptions, observational field notes, or pertinent passages from institutional documents. However, there is not a specific system or formula to follow for coding. Qualitative coding is termed *heuristic,* meaning "to discover" (Hatch, 2002; Miles & Huberman, 1994; Saldana, 2013). Coding begins by looking for patterns such as similarities, differences, frequencies, sequences, relationships, or causations from collected

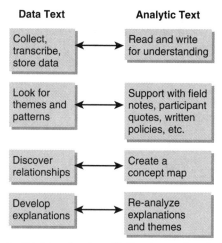

FIGURE A.1 Overview for thinking about qualitative data and analyzing the data.

data. Coding is filtered by how the project participants or you, the evaluator, perceive and interpret your observations and experiences. Coding also reflects the assumptions or framework brought to your project and the qualitative philosophical design selected (Saldana, 2013).

Coding is a process that may be organized as follows (Saldana, 2013):

1. Identifying salient points or quotations from your collected data

2. Putting a label or code (one word or a short sentence) on the quotation

3. Grouping the labels or codes into a category and subcategories, as needed

4. Identifying common themes or concepts

Suggested categories for organization of coding are presented in Box A.2.

Helpful Hints for Coding

- As you collect and identify potentially useful qualitative data, write your ideas or analytical thoughts next to the quotation. Your ideas or thoughts should be bracketed to differentiate them from your interview, document, or observation data.

- Be organized.

BOX A.2 Suggested Categories for Organizing a First Round
              of Coding

- Magnitude: enormity or seriousness

- Frequency: repetitiveness

- Structures and processes

  - Emotion

  - Values

  - Comparison

  - Descriptive

  - Process

  - Causes

  - Consequences

- Patterns

  - Causes and consequences

From Saldana, 2013.

- Persevere. Coding is challenging and time consuming.

- Be able to deal with uncertainty.

- Be flexible. Coding is cyclical, and coding schemes evolve throughout the analysis process.

- Be creative.

- Be rigorously ethical (Saldana, 2013).

Remember that sufficient *quality* data is the goal of *qualitative* data collection, and there are no limitations on the number of codes, categories, or concepts that may arise from your collected data. You may choose to initially code manually to learn the basics. Computer-assisted qualitative data analysis software (CAQDAS) is also available, if desired. Popular software programs include ATLAS, MSCQDA, and NVivo (Saldana, 2013). Table A.2 is an example of a coding schema.

TABLE A.2 Example of a Coding Scheme

Purpose of evaluation: Describe and differentiate roles of peer health adviser and certified medical interpreter.

Framework: Phenomenology

Participants: Seven women fluent in English and a refugee patient's preferred spoken language.

Definitions: Peer health adviser—a person who contributes to the health status of refugee mothers, infants, and families through comprehensive case coordination and outreach to increase access to maternal and child health and family services and to assist healthcare providers to deliver culturally safe care responsive to refugee maternity and pediatric patients' unique needs (Reavy, Hobbs, Hereford, & Crosby, 2012). *Certified medical interpreter*—a person who renders orally into one language a message spoken in a different language. An appropriate interpreter for a healthcare setting is an adult who (1) is a fluent speaker of both languages in question, (2) is not a relative of the patient, and (3) has received professional training and certification as an interpreter (CCHCP, 2010).

Focus group questions: A. How would you describe your role as a Culturally Appropriate Resources and Education (C.A.R.E) clinic health advisor? B. How would you describe your role as a certified medical interpreter?

Specific	Deductive Reasoning		General
Salient point:	Code or Label	Code or Label	Concepts or Themes
Quotation (in italics)	Round 1	Round 2	
Field note or Observation			

Focus Group Discussion

A1. *C.A.R.E. clinic health advisors help the healthcare workers understand different cultures and make the refugee's voice stronger.*	[1]Stronger voice for refugee [2]Cultural understanding		
A2. Being fluent in speaking English and a refugee's preferred spoken language provided community recognition for the health advisors as leaders for the women.	[3]Status [4]Community	1. Communication 1a. Empowerment	Building trust
A3. *You work with the same person; you know their issues. People do not have to wonder where to go.*	[1]Voice/ Communication [4]Community	2. Community	Valuing self

Continued

TABLE A.2 Example of a Coding Scheme—cont'd

Specific	Deductive Reasoning	General
A4. *People call me asking what I think. They think that you can solve everything and it's hard for them to see if they are talking to you as a friend or a health advisor.*	[4]Community [1]Communication [5]Role confusion	3. Navigating the system
A5. Many of the health advisors are refugees and have experienced traumatic events similar to those of the current patients. It is the health advisor who understands and encourages those questions that a patient may be embarrassed to ask.	[1]Communication [6]Empowered	
B1. *If you are not an interpreter, then you cannot go into the room with the doctor and patient, and the doctor can't share information with you. Many times refugees don't understand what the doctor is saying and will say "yes" to everything.*	[5]Communication [6]Disempowered [7]Feelings of frustration	
B2. *When you are only a health advisor you can't translate in the hospital, so there is a breakdown in communication because the healthcare worker can't tell, and the patient is usually confused. You need a health advisor for all refugees because the case managers cannot do that job.*	[4]Community [1]Communication [6]Disempowered [7]Feelings of frustration	

Data from Reavy, Hobbs, Hereford, & Crosby, 2012; Saldana, 2013.

RIGOR AND INTEGRITY FOR QUALITATIVE METHODS

Rigor and integrity are important criteria in both qualitative and quantitative evaluation because they contribute to development of the reader's *trust* in the *truthfulness* of the evaluation results. Recall that qualitative evaluation focuses on interpretation and description. Four criteria are generally recognized for evaluating qualitative rigor: *credibility, dependability, confirmability,* and *transferability* (Lincoln & Guba, 1985). Self-assessment of strengths and weaknesses is classically performed using these criteria of truthfulness.

Credibility is the aim of qualitative researchers because credibility represents the researcher's effort to enhance the believability of the collected data and subsequent analysis or interpretations. *Dependability* is similar to the quantitative criteria of reliability and answers the question, "Would the researcher get similar results if it were repeated with similar participants and context?" Remember: without dependability, there is no credibility. *Confirmability* is about objectivity and implies that the collected data and interpretations represent the participants' voice and are not biased by the researcher. *Transferability* means that the findings of the qualitative study are adequately described for another person to reach a conclusion whether or not the findings may be useful to his or her context (Beck, 1993; Lincoln & Guba, 1985; Polit & Beck, 2012).

Demonstrations of rigor in data collection and evaluation include the following: *saturation, audit trail, confirmability, triangulation,* and *multiple raters.* These actions contribute to ensuring that the criteria for rigor are met. *Saturation* occurs when no new information is obtained from data collection. Stated another way, saturation occurs when the researcher hears repetitive stories from multiple participants and the information is redundant. Saturation therefore contributes to limiting participant or sample size while ensuring that adequate amounts of data have been collected. *Participant verification* is a means of confirmability because it implies that participants are presented with evaluation findings and are able to recognize themselves and confirm the accuracy of the findings. *Member checking* is similar to participant verification, but it implies that the evaluator engages the participant in interpretation of data. Member checking is generally an ongoing activity for the purpose of confirming accuracy of data interpretation. *Multiple raters* contribute to confirmability and credibility by acting as a second investigator who reads the transcripts and assists in coding. *Triangulation* is important in credible data collection. Triangulation means that data are collected with multiple methods or from multiple participants or multiple evaluations. An example of triangulation is the new adjunct teacher who stated in a structured interview that she used group work, yet in multiple observations of her class there was no evidence to support her teaching strategy. In an unstructured interview after the class, the teacher acknowledged that students complained about group work and did not want to participate. The students' actions were initially intimidating to the new teacher. Using multiple methods to evaluate a teaching strategy brought to light an issue for further assessment. An *audit trail* is a careful and detailed documentation of the evaluator's conceptual development of data. Documentation in the audit trail should include raw data, coding (deconstruction to reconstruction), process notes, field notes, resources, and materials (Denzin & Lincoln, 1994; Grove et al., 2013; Polit & Beck, 2012).

In closing, evaluation of the DNP project is a vital element in the cycle of using and creating practice evidence. Expert use of qualitative methods and diligent attention to credibility lead to trust in the truthfulness of findings. The quality of your project's implementation and evaluation speaks firmly to the importance of the DNP role.

WRITING REMINDERS...

Writing a qualitative report or manuscript for publication must be convincing. To accomplish this goal, compose an argument that systematically presents data "to support the evaluator's case and to refute alternative explanations" (Morse, 1994, p 231).
  Reminders about qualitative writing (Morse, 1994, pp 231–232):

- "Write the article as if the reader is solving the puzzle with the [evaluator]."
and

- "Present a summary of the major findings and then present the findings that support the conclusion."

REFERENCES

Agency for Healthcare Research and Quality (AHRQ). (2013). *Contextual factors: The importance of considering and reporting on context in research on the patient-centered medical home.* AHRQ publication no. 130045-EF. Retrieved from http://pcmh.ahrq.gov/sites/default/files/attachments/ContextualFactors.pdf

Aitken, L.M., & Mardegan, K.J. (2000). "Thinking aloud": Data collection in the natural setting. *Western Journal of Nursing Research, 22*(7), 841-853.

Baum, F., MacDougall, C., & Smith, D. (2006). Participatory action research. *Journal of Epidemiological Community Health, 60*(10), 854-857.

Beck, C.T. (1993). Qualitative research: The evaluation of its credibility, fittingness, and auditability. *Western Journal of Nursing Research, 15*(2), 263-266.

Blackburn, S. (1994). *The Oxford dictionary of philosophy.* Oxford, United Kingdom: Oxford University Press.

Bohman, J., & Rehg, W. (2005). Jurgen Habermas. In *Stanford encyclopedia of philosophy.* Retrieved from http://plato.stanford.edu/entries/critical-theory/

Bourdeau, M. (2013). August Comte. In *Stanford encyclopedia of philosophy.* Retrieved from http://plato.stanford.edu/entries/comte/

Burns, S.K., & Grove, N. (2011). *Understanding nursing research: Building an evidence-based practice* (5th ed.). St. Louis, MO: Elsevier Saunders.

Centers for Disease Control and Prevention (CDC). (2009). *Data collection methods for evaluation: Document review, no. 18.* Retrieved from http://www.cdc.gov/healthyyouth/evaluation/pdf/brief18.pdf

Cross Cultural Health Care Program (CCHCP). (2010). *The cross cultural health care program.* Retrieved from http://xculture.org/medical-interpreter-training/bridging-the-gap-training-program/

Denzin, N.K., & Lincoln, Y.S. (Eds.). (1994). *Handbook of qualitative research.* Thousand Oaks, CA: SAGE Publications.

Dougal, R.L., Anderson, J.H., Reavy, K., & Shirazi, C.C. (2011). Family presence during resuscitation and/or invasive procedures in the emergency department: One size does not fit all. *Journal of Emergency Nursing, 37*(2), 152-157.

Ericsson, K.A., & Simon, H.A. (1993). *Protocol analysis: Verbal reports as data.* Cambridge, MA: MIT Press.

Friere, P. (1970; reissued 2000). *Pedagogy of the oppressed.* New York, NY: Bloomsbury Academic.

Grove, S.K., Burns, N., & Gray, J.R. (2013). *The practice of nursing research: appraisal, synthesis, and generation of evidence* (7th ed.). St. Louis, MO: Elsevier Saunders.

Guba, E.G. (1990). The alternative paradigm dialog. In E.G. Guba (Ed.), *The paradigm dialog* (pp 17-30). Thousand Oaks, CA: SAGE Publications.

Hatch, J.A. (2002). *Doing qualitative research in education settings.* Albany, NY: SUNY Press.

Huberman, A.M., & Miles, M.B. (1994). Data management and analysis methods. In N.K. Denzin & Y.S. Lincoln (Eds.), *Handbook of qualitative research* (pp 428-444). Thousand Oaks, CA: SAGE Publications.

Joanna Briggs Institute (JBI). (2014). *Reviewers' manual (2014 Ed.).* University of Adelaide, South Australia: Joanna Briggs Institute. Retrieved from http://joannabriggs.org/assets/docs/sumari/ReviewersManual-2014.pdf

Johnson, B.D., Dunlap, E., & Benoit, E. (2010). Structured qualitative research: organizing "mountains of words" for data analysis, both qualitative and quantitative. *Substance Use and Misuse, 45*(5), 648-670.

Kitson, K. (2002). Recognizing relationship: Reflections on evidence-based practice. *Nursing Inquiry, 9*(3), 179-186.

LeCompte, M.D., Millroy, W.L., & Preissis, J. (Eds.). (1992). *The handbook of qualitative research in education.* San Diego, CA: Academic Press.

Leeman, J., & Sandelowski, M. (2012). Practice-based evidence and qualitative inquiry. *Journal of Nursing Scholarship, 44*(2), 171-179.

Leininger, M.M., & McFarland, M. (2006). *Culture care diversity and universality: a worldwide nursing theory* (2nd ed.). Sudbury, MA: Jones & Bartlett.

Lincoln, Y.S., & Guba, E.G. (1985). *Naturalistic inquiry.* Thousand Oaks, CA: SAGE Publications.

LoBiondo-Wood, G., & Haber, J. (2010). *Nursing research: Methods and critical appraisal for evidence-based practice* (7th ed.). St. Louis, MO: Mosby Elsevier.

Miles, M.B., & Huberman, A.M. (1994). *Qualitative data analysis* (2nd ed.). Thousand Oaks, CA: SAGE Publications.

Morse, J.M. (1994). Designing funded qualitative research. In N.K. Denzin & Y.S. Lincoln (Eds.), *Handbook of qualitative research* (pp 220-235). Thousand Oaks, CA: SAGE Publications.

Noiseux, S., & Ricard, N. (2008). Recovery as perceived by persons with schizophrenia, family members, and health professionals; a grounded theory. *International Journal of Nursing Studies, 45*(8), 1148-1162.

Oxford Dictionaries. (2014). Retrieved from http://www.oxforddictionaries.com

Polit, D.F., & Beck, C.T. (2012). *Nursing research: Generating and assessing evidence for nursing practice* (9th ed.). Philadelphia, PA: Wolters Kluwer/Lippincott Williams & Wilkins.

Reavy, K., Hobbs, J., Hereford, M., & Crosby, K. (2012). A new clinic model for refugee health care: Adaptation of cultural safety. *Journal of Rural and Remote Health, 12*, 1826.

Sackett, D.L., Straus, S., Richardson, S., Rosenberg, W., & Haynes, R.B. (2000). *Evidence-based medicine: How to practice and teach EBM* (2nd ed.). London, United Kingdom: Churchill Livingstone.

Saldana, J. (2013). *The coding manual for qualitative researchers* (2nd ed.). Thousand Oaks CA: SAGE Publications.

Sandelowski, M. (2010). What's in a name? Qualitative description revisited. *Research in Nursing and Health, 33*, 77-84.

Spindler, G., & Spindler, L. (1992). Cultural process and ethnography: An anthropological perspective. In M.D. LeCompte, W.L. Millroy, & J. Preissle (Eds.), *The Handbook of Qualitative Research in Education* (pp 53-92). Thousand Oaks, CA: SAGE Publications.

Stake, R. (1994). Case studies. In N.K. Denzin & Y.S. Lincoln (Eds.), *Handbook of Qualitative Research* (pp 236-246). Thousand Oaks, CA: SAGE Publications.

Titler, M.G., Kleiber, C., Steelman, V., Rakel, B.A., Budreau, G., Everett, L.Q., Buckwalter, K.C., Tripp-Reimer, T., & Goode, C.J. (2001). The Iowa model of evidence-based practice to promote quality care. *Critical Care Nursing Clinics of North America, 13*(4), 497-509.

Tripp-Reimer, T., & Doebbeling, B. (2004). Qualitative perspectives in translational research. *Worldviews on Evidence-Based Nursing, 1*(S1), S65-S72.

University of Utah. (2014). *What is qualitative research?* Retrieved from http://nursing.utah.edu/research/quality-research-network.php

IF YOU WANT TO READ MORE...

If you need additional resources for greater detail related to qualitative methods, the following list is helpful.

• Denzin, N.K., & Lincoln, Y.S. (Eds.). (1994). *Handbook of qualitative research*. Thousand Oaks, CA: SAGE Publications.

- Glaser, B., & Strauss, A. (1999). *The discovery of grounded theory: Strategies for qualitative research*. New Brunswick, CT: Aldine Transaction.
- Miles, M.B., & Huberman, A.M. (1994). *Qualitative data analysis* (2nd ed.). Thousand Oaks, CA: SAGE Publications.
- Saldana, J. (2013). *The coding manual for qualitative researchers* (2nd ed.). Thousand Oaks, CA: SAGE Publications.

B

Appendix: Review of Quantitative Evaluation for Practice Projects

Evidence-based practice has resulted in changes in thinking about statistical analysis as a tool for generating, evaluating, and using evidence in clinical decisions.

DENISE F. POLIT, 2010

The influence of Florence Nightingale on today's hospitals and nurses runs deep. In addition to *Notes on Nursing* (1860), Nightingale wrote *Notes on Hospitals* (1863). These and other publications have influenced hospital architecture and professional nursing care for more than a century. Nightingale evaluated her written notes regarding conditions during the Crimean War where the sick and dying were cared for. She was one of the first to analyze her data with statistics, beginning with statistics on hospital mortality. Statistical analysis was a new social phenomenon during Nightingale's life, and she incorporated it into her practice. She displayed her statistical findings in a form called a *coxcomb*, a variation on the modern pie graph. Nightingale's observations of military hospital conditions from 1854 to 1856 during the Crimean War documented that soldiers were dying at twice the rate of civilians. Data collected by Nightingale included average size of the army, deaths from preventable diseases, wounds, and injuries, and all other causes. Following the war, Nightingale wrote an 830-page report with statistical graphics, identifying reasons for the increased number of deaths in military hospitals. Her use of visual graphics helped convince Queen Victoria of the need for social change in the area of public health (Nightingale's Coxcombs, 2008; Rehmeyer, 2008; Sweet, 2014).

Statistical skills needed by DNP students follow in the steps of Nightingale because the focus is the practice setting. Today's DNP students use knowledge of statistics for (1) critiquing quantitative research publications to establish trust in the findings and (2) evaluating implementation of evidence-based practice (EBP) guidelines or recommendations for practice. Application of statistical methods by DNP leaders for implementation of a quality improvement project, policy revision, or intervention project will vary according to context, population, and recommendation for change. Statistics for EBP projects may focus on the following: aspects of incident prevalence and association; patients' satisfaction with care; information technology; and process, outcomes, and/or actions associated with implementation. Patient-centered care and safety remain the foci of the scholarly project (Joanna Briggs Institute, 2014).

Quantitative evaluation for practice implies that variables identified from your EBP guidelines or recommendations are observed, surveyed, evaluated, and shared with stakeholders, peers, patients, and other identified healthcare audiences in the practice setting. The implication is that evaluation for decision making and findings should be presented using terms and graphics that are understandable and practical for end users. Appendix B is a review of terminology and rationale and an overview of quantitative statistical tests. For in-depth understanding of calculating statistics and evaluating findings, you are directed to a statistical text of your choice because the intent of this book is *not* to replicate a required statistical and/or research course or textbook. Additional reading recommendations for understanding and using statistics are found at the end of this appendix.

PHILOSOPHICAL PARADIGM OF QUANTITATIVE ANALYSIS

Positivism was the research paradigm or worldview prominent in the 19th century following the Industrial Revolution. Positivism is a philosophy wherein logical, disciplined reasoning is scientifically or mathematically verified. The post-Industrial Revolution era was a historic time when sustained growth implied a positivistic view that itself implied an objective reality of the world. Put another way, positivism implies that observation is *not* affected by human interpretations, beliefs, and biases. The absoluteness of positivism was challenged because total objectivity was not always possible. *Postpositivism* was born. Whereas a positivist's worldview was to understand the world adequately to predict and control it, a *postpositivist's view* recognized the impossibility of total objectivity and strived for *probabilistic* evidence (Polit & Beck, 2012; Trochim, 2006).

In today's world of research, quantitative methodology is considered *probabilistic* within the postpositivistic paradigm. Quantitative designs within the postpositivistic paradigm include *experimental, quasiexperimental,* and *nonexperimental*. These designs are discussed in the next section.

QUANTITATIVE METHODS FOR EVALUATION

The methodology of quantitative evaluation begins with understanding the broad designs of postpositivism.

An **experimental design** requires all three of the following components.

1. *Random assignment* to a control group or an intervention group is imperative for a design to be called experimental. Note that the term *randomization* connected with research *method* (i.e., random assignment to a control group or a manipulation group) is different from *randomization* connected with *sampling* (i.e., random sampling of eligible participants for the study) (LoBiondo-Wood & Haber, 2010; Polit & Beck, 2012).

2. *Control* in an experimental design means that those randomly assigned to the control group receive either the usual or standard treatment or a placebo. The control group is not manipulated (LoBiondo-Wood & Haber, 2010; Polit & Beck, 2012).

3. *Manipulation* means that something is done to the sample that was randomly assigned to the experimental or intervention group. "Doing something" to the experimental group may be a new treatment, new medical device or medication, new intervention, or new process for delivery of patient care (LoBiondo-Wood & Haber, 2010; Polit & Beck, 2012).

Quasiexperimental methods are similar to experimental designs except sample subjects are not randomly assigned to groups. Quasiexperimental methods are often used by nurses because the evaluation method is a better fit for the realities of the practice setting including access to patients, costs, feasibility, and patient safety (LoBiondo-Wood & Haber, 2010; Polit & Beck, 2010; Trochim, 2006).

Nonexperimental quantitative methods may also be called *quantitative descriptive*. As the name implies, nonexperimental methods do not randomly assign participants to a control group or manipulation group because there is no intervention or manipulation of the sample (LoBiondo-Wood & Haber, 2010). Nonexperimental studies may describe actions, context, or process (Rehmeyer, 2008; Sweet, 2014).

Examples of quantitative methods include the following (LoBiondo-Wood & Haber, 2010; Polit, 2010; Polit & Beck, 2012):

- *Randomized controlled trial (RCT)* is an experimental test of interventions.

- *Postgroup only* means that data about the intervention (dependent variable) are collected only one time after completion of randomization and intervention. (This design is classified as nonexperimental if there is no control group.)

- A *crossover design* is a "within-subjects" design, meaning that the same people are exposed to more than one intervention but in different orders. Crossover designs are classified as experimental but may also be classified as quasiexperimental if one sample serves as its own control group between the two exposures.

- *Time series* or interrupted time series designs collect data over time to evaluate change (Speroff & O'Connor, 2004).

- *One-group pretest/post-test* implies that there is no control group (quasiexperimental).

- *Retrospective studies* use nonexperimental methods to identify a phenomenon from the past to find a cause in the present. Epidemiologists use retrospective quantitative methods and qualitative case studies to identify causes of epidemic outbreaks.

- *Prospective* or *longitudinal studies* identify a problem and a presumed cause and then look ahead to test the presumed effect. This is a quasiexperimental design.

- *Comparative studies* assess differences or similarities to increase understanding or demonstrate effectiveness. Comparative studies are experimental but do not show causation, (i.e., comparison groups instead of control groups)

An experimental or quasiexperimental researcher is not a passive observer but actively participates with an intervention and a control. This differs markedly from the nonexperimental researcher who explores relationships or differences and looks for correlations (Polit, 2010; Pyrczak, 2010).

PRACTICE AND QUANTITATIVE EVALUATION

Praxis implies practical use and application. Recall the differences between the foci of a DNP project and those of a PhD dissertation. The focal point of a PhD dissertation is to revise or contribute to a body of knowledge, whereas the center of interest for a DNP project is to (1) find and synthesize best available evidence for the purpose of making decisions that affect healthcare delivery and systems (Hickey & Brosnan, 2012) and then (2) implement and evaluate the project. The practice context is more concrete in its structure versus the more abstract thinking accompanying a research study (Grove, Burns, & Gray, 2013). Statistical focus on a traditional hypothesis-testing framework "has all but been abandoned" by the medical community in the immediate practice setting (Polit, 2010, p vii).

Descriptive statistical evaluations and risk indexes are recommended as best quantitative evaluations for your project. DNP projects generally occur in one setting with a small sample size because the purpose for the project directly relates to decision making in practice. Pilot projects or studies are therefore recommended. Convenient, small sample sizes and settings limit generalizability of findings. Conversely, the integration of best evidence into the healthcare setting fulfills the expectations of translational science phase 2 in addition to meeting identified needs in your practice setting. Practice projects are designed and implemented to evaluate practice outcomes, practice patterns or processes, healthcare systems such as information technology, quality standards against national benchmarks, cost analyses, and quality improvement reviews for evaluation of safe, timely, effective, equitable, and patient-centered care (Lauver & Phalen, 2012).

DATA COLLECTION OF QUANTITATIVE DATA

Collection of quantitative data should provide meaningful information about identified project variables to be measured. Quantitative tools are structured with predetermined categories of responses to provide information about the identified variable. Examples of data tools and collection include observation and recording of well-defined actions. Quantitative patient information from electronic health records (EHRs) and biological and physiological measurements measured with technical devices are other sources of data that can be quantified. Questionnaires with closed-ended questions use different types of quantitative formats. The following list provides examples of questions for collection of quantitative data (Norwood, 2010; University of Wisconsin Eau Claire, n.d.):

- *Dichotomous items* are yes/no answers that provide nominal-level data.

- *Forced-choice items* are similar to dichotomous items. They force a sample participant to respond to one of two options and provide nominal-level data.

- *Multiple-choice items* assess knowledge, perceptions, or viewpoints that provide nominal-level data.

- *Rank order* items reflect perception or preference and provide ordinal-level data.

- *Rating scale items* force a response along a continuum and provide ordinal-level data.

- *Likert scale items* provide a continuum of responses, but the sample participant selects only one response. This tool provides interval-level data.

- *Analog scale items*, whether visual or numerical, yield responses that reflect the magnitude of experience, pain, or belief. Analog scales are measured beginning from zero. Data are measured by ratios.

- *Checklists* ask sample participants to select all choices that apply and provide nominal-level data.

STATISTICAL ANALYSIS FOR QUANTITATIVE DATA

Analyses of quantitative data imply statistical evaluation. The ***purposes of statistics*** are to describe and predict for the purpose of making practice decisions. The possibilities of *probably* capturing reality with a high degree of confidence are realized with statistics (Polit & Beck, 2012). A review of statistical tests and terminology is hereafter presented.

Scales of Measurement

- *Nominal* means *naming* categories and is a relative standing. For example, asking patients to name their religious preference becomes a data point represented by a number associated with a name.

- *Ordinal* means *rank order* and is also a relative standing. For example, staff nurses are asked to rank in order of preference five topics of interest for in-service meetings.

- *Interval* is a ranking measurement that has a floating zero. An example is temperature. Degrees of heat are ranked, but zero may change depending on Celsius or Fahrenheit measurement tools.

- *Ratio* is also a ranking measurement but has an absolute zero. Weight and height are examples of ratio measurements (Kim & Mallory, 2014; Polit, 2010; Pyrczak, 2010).

Descriptive Statistics

Descriptive statistics are used to describe, compare, or characterize context, process, or actions of a specific practice population or system. Descriptive statistics often lead to a better understanding of important variables for both practitioners and scientists by describing and summarizing collected data. Means, standard deviations (SDs), frequencies, and percentages describe one variable at a time and are generally calculated and understood before calculating and analyzing two or more variables by using more complex statistical tests (Polit, 2010).

Univariate descriptive statistics measure one variable at a time. Put another way, univariate analysis is one measurement made on each observation (Johnson, Kemp, & Kotz, 2004). In this appendix, univariate statistics are grouped into three classes or categories: frequency distributions, measures of central tendency, and measures of variability.

Frequency Distributions

Frequency distributions are about tabulating and displaying data. An *absolute frequency* is the number of times a value is observed (f) by the number of participants or cases (N) (Polit, 2010; Pyrczak, 2010). Table B.1 is an example of a frequency distribution table.

Percentage (%) demonstrates the number per 100 who have a certain attribute or characteristic and is termed *relative frequency*. Proportion is the same as percentage but is not multiplied by 100. (Polit, 2010; Pyrczak, 2010). Box B.1 is an example of a relative frequency.

Statistical software programs for computers have options for preparing tables and figures, including a frequency distribution table that displays both absolute

---

BOX B.1 Example of Relative Frequencies: Proportion and Ratio

3/32 is a proportion: 3 divided by $32 = 0.094 \times 100 = 9.4\%$

TABLE B.1 Example of an Absolute Frequency Distribution Table

Test	Frequency (f)	Percentile
83	3	9.4%
85	4	12.5%
88	3	9.4%
90	5	15.6%
91	4	12.5%
93	3	9.4%
96	3	9.4%
97	1	3%
99	6	18.8%
Total	**N = 32**	**100%**

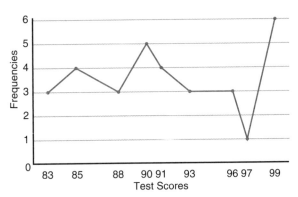

FIGURE B.1 Example of a frequency polygon.

and relative frequencies. Statistical software programs are discussed later in this chapter.

Frequency polygons are used with continuous variables. An example of a frequency polygon is a patient's temperature on the Y-axis (vertical dimension) and time on the X-axis (horizontal dimension) (Polit, 2010; Pyrczak, 2010). Figure B.1 is an example of a frequency polygon.

Bar graphs are other means of showing frequency information. The X-axis displays age categories, and the Y-axis displays frequency as a percentage (Polit, 2010; Pyrczak, 2010). Figure B.2 is an example of a bar graph.

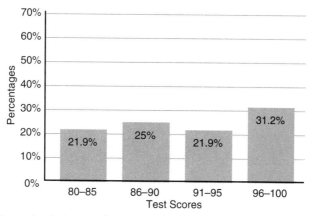

FIGURE B.2 Example of a bar graph.

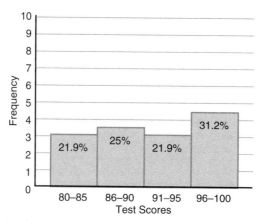

FIGURE B.3 Example of a software-generated histogram.

Histograms are similar to bar graphs except the bars touch each other. Histograms are also similar to polygons. A polygon displays continuous variability, whereas a histogram displays individual data for the variable (Polit, 2010; Pyrczak, 2010). Figure B.3 is an example of a histogram with the same information as the bar graph.

A *pie chart* is an alternative to a bar graph and is sometimes called a circular bar graph. Percentiles are arranged from largest to smallest (Polit, 2010; Pyrczak, 2010). Figure B.4 is an example of a pie chart.

Measures of Central Tendency

Measures of central tendency represent the middle of data distribution. For example, the mean, median, and mode are central tendency measures and are

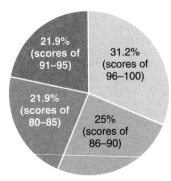

FIGURE B.4 Example of a computer software–generated pie chart.

TABLE B.2 Example of Measures of Central Tendency

Measure	Value
N	32
Test scores	83, 83, 83, 85, 85, 85, 85, 88, 88, 88, 90, 90, 90, 90, 90, 91, 91, 91, 91, 93, 93, 93, 96, 96, 96, 97, 99, 99, 99, 99, 99, 99
Mean: The mean is the sum of each score divided by the total N	$\dfrac{2,925}{32} = 91.4$
Median	91 is the score with 50% above it and 50% below it
Mode	99 is the score that occurs most frequently

considered alternative types of measuring the *average*. An example of a measurement of central tendency is displayed in Table B.2.

- *Mean* is the most commonly used and understood central tendency index. The mean is an arithmetic average that is calculated by summing each individual data value by the number of participants. Mean is represented as $\bar{x}$ and is pronounced x-bar.

- The *median* is the middle point in a distribution. Put another way, the median divides the data points into equal halves or is the average *location*. An outlier (a data point with a numerical point much larger or smaller than the nearest data point) does not affect the median.

- *Mode* is the numerical value occurring most frequently. Mode is the least used measure of central tendency because a single distribution may have two or more modes, and the values fluctuate between samples, thus making the mode *unstable* (Polit, 2010; Pyrczak, 2010). Table B.2 is an example of *measures of central tendency*, specifically mean, median, and mode.

Measures of Variability

Measures of variability gauge the distribution of scores from the middle of the distribution.

- *Range* is the most understandable measure of dispersion because it simply measures the difference between the lowest and highest scores. Range, however, may not accurately indicate variability. For example, if the range is small, it may indicate that grades on a midterm examination had little variability. If the range is wide, it could indicate wide variability on test scores or it could be one person who did poorly. The *interquartile range* measures variability of only the middle 50%, thereby decreasing the influence of outliers. Interquartile range has been described "as a first cousin to the median" (Pyrczak, 2010, p 47).

- *Standard deviation (SD)* is the most widely used measure of variability. Like the mean, SD uses all of the collected scores or values. The SD provides information about differences—specifically differences between every score or value and the mean value. In a distribution that is normally distributed, fixed percentages identify distance from the mean, but SDs are seldom normal. Written reports of findings generally describe findings using mean and SD because it is easier for your audience to perceive the variability (Polit, 2010).

- Displaying measurement variability is best accomplished by showing the shapes of distributions using a *curve*. In a *normal distribution* or bell-shaped curve, 1 SD is 68% of the distance from the mean. That means 34% is above the mean and 34% is below the mean. Ninety-five percent falls within 2 SDs of the mean, and 99.7% falls within 3 SDs. A small percentage (approximately 2.3% of scores) is estimated to fall 3 SDs from the mean (Polit, 2010). Figure B.5 illustrates a normal distribution based with the bell curve.

- Curves are not necessarily symmetrical. *Asymmetrical distributions* are described as skewed, meaning that one end of the curve may have a tail as a result of data outliers. A *positively skewed distribution* has a longer tail to the right. A *negatively skewed distribution* has a longer tail to the left (Polit, 2010). Figure B.6 shows asymmetrical curves.

- The *modality* of a curve may have two (bimodal) or more (multimodal) peaks. Modality shows asymmetry of modes. Note the root word *mode* in bimodal

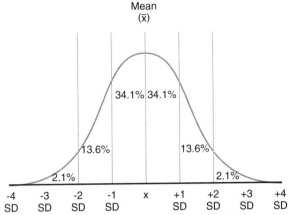

FIGURE B.5 Example of a bell curve demonstrating a normal distribution.

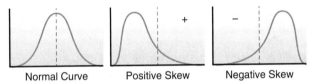

FIGURE B.6 Comparative example of a normal curve, a positive skew, and a negative skew.

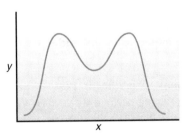

FIGURE B.7 Example of a bimodal curve.

and multimodal (Polit, 2010). Figure B.7 illustrates the variability demonstrated when bimodal peaks are curved.

Bivariate descriptive statistics show bonds or relationships of two variables. Put another way, bivariate analysis means that two measurements are made on each observation. The two paired observations are called X and Y. Examples are height and weight. Note that bivariate statistics are not two samples or two groups; a bivariate statistic indicates a pair of values (X_1, X_2) (Hedden, n.d.; Stark, 2013).

A *scatterplot* shows a linear relationship using an X-axis and a Y-axis. A scatterplot shows a positive or negative association. It does not provide information about the strength of the relationship (Hedden, n.d.; Stark, 2013).

Numerical quantification of a scatterplot is called *Pearson's r.* Pearson's *r* is not a bivariate statistic; it is a **correlation coefficient** and is useful in quantitative research studies. However, scatterplots are helpful for interpretation of Pearson's *r.* Relationships of bivariate descriptive statistics and Pearson's *r* address the following questions (Hedden, n.d.; Pyrczak, 2010):

1. Existence: Is there a relationship?

2. Magnitude: How strong is the relationship?

3. Precision: How accurate is the estimate?.

Correlation coefficients demonstrate direction and strength or degree of a *relationship* between two variables measured on an interval or ratio scale. Pearson's *r* provides information about tilt (up or down) and how tightly the data are grouped around the axis (Stark, 2013). The *Pearson's r* range is from −1.00 (strong negative correlation) to 1.00 (strong positive correlation). This means that −1.00 or 1.00 is a perfect relationship, and findings closer to the perfect score indicate a stronger relationship; 0.00 indicates total absence of a relationship. Interpretation of findings is reported as a value, and findings are interpreted as *strong, moderate,* or *weak* (Hedden, n.d.; Polit, 2010; Pyrczak, 2010). Figure B.8 illustrates strength and direction of correlation.

Risk Indexes

A **contingency table** is a cross-tabulation generally using nominal data but occasionally ordinal data. A contingency table, best described as a "two-dimensional distribution table" (p 61), shows one variable in rows and another in columns for the purpose of examining relationships between variables (Polit, 2010). Risk indexes are displayed on contingency tables.

Risk indexes interpret risk and risk reduction within a specified context for the purpose of answering questions about a relative risk or benefit of an intervention or exposure (Polit, 2010). Risk indexes are particularly useful in the practice setting and contribute to decision making. An **effect size** can be derived from risk indexes but is also calculated with the following formula:

$$ES = (\bar{x} \text{ experimental group} - \bar{x} \text{ control group}) \div SD \text{ control group}$$

Effect size (ES in the equation) is the amount of change that occurs because of an intervention or treatment compared with not receiving an intervention or treatment. Effect size is an important figure in the calculation of a power

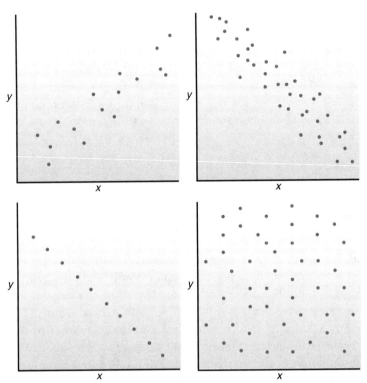

FIGURE B.8 A to D, Scatterplots indicating direction and strengths of correlation. Top left: weak positive relationship; Top right: strong negative relationship; Bottom left: perfect negative relationship; Bottom right: no relationship.

analysis in RCTs (Agency for Healthcare Research and Quality [AHRQ], 2014; Polit, 2010). Box B.2 gives an overview of risk indexes and calculations.

Types of risk indexes include *absolute risk, absolute risk reduction, relative risk, relative risk reduction, odds ratio,* and *number needed to treat (NNT).*

- *Absolute risk* or *absolute risk reduction* is the probability, or chance (presented as a percentage) of having an identified healthcare issue divided by all the sampled people who could have been exposed (but were not) to the identified healthcare issue (AHRQ, 2014; Polit, 2010). The AHRQ (2014) gives an example of 1,000 people who are more than 75 years old and who take ibuprofen for osteoarthritis pain. Of those 1,000 people, 2 will die of stomach bleeding. The absolute risk of dying from stomach bleeding is 2 in 1,000, or 0.2% of people taking ibuprofen for osteoarthritis pain (AHRQ, 2014; Polit, 2010).

- *Relative risk* or *risk ratio* compares the absolute risks in two groups of people. Put another way, relative risk is the probability of a poor outcome for people exposed to a risk compared with the probability of a similar poor outcome without the risk exposure. Relative risk presents outcome in one group compared with outcome in a second, comparable group (AHRQ, 2014; Polit, 2010). Box B.2 shows calculation of relative risk.

BOX B.2 Examples of Risk Indexes (Examples use Fictitious Data and Sample Information)

	Diagnosed With Influenza		
	Yes	No	Total
Group who did *not* receive influenza vaccine	22 a	12 b	34
Group who received influenza vaccine	6 c	30 d	36
Total	28	42	70

Absolute risk is the proportion of people who experience an undesirable effect in each group.

Absolute risk (not vaccinated): a / (a + b)

   Example: 22 / (22 + 12) = 22 / 34 = 0.647 (64.7%)

Absolute risk (vaccinated): c / (c + d)

   Example: 6 / 6 + 30) = 6 / 36 = 0.167 (16.7%)

Absolute risk reduction (risk difference) is an estimated proportion of the people who would contract the flu if they did not receive the influenza vaccine.

Absolute risk reduction: [a / (a + b)] − [c / (c + d)]

   Example: 0.647 − 0.167 = 0.48 (48%)

Relative risk (risk ratio) is a ratio of the absolute risks of the two groups (vaccinated and not vaccinated).

Relative risk: [a / (a + b)] / [c / (c + d)]

   Example: 0.647 / 0.167 = 3.874

Continued

> **BOX B.2** Examples of Risk Indexes (Examples use Fictitious Data and Sample Information)—cont'd
>
> Interpretation: When the *relative risk* is close to 1, there is no relationship between the risk of no vaccination and contracting the flue. A relative risk of 3.874 indicates a substantial relationship of contracting the flu when the person was not vaccinated.
>
> ***Relative risk reduction*** estimates the proportion of risk that is reduced with treatment or intervention.
>
> *Relative risk reduction*, also called *absolute risk reduction* divided by the absolute risk of people who received the intervention (influenza vaccine): [a / (a + b)] − [c / (c + d)] / [c / (c + d)]
>
> Example: 0.48 / 0.167 = 2.874
>
> Interpretation: A *relative risk reduction* of 2.874 indicates a substantial decreased risk of not contracting the flu for people who received the influenza vaccine.

- *Relative risk reduction or risk ratio* is the estimated risk of poor health when one group receives an exposure to the risk and another group does not. Put another way, relative risk reduction may be the comparison of an experimental group whose members receive an exposure to a health risk in addition to an intervention or medication to reduce the health risk *and* a control group whose members receive an exposure to the same health risk and receive no intervention or medication (AHRQ, 2014; Polit, 2010). Box B.2 demonstrates calculation of relative risk reduction.

- An *odds ratio* is similar to a risk ratio, but it is less intuitive even though it is an accepted term for gambling. An odds ratio is a good test for comparing the chance of an event occurring in one group compared with another group without the event. AHRQ (2014) provides a good example of an odds ratio. In a comparative study, two groups of pregnant diabetic women were treated with either metformin or insulin. The odds ratio of an early delivery (less than 37 weeks) was 1.06 for metformin, meaning that women taking metformin had a small (1.06) increase in the odds of delivering early compared with the women controlling their diabetes with insulin (AHRQ, 2014; Polit, 2010). Box B.3 shows an odds ratio. What is the difference between a risk

---

BOX B.3 Examples of Odds and an Odds Ratio (Examples Use Fictitious Data and Sample Information)

Odds are the proportion of people in each group (i.e., received the flu vaccine and did not receive the vaccine) who were subsequently diagnosed with the flu.

Odds of people contracting the flu who did not receive the flu vaccine: a/b

Example: 22 / 12 = 1.83

Odds of people contracting the flu who received the flu vaccine

Example: 6 / 20 = 0.02

Odds ratio is the ratio of the two odds: (a / b) / (c / d)

Example: 1.83 / 0.02 = 91.5

Interpretation: The odds of contracting the flu are estimated at 91.5 times higher in the group that was not vaccinated. When the odds ratio is close to 1, the interpretation is similar to the risk ratio meaning that there is no relationship.

---

ratio and an odds ratio? A risk ratio is easier to understand than an odds ratio because a risk ratio is more intuitive in understanding the measure of association. Odds ratios are useful in measuring exposure and outcome. When the exposure occurs in less than 10% of the unexposed population, the odds ratio and risk ratio are comparable or have a reasonable approximation. When the exposure rate is greater than 10%, the odds ratio will exaggerate the risk ratio (Polit, 2010; Vera, 2008). There remains an ongoing debate regarding whether an odds ratio or a risk ratio is better. The answer is complex, and an argument can be made on both sides. The intent of this appendix is to present useful tools for evaluation of your DNP project. The article by Cummings (2009) is useful to understand the arguments for odds ratios and risk ratios more fully.

- *Number needed to treat (NNT)* is a useful tool for making decisions related to how many people need to be treated for an improved outcome. Stated another way, NNT is the number of patients who need to be treated to prevent one additional unfavorable outcome such as a stroke or death. The

---

BOX B.4 Number Needed to Treat Estimating How Many People Need to Receive Treatment to Prevent One Undesirable Outcome

NNT for prevention of 1 person contracting the flu:

1 / ARR

or

1 / [a / (a + b)] − [c / (c + d)]

Example: 1 − 0.48 = 0.52

Interpretation: Between 0 and 1 people not currently vaccinated need to receive the flu vaccine to decrease 1 additional person from contracting the flu. Decision makers can use this estimate to evaluate yearly cost expenditures to sustain influenza vaccinations among healthcare workers and advertising to communities.

ARR, absolute risk ratio; NNT, number needed to treat.

Centre for Evidence-Based Medicine (CEBM) has a table for converting odds ratios into NNT (CEBM, 2014). The NNT table can be accessed at http://www.cebm.net/number-needed-to-treat-nnt/. NNT is useful for making decisions about monetary information comparing cost effectiveness of interventions (CEBM, 2014) (Box B.4).

Inferential Statistics

Recall that *descriptive statistics* are important for practice because the statistical tests evaluate characteristics, circumstances, and behaviors of your sample. Descriptive statistics and graphics are more easily understood by your intended audience when disseminating findings.

    Inferential statistics focus on the probability of an identified outcome occurring in the real world. Stated another way, inferential statistics are calculated from data collected from samples, not the entire population. To make inferences to the population of focus, however, estimation of population parameters is needed (Grove et al., 2013; Polit, 2010).

    Whereas descriptive statistics summarize your current data set, inferential statistics make predictions about the population of focus (My Market Research

Methods, 2011). Understanding inferential statistics is important for evaluating your practice project as well as for critiquing research publications (see Section II) and thinking about your postgraduation scholarly trajectory (see Section IV).

Helpful hint: Consult a statistician during your project's planning stage, analysis stage, and at other times of need whenever you intend to use inferential statistics.

Inferential statistics are grounded in *laws of probability.* Inferential tests provide statistical possibilities of *probably* capturing reality with a high degree of confidence. Probability has its origins in observation and games of chance. The classic coin toss test describes the probability of an event or consecutive events occurring in the real world. Before discussing inferential statistical tests, however, *probability* as a statistical sampling method is essential information.

Statistical Sampling

Sampling within a statistical context creates the basic or individual unit that represents a *population.* The sample then becomes the target for collection of data. Characteristics of the population of interest are identified from your EBP practice recommendations. Based on those characteristics, *inclusion and exclusion criteria* are identified for sampling (LoBiondo-Wood & Haber, 2010; Polit & Beck, 2012; Grove et al., 2013). For example, if the project evaluation focuses on change in body fat composition of participants in a community-based program for obesity, then the inclusion criteria may be adult men and women between the ages of 21 and 35 years who measure 50% or greater than a normal body mass index. Exclusion criteria would be men, women, and children younger than 21 years of age and older than 35 years of age or men and women who measure less than 50% of a normal body mass index. Inclusion and exclusion criteria are established to control for variability that would limit the strength of evidence.

Probability sampling is a term that describes strength of the sampling process because it represents the identified target population. Probability sampling is random sampling and contributes to decreasing bias in research studies. Pyrczak (2010) reminds us that using a large sample does not correct for bias; random sampling corrects for bias. Probability sampling therefore is considered rigorous and representative of the target population. Examples of probability sampling include random selection, simple random sampling, stratified sampling, and cluster sampling (Grove et al., 2013; LoBiondo-Wood & Haber, 2010; Polit & Beck, 2012).

The opposite of probability sampling is *nonprobability sampling.* Nonprobability sampling is nonrandom sampling and is considered biased because it is unknown whether or not the sample is representative of the population of study. Nonprobability sampling is not a statistical test. Examples of nonprobability sampling include convenience, quota, purposive, and snowball. Convenience sampling has the greatest risk of bias over any form of sampling because the selection process is rooted in convenient access to people or units for sample data (Grove et al., 2013; LoBiondo-Wood & Haber, 2010; Polit & Beck, 2012). An example of convenience sampling is when a data collector attends a nursing conference for the purpose of distributing and collecting questionnaires from the attendees. The conference attendees may or may not fit the inclusion criteria for the study's purpose and *probably* are not representative of the target population. *Purposive sampling* implies that the evaluator purposefully selects the sample specific to the needs of the project. Purposive sampling for collection of both qualitative and quantitative data is useful because the sample is purposefully selected based on the specific needs of the project and the evaluator's judgment that the sample participants meet the identified criteria (Grove et al., 2013; LoBiondo-Wood & Haber, 2010; Polit & Beck, 2012).

In the practice setting, most samples are nonprobability sampling—usually purposive or convenience. Does this mean that project evaluators cannot use inferential statistical tests because the sampling is nonprobability? The answer is a resounding *no*. "The tests are robust enough to not seriously affect the results unless the data are skewed in unknown ways" (LoBiondo-Wood & Haber, 2010, p 321).

Rationale about probability or random sampling relates to the concept of *probability distribution* or *sampling distribution*. The *central limit theorem* implies the following: (1) the mean of the sampling distribution is identical to the population mean; and (2) if the scores of the population are normally distributed, the sample distribution will be normal. Recall that a normal distribution is graphically presented as a bell curve and is based on mean and SD. Therefore, the SD of the sample distribution needs to be determined. The SD of a sampling distribution of the mean is called *standard error of the mean*. Error implies that the sample from the population contains differences from the population mean. The smaller the standard error of the mean, the more accurate is the estimate that the sample mean is similar to the population mean. The larger the standard error of the mean, the greater is the probability that the sample mean is a poor estimate of the population mean (LoBiondo-Wood & Haber, 2010; Polit, 2010; Sampling Distributions, 2015).

Inferential Statistical Tests

Parametric statistics are useful for project evaluations because parametric estimation infers that statistics from a sample are used to make decisions about the target population. When selecting a statistical test for evaluation, therefore, choose the test based on the appropriateness for the type of data collected (LoBiondo-Wood & Haber, 2010; Polit, 2010). The inferential statistical tests identified in Box B.5 are explained here:

A *t-test* is a commonly used statistical test for project evaluation and research analysis because it demonstrates differences between two groups. The *t*-test

---

BOX B.5 Overview of Inferential Statistical Tests

Tests of Difference Between Means

- *Parametric statistics*
  - Conducted on interval or ratio
  - Grounded in the estimation of at least one population parameter
  - Common inferential statistics: *t*-tests, ANOVA
- *Nonparametric statistics*
  - Conducted on nominal or interval
  - Less restrictive assumptions about sampling distribution
  - Common inferential statistics: chi square, Fisher exact probability

Tests of Association

- *Parametric statistics*
  - Conducted on interval or ratio
  - Relationship between two or more variables
  - Common inferential statistics: Pearson's *r*
- *Nonparametric statistics*
  - Conducted on nominal or interval
  - Less restrictive assumptions about sampling distribution
  - Common inferential statistics: Spearman's rho, correlation coefficient

---

ANOVA, analysis of variance.
Adapted from LoBiondo-Wood & Haber, 2010, p 324.

assesses the difference between two group means. Ideally, the two groups should be unmatched or independent from each other and the identified variable measured on an interval or ratio level. If the groups are matched and evaluation of differences is still desired, a *paired t-test* should be used (LoBiondo-Wood & Haber, 2010). If the sample size is small, such as a pilot study or implementation of your project in one setting, the true standard error of the mean may be estimated because of the small numbers of participants and the single setting. The small sample size is recognized as the source of sample data. The theoretical distribution then uses a *t* distribution to estimate standard error of the mean. The shape of a *t* distribution depends on the sample size. Note that *t* distribution tables have been developed for different sample sizes and probability levels (Polit, 2010).

ANOVA or analysis of variance is similar to a *t*-test except there are more than two groups. ANOVA does not test the means separately but considers variation between and within groups (LoBiondo-Wood & Haber, 2010).

Chi-square statistics are at the nominal level. Chi-square is a nonparametric test and assesses difference in frequency between two groups (LoBiondo-Wood & Haber, 2010).

Fisher exact probability test is used when the chi-square test has less than six frequencies in each group (LoBiondo-Wood & Haber, 2010).

Pearson's r is an example of a parametric test of relationship or correlation. Once the value of the Pearson's *r* is calculated, a distribution table specific to the test determines whether the value is significant (LoBiondo-Wood & Haber, 2010).

Spearman's rho is a nonparametric test to assess strength of relationship between two pairs of ranks (LoBiondo-Wood & Haber, 2010).

A *contingency coefficient* is similar to a *correlation coefficient.* With correlation coefficients, parametric data levels are nominal and ordinal, and values range from −1.0 to +1.0, meaning either a perfect negative correlation or a perfect positive correlation. A zero means no correlation of variables (LoBiondo-Wood & Haber, 2010).

A *confidence interval (CI)* is a calculation that the population value lies within an interval around the point estimate. The degree of confidence of *probably* being right is higher because estimating the parameter describes a range of values, not a single value point. A CI around a mean value is calculated using the standard error of the mean. For example, 95% of scores in a normal distribution curve lie within 2.5 SDs from the mean. Although a 95% confidence level is the default percentage or most commonly used CI, less risk can be established with 99%.

Calculation example: 95% CI = x̄ ± (1.96 × SEM)

CIs can also be calculated with the bivariate descriptive statistics of percentages and risk indexes. A binomial (normal and dichotomous) curve is built around a proportion. Computations are complex, and recommendations are that you use a statistical software program. Hints about CIs built around proportions note that (1) CI parameters are rarely symmetric around the sample proportion, and (2) width of the CI depends on both sample size and value of the proportion (Grove et al., 2013; Polit, 2010; Polit & Beck, 2012).

Statistical Significance and Clinical Importance

Statistical significance, represented by a *p value,* implies that the finding is unlikely to have happened by chance. Statistical significance is the estimated measure of the degree of truth that the findings are representative of the population. A finding, however, may be statistically significant yet have no *clinical importance.* For example, a finding that blood pressures between two groups of 16-year-old female subjects were statistically significant may be insignificant for clinical decision making when the actual scores reflect that blood pressure in one group averaged 113/55 mm Hg and blood pressure in the other group averaged 109/58 mm Hg. In other words, the magnitude or size of the effect is not evident in a p value and is therefore not helpful in making decisions. A more informative statistical analysis regarding clinical importance may be two CIs comparing the two groups (Grove et al., 2013; LoBiondo-Wood & Haber, 2010).

Advanced Statistical Calculations

Translational science is a masterful model for collaboration between practice and science. The rigor involved in implementation and evaluation of EBP recommendations for practice produces valuable results for decision making in the practice setting. Postgraduate collaboration with nurse scientists can lead to construction of RCTs and meta-analyses to validate and disseminate your project findings further.

Advanced research methods require advanced statistical calculations that are within the purview of nurse scientists. Examples of advanced statistical calculations include multivariate statistics, multiple regression, and factor analysis. These statistical tests delve deeper into relationships or correlations by looking at factors and levels that increase understanding. Advanced statistics are also useful for statistical modeling (Grove et al., 2013; LoBiondo-Wood & Haber, 2010; Polit, 2010).

RIGOR: VALIDITY AND RELIABILITY

Validity and reliability are the foundations of *rigor* in quantitative evaluation. *Validity* implies that the measurement tool or instrument (e.g., questionnaire) measures what it is designed to measure. However, validity is a *matter of degree,* meaning that it is not *whether* the measurement tool is valid but rather to what degree it is valid. Indeed, some characteristics such as *joy* are difficult to measure. Three major types of measurement validity may vary according to the information provided and the purpose of the investigator. When you critique a research publication, evaluate whether it has sufficient evidence to demonstrate validity (e.g., consistency and accuracy) in measurement (LoBiondo-Wood & Haber, 2010; Patten, 2012). Validity is difficult to measure. LoBiondo-Wood & Haber (2010) wrote that "adequate validity is frequently claimed, but rarely is the method specified" (p 288).

Reliability implies consistency, accuracy, precision, stability, equivalence, and homogeneity. The common definition of *reliability* means that a study would produce the same or similar results if the same tool was used again in the same way. There are several tools to measure reliability. *Stability* (instrument's ability to produce same results) can be measured with *test-retest reliability* and *parallel or alternate form.* *Homogeneity* (all items in measurement tool measure the same concept) can be evaluated with *split-half reliability, Cronbach's alpha,* or the *Kuder-Richardson coefficient.* *Equivalence* (equivalent tests produce same results) is assessed with *interrater reliability* (LoBiondo-Wood & Haber, 2010).

The relationship between validity and reliability leads to the principle that *validity is more important than reliability.* This makes intuitive sense. For example, reliability of an instrument can obtain the same or similar results because the measurement items do not change, thereby leading to positive reliability coefficients (Grove et al., 2013; LoBiondo-Wood & Haber, 2010; Patten, 2012; Polit & Beck, 2012; Pyrzcak, 2010). However, evaluation about patient care that collects data only on the number of patients' falls does not reflect the quality of care performed by nurses. In other words, measurement validity is not demonstrated when patient safety is evaluated only on the number of patients' falls.

COMPUTER SOFTWARE FOR DATA ANALYSIS

What can computer software for data analysis (also called analytics) do for you and your scholarly project?

- Reduce calculation errors

- Manage data

- Create visual graphics for effective delivery of findings

- Easily share data with others

- Perform analyses faster and more efficiently (Carolan, n.d.)

Multiple marketable and free resources exist for computer software programs. The most recognized name is SPSS. IBM (Armonk, NY) acquired SPSS in 2009 and changed the official name to *IBM SPSS Statistics.* The acronym SPSS stands for Statistical Package for the Social Sciences. Java (Oracle, Redwood Shores, CA) and SAS (SAS Institute, Cary, NC) follow in popularity (Muenchen, 2014). Each program differs in function. Their use, however, remains the same: confidence in computing, predicting, and presenting data analyses. Microsoft Excel (Microsoft, Redmond, WA) also has data analysis functions. You, the consumer, select the software program that best meets your needs regarding usability and cost. Check with your library, college, or university for available programs. For your personal computer, student prices may be available to purchase an analytics program. Free access to online analytics programs may also be available for some programs. Remember that *you,* the consumer, select the software program that best meets your needs regarding usability and cost.

In summary, remember the importance of distinguishing between practice projects and research studies. Practice evaluation and interpretation of findings contribute to decision making about improvement or change for patient safety or healthcare quality. Research analysis implies contributions or revisions of new evidence. Indeed, collaboration and respect for different scholarly roles provide creative opportunities and growth of nursing knowledge.

WRITING REMINDERS...

Quantitative Data and the Written Report

The following guidelines are provided to assist you when writing about and illustrating analyzed data. Quantitative statistical data can be presented as text, table, or figure. If you choose to use all three forms, carefully include only information that adds clarification and support to your written report.

- *Tables* are the best option for presentation of numerical and nominal information. Tables organize numbers or words in columns with a label or title for each column. Consider using appendices if you plan to display numerous tables.

- **Figures** include different types of graphs (e.g., bar graph, pie graph, histogram, scatterplot, X,Y line graphs, drawings, or photographs). Figures are a sensible option for illustrating trends, comparisons, or relationships.

- **Tables and figures** should be easy for your reader to understand. Clarity can be enhanced with good labeling. For example, rows and columns on contingency tables or X- and Y-axes on scatterplots must be labeled clearly.

- Placements differ regarding the explanation or legend describing the **table or figure.** Table explanations or legends go above the table because tables are read from the top down.

- Not all analyzed data need to be presented in a table or figure. Easily understood data can be presented in a single sentence within the **text** by presenting key statistical points within parentheses.

- When presenting whole numbers within a **text,** the numbers nine or less should be written as words; numbers 10 and greater are written as digits. The number of digits used for presenting decimals should be consistent throughout your written report. Depending on your need, one or two digits past the decimal point are adequate.

Data from Bates College, 2012; Vanderbilt Institutional Research Group, 2010.

REFERENCES

Agency for Healthcare Research and Quality (AHRQ). (2014). *Glossary of terms.* Retrieved from http://www.ahrq.gov/patients-consumers/patient-involvement/ask-your-doctor/tips-and-tools/glossary.html

Bates College. (2012). *Almost everything you wanted to know about making tables and figures.* Lewiston, ME: Bates College, Department of Biology. Retrieved from http://abacus.bates.edu/~ganderso/biology/resources/writing/HTWtablefigs.html

Carolan, B.V. (n.d.). *Using computer programs for quantitative data analysis.* Montclair, NJ: Montclair State University. Retrieved from http://www.montclair.edu/media/montclairedu/graduateschoolthe/students/graduateconference9-17docs/dataanalysis.pdf

Centre for Evidence-Based Medicine (CEBM). (2014). *Number needed to treat.* Retrieved from http://www.cebm.net/number-needed-to-treat-nnt

Cummings, P. (2009). The relative merits of risk ratios and odds ratios. *JAMA Pediatrics, 163*(5), 438-445.

Grove, S.K., Burns, N., & Gray, J.R. (2013). *The practice of nursing research: appraisal, synthesis, and generation of evidence* (7th ed.). St. Louis, MO: Elsevier Saunders.

Hedden, K.S. (n.d.). *Introduction to bivariate statistics.* Retrieved from http://dept.stat.lsa.umich.edu/~kshedden/Courses/Stat401/Notes/401-bivariate-slides.pdf

Hickey, J.V., & Brosnan, C.A. (2012). *Evaluation of health care quality in advanced practice nursing.* New York, NY: Springer Publishing.

Joanna Briggs Institute. (2014). Economic evidence and evidence-based practice. In *Joanna Briggs Institute reviewers' manual 2014.* Retrieved from http://joannabriggs.org/assets/docs/sumari/ReviewersManual-2014.pdf

Johnson, L., Kemp, A.W., & Kotz, S. (2004). *Univariate discrete distributions* (3rd ed.). Hoboken, NJ: John Wiley & Sons.

Kim, M., & Mallory, C. (2014). *Statistics for evidence-based practice in nursing.* Burlington, MA: Jones & Bartlett Learning.

Lauver, L., & Phalen, A.G. (2012). An example of a statistics course in a Doctor of Nursing Practice (DNP) program. *Nurse Educator, 37*(1), 36-41.

LoBiondo-Wood, G., & Haber, J. (2010). *Nursing research: methods and critical appraisal for evidence-based practice* (7th ed.). St. Louis, MO: Mosby Elsevier.

Muenchen, R. (2014). *The popularity of data analysis software.* Retrieved from http://r4stats.com/articles/popularity/

My Market Research Methods. (2011). *Descriptive vs. inferential statistics. What's the difference?* Retrieved from http://www.mymarketresearchmethods.com/descriptive-inferential-statistics-difference/

Nightingale, F. (1860). *Notes on nursing.* New York, NY: D. Appleton and Company.

Nightingale, F. (1863). *Notes on hospitals.* London: Longman, Roberts, and Green.

Nightingale's coxcombs. (2008). *Understanding Uncertainty.* Cambridge, United Kingdom: University of Cambridge. Retrieved from http://understandinguncertainty.org/coxcombs

Norwood, S. (2009). *Research essentials: foundations for evidence-based practice.* Upper Saddle River, NJ: Pearson.

Patten, M.L. (2012). *Understanding research methods: an overview of the essentials* (8th ed.). Glendale, CA: Pyrczak Publishing.

Polit, D.F. (2010). *Statistics and data analysis for nursing research* (2nd ed.). Upper Saddle River, NJ: Pearson.

Polit, D.F., & Beck, C.T. (2012). *Nursing research: Generating and assessing evidence for nursing practice* (9th ed.). Philadelphia, PA: Wolters Kluwer Health/Lippincott Williams & Wilkins.

Pyrczak, F. (2010). *Making sense of statistics: a conceptual overview* (5th ed.). Glendale, CA: Pyrczak Publishing.

Rehmeyer, J. (2008). Florence Nightingale: The passionate statistician. *Science News.* Retrieved from https://www.sciencenews.org/article/florence-nightingale-passionate-statistician

Speroff, T., & O'Connor, G.T. (2004). Study designs for PDSA quality improvement research. *Quality Management Health Care, 13*(1), 17-32.

Stark, P.B. (2013). *SticiGui: statistical tools for Internet and classroom instruction.* Retrieved from http://www.stat.berkeley.edu/~stark/SticiGui/Text/testing.htm

Stat Trek. Sampling distributions. (2015). Retrieved from http://stattrek.com/sampling/sampling-distribution.aspx

Sweet, V. (2014). Far more than a lady with a lamp. *The New York Times,* March 4, p D3.

Trochim, W.M.K. (2006). Positivism and post-positivism. *Research Methods Knowledge Base.* Retrieved from http://www.socialresearchmethods.net/kb/positvsm.php

University of Wisconsin Eau Claire. (n.d.). *Data collection methods.* Retrieved from http://people.uwec.edu/piercech/researchmethods

Vanderbilt Institutional Research Group. (2010). *General practices in reporting quantitative data.* Nashville, TN: Vanderbilt University. Retrieved from http://virg.vanderbilt.edu/AssessmentPlans/Results/Reporting_Results_Quantitative.aspx

IF YOU WANT TO READ MORE...

Grove, S.K., Burns, N., & Gray, J.R. (2013). *The practice of nursing research: Appraisal, synthesis, and generation of evidence* (7th ed.). St. Louis, MO: Elsevier Saunders.

LoBiondo-Wood, G., & Haber, J. (2014). *Nursing research: Methods and critical appraisal for evidence-based practice* (8th ed.). St. Louis, MO: Elsevier.

Polit, D.F. (2010). *Statistics and data analysis for nursing research* (2nd ed.). Boston, MA: Pearson.

Polit, D.F., & Beck, C.T. (2012). *Nursing research: Generating and assessing evidence for nursing practice* (9th ed.). Philadelphia, PA: Wolters Kluwer/Lippincott Williams & Wilkins.

Pyrczak, F. (2014). *Making sense of statistics: A conceptual overview* (6th ed.). Glendale, CA: Pyrczak Publishing.

Index

Page numbers followed by "t" denote tables; page numbers followed by "f" denote figures.